# Lecture Notes in Computer Science 8401

*Commenced Publication in 1973*
Founding and Former Series Editors:
Gerhard Goos, Juris Hartmanis, and Jan van Leeuwen

Andreas Holzinger    Igor Jurisica (Eds.)

# Interactive Knowledge Discovery and Data Mining in Biomedical Informatics

## State-of-the-Art and Future Challenges

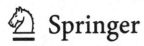
Springer

Volume Editors

Andreas Holzinger
Research Unit Human-Computer Interaction
Austrian IBM Watson Think Group
Institute for Medical Informatics, Statistics and Documentation
Medical University of Graz
Auenbruggerplatz 2/V, 8036 Graz, Austria
E-mail: a.holzinger@hci4all.at

Igor Jurisica
Princess Margaret Cancer Centre
University Health Network
IBM Life Sciences Discovery Centre
TECHNA for the Advancement of Technology for Health
TMDT Room 11-314, 101 College Street, Toronto, ON, M5G 1L7, Canada
E-mail: juris@ai.utoronto.ca

ISSN 0302-9743                                e-ISSN 1611-3349
ISBN 978-3-662-43967-8                         e-ISBN 978-3-662-43968-5
DOI 10.1007/978-3-662-43968-5
Springer Heidelberg New York Dordrecht London

Library of Congress Control Number: 2014941875

LNCS Sublibrary: SL 3 – Information Systems and Application, incl. Internet/Web and HCI

*Typesetting:* Camera-ready by author, data conversion by Scientific Publishing Services, Chennai, India

Printed on acid-free paper

Springer is part of Springer Science+Business Media (www.springer.com)

# Preface

One of the grand challenges in our digital world are the large, complex, high-dimensional and often weakly structured data sets and massive amounts of unstructured information. This "big data" challenge (V4: volume, variety, velocity, veracity) is most evident in biomedical informatics: The trend toward precision medicine (P4 medicine: predictive, preventive, participatory, personalized) has resulted in an explosion in the amount of generated biomedical data sets, not only from traditional patient data, but additionally also due to more and more "omics" data (e.g., from genomics, proteomics, metabolomics, lipidomics, transcriptomics, epigenetics, microbiomics, fluxomics, phenomics, etc.). Neither the medical doctor nor the biomedical researcher of today is capable of memorizing all these data. Therefore, modern biomedicine simply will not develop any further without computational solutions for analyzing these data.

With steady progress in analyzing these data, the direction is toward *integrative approaches* that combine data sets using rich networks of specific relationships, such as physical protein interactions, transcriptional regulatory networks, microRNA, gene regulatory networks, metabolic and signaling pathways, to name just a few. However, several challenges remain open.

A synergistic combination of methodologies and approaches from two areas offer ideal conditions for solving these aforementioned problems: human–computer interaction (HCI) and knowledge discovery and data mining (KDD). The central goal is to support human intelligence with machine learning, in order to interactively gain new and previously unknown insights into these data.

Consequently, the objective of the HCI-KDD task force is to combine the best of both worlds—HCI, with the emphasis on human issues including perception, cognition, interaction, reasoning, decision making, human learning and human intelligence; and KDD, encompassing data integration, fusion, preprocessing, data mining, and visualization, concerting computational statistics, machine learning, and artificial intelligence – while always considering the privacy, data protection, and safety and security issues.

The mission of the HCI-KDD task force is to form a network of excellence by bringing together professionals from diverse areas with various backgrounds who share a common vision: making sense of complex data.

The HCI-KDD expert network organizes special sessions at least twice a year; the first took place in Graz (Austria), the second in Macau (China), the third in Maribor (Slovenia), the fourth in Regensburg (Germany), the fifth in Lisbon (Portugal), the sixth in Warsaw (Poland), the seventh in Vienna (Austria) and the eighth is planned to take place at the international research station for mathematical innovation and discovery in Banff (Canada) in summer 2015.

Volume 8401 of the *Lecture Notes in Computer Science* is a state-of-the-art volume focusing on hot topics from interactive knowledge discovery and data mining in biomedical informatics. Each paper describes the state of the art and focuses on open problems and future challenges in order to provide a research agenda to stimulate further research and progress.

To acknowledge here all those who contributed to all our efforts and stimulating discussions would be impossible. Many people contributed to the development of this book, either directly or indirectly, so we will use the plural form here: First of all we thank the HCI-KDD expert network for their expertise and reviews on the papers collected in this book – we are grateful for the comments and discussions from the members of the international scientific board, the clinical advisory board, and the industrial board and the international students committee. We thank multiple funding agencies, industry, and governments for supporting this international effort, and our institutes for the academic freedom we enjoy, the intellectual environments, and opportunity for carrying out such scientific enterprises. We thank our families, our friends, and our colleagues for their nurturing and positive encouragement. Last but not least we thank Springer's management team and production team for their smooth support.

March 2014                                              Andreas Holzinger
                                                             Igor Jurisica

# About the Editors

Andreas Holzinger is head of the Research Unit HCI, Institute for Medical Informatics, Statistics and Documentation at the Medical University Graz, lead at the HCI-KDD network, head of the first Austrian IBM Watson Think Group in close cooperation with the Software Group of IBM Austria, Associate Professor of Applied Informatics at the Faculty of Computer Science, Institute of Information Systems and Computer Media, and lecturer at the Bioinformatics Group at Graz University of Technology. He serves as consultant for the Canadian, Swiss, French, and Dutch Government, for the German Excellence Initiative, and as a national expert in the European Commission (Lisbon delegate). Andreas was Visiting Professor in Berlin, Innsbruck, Vienna, London, and Aachen. Andreas and his team are passionate about bringing together human–computer interaction and knowledge discovery/data mining, with the goal of supporting human intelligence with machine learning – to gain new, previously unknown insights into complex biomedical data. http://www.hci4all.at

Igor Jurisica is Tier I Canada Research Chair in Integrative Cancer Informatics, and is a senior scientist at the Princess Margaret Cancer Centre, professor at the University of Toronto, and visiting scientist at the IBM Centers for Advanced Studies. Igor is head of the IBM Life Sciences Discovery Center at the Ontario Cancer Institute at the Princess Margaret Hospital and also an adjunct professor at the School of Computing, Department of Pathology and Molecular Medicine at Queen's University and Department of Computer Science and Engineering at York University in Toronto. Igor's research focuses on integrative computational biology and the representation, analysis, and visualization of high-dimensional data to identify prognostic and predictive signatures, drug mechanisms of action, and the in-silico repositioning of drugs. His interests include comparative analysis for mining different integrated complex data sets, for example protein–protein interactions, high-dimensional cancer data, and high-throughput screens for protein crystallization. http://www.cs.toronto.edu/~juris.

# HCI-KDD Network of Excellence

We are grateful for the support and help of all members of the expert group HCI-KDD, see http://www.hci4all.at/expert-network-hci-kdd

## International Scientific Committee

| | |
|---|---|
| Beatrice Alex | Institute for Language, Cognition and Computation, School of Informatics, University of Edinburgh, UK |
| Amin Anjomshoaa | Information and Software Engineering Group, Vienna University of Technology, Austria |
| Matthieu d'Aquin | Knowledge Media Institute, The Open University, Milton Keynes, UK |
| Joel P. Arrais | Centre for Informatics and Systems, University of Coimbra, Portugal |
| John A. Atkinson-Abutridy | Department of Computer Science, Universidad de Concepcion, Chile |
| Alexandra Balahur | Institute for the Protection and Security of Citizen, European Commission Joint Research Centre, Ispra, Italy |
| Smaranda Belciug | Department of Computer Science, Faculty of Mathematics and Computer Science, University of Craiova, Romania |
| Mounir Ben Ayed | Research Group Intelligent Machines, Ecole Nationale d'Ingenieurs de Sfax, Tunisia |
| Miroslaw Bober | Department of Electronic Engineering, University of Surrey, Guildford, UK |
| Matt-Mouley Bouamrane | Institute of Health and Wellbeing, University of Glasgow, UK |
| Mirko Cesarini | Department of Statistics and Quantitative Methods, Università di Milano Bicocca, Milan, Italy |
| Polo Chau | School of Computational Science and Engineering, College of Computing, Georgia Tech, USA |
| Chaomei Chen | College of Information Science and Technology, Drexel University, USA |
| Elizabeth S. Chen | Center for Clinical and Translational Science, Department of Medicine, University of Vermont, USA |

Nitesh V. Chawla                    Data, Inference, Analytics and Learning Lab,
                                    University of Notre Dame, USA
Matthias Dehmer                     Universität für Gesundheitswissenschaften,
                                    Medizinische Informatik and Technik,
                                    Austria
Alexiei Dingli                      Intelligent Systems Technologies Research
                                    Group, University of Malta, Malta
Tomasz Donarowicz                   Institute of Mathematics and Computer
                                    Science, Wroclaw University of
                                    Technology, Poland
Achim Ebert                         Fachbereich Informatik, AG Computergrafik
                                    und HCI, TU Kaiserslautern, Germany
Max J. Egenhofer                    Center for Geographic Information and
                                    Analysis, University of Maine, USA
Kapetanios Epaminondas              Computer Science and Software Engineering
                                    Department, University of Westminster,
                                    London, UK
Massimo Ferri                       Department of Mathematics, University of
                                    Bologna, Italy
Alexandru Floares                   Artificial Intelligence Department, Cancer
                                    Institute Cluj-Napoca, Romania
Ana Fred                            Communication Theory and Pattern
                                    Recognition Group, IST – Technical
                                    University of Lisbon, Portugal
Adinda Freudenthal                  Faculty Industrial Design Engineering,
                                    Technical University Delft, The Netherlands
Bogdan Gabrys                       Smart Technology Research Centre,
                                    Computational Intelligence Group,
                                    Bournemouth University, UK
Marie Gustafsson Friberger          Computer Science Department,
                                    Malmö University, Sweden
Randy Goebel                        Centre for Machine Learning, Department of
                                    Computer Science, University of Alberta,
                                    Edmonton, Canada
Venu Govindaraju                    Center for Unified Biometrics and Sensors,
                                    University of Buffalo State New York,
                                    USA
Gary Gorman                         Asia-New Zealand Informatics Associates,
                                    Faculty of Computer Science and IT,
                                    University of Malaya, Malaysia
Michael Granitzer                   Media Computer Science, University Passau,
                                    Germany
Dimitrios Gunopulos                 Knowledge Discovery in Databases
                                    Laboratory, Department of Informatics,
                                    University of Athens, Greece

Siegfried Handschuh          Semantic Information Systems and Language
                             Engineering Group, Digital Enterprise
                             Research Institute, Ireland
Helwig Hauser                Visualization Group, University of Bergen,
                             Norway
Julian Heinrich              Visualization Research Centre, University
                             of Stuttgart, Germany
Kristina Hettne              BioSemantics group, Department of Human
                             Genetics, Leiden University Medical Center,
                             The Netherlands
Andreas Hotho                Data Mining and Information Retrieval Group,
                             University of Würzburg, Germany
Jun Luke Huan                Computational Knowledge Discovery Lab,
                             University of Kansas, Lawrence,
                             USA
Anthony Hunter               Intelligent Systems Group, Department of
                             Computer Science, UCL University College
                             London, UK
Beatriz De La Iglesia        Knowledge Discovery and Data Mining Group,
                             School of Computing Sciences, University
                             of East Anglia, Norwich, UK
Alfred Inselberg             School of Mathematical Sciences, Tel Aviv
                             University, Israel
Kalervo Jaervelin            School of Information Science, University of
                             Tampere, Finland
Andreas Kerren               ISOVIS Group, Department of Computer
                             Science, Linnaeus University, Växjö, Sweden
Kinshuk                      Technology Enhanced Knowledge Research
                             and Learning Analytics, Athabasca
                             University, Canada
Jiri Klema                   Department of Cybernetics, Faculty of
                             Electrical Engineering, Czech Technical
                             University, Prague, Czech Republic
Gudrun Klinker               Computer Aided Medical Procedures and
                             Augmented Reality, Technische Universität
                             München, Germany
Lubos Klucar                 Laboratory of Bioinformatics, Institute of
                             Molecular Biology, Slovak Academy of
                             Sciences, Bratislava, Slovakia
David Koslicki               Mathematics Department, Oregon
                             State University, Corvallis, USA
Patti Kostkova               eHealth Research Centre, City University
                             London, UK

Damjan Krstajic                 Research Centre for Cheminformatics,
                                Belgrade, Serbia
Natsuhiko Kumasaka              Center for Genomic Medicine (CGM), Tokyo,
                                Japan
Robert S. Laramee               Data Visualization Group, Department of
                                Computer Science, Swansea University, UK
Nada Lavrac                     Department of Knowledge Technologies, Joszef
                                Stefan Institute, Ljubljana, Slovenia
Sangkyun Lee                    Artificial Intelligence Unit, Dortmund
                                University, Germany
Matthijs van Leeuwen            Machine Learning Group, KU Leuven,
                                Heverlee, Belgium
Alexander Lex                   Graphics, Vision and Interaction, Harvard
                                University, Cambridge (MA), USA
Chunping Li                     School of Software, Tsinghua University, China
Luca Longo                      Knowledge and Data Engineering Group,
                                Trinity College Dublin, Ireland
Lenka Lhotska                   Department of Cybernetics, Faculty of
                                Electrical Engineering, Czech Technical
                                University Prague, Czech Republic
Andras Lukacs                   Institute of Mathematics, Hungarian Academy
                                of Sciences and Eoetvos University,
                                Budapest, Hungary
Avi Ma' Ayan                    Systems Biology Center, Mount Sinai Hospital,
                                New York, USA
Ljiljana Majnaric-Trtica        Department of Family Medicine, Medical
                                School, University of Osijek, Croatia
Martin Middendorf               Institut für Informatik, Fakultät für
                                Mathematik und Informatik, University of
                                Leipzig, Germany
Silvia Miksch                   Centre of Visual Analytics Science and
                                Technology, Vienna University of
                                Technology, Vienna, Austria
Antonio Moreno-Ribas            Intelligent Technologies for Advanced
                                Knowledge Acquistion, Universitat Rovira i
                                Virgili, Tarragona, Spain
Katharina Morik                 Fakultät Informatik, Lehrstuhl für Künstliche
                                Intelligenz, Technische Universität
                                Dortmund, Germany
Abbe Mowshowitz                 Department of Computer Science, The City
                                College of New York, USA
Marian Mrozek                   Institute of Computer Science, Jagiellonian
                                University, Krakow, Poland

Zoran Obradovic

Data Analytics and Biomedical Informatics
Center, Temple University, USA

Daniel E. O'Leary

School of Business, University of Southern
California, Los Angeles, USA

Patricia Ordonez-Rozo

Clinical and Translations Research
Consortium, University of Puerto Rico Rio
Piedras, San Juan, Puerto Rico

Ant Ozok

Department of Information Systems, UMBC,
Baltimore, USA

Vasile Palade

Department of Computer Science, University of
Oxford, UK

Jan Paralic

Department of Cybernetics and Artificial
Intelligence, Technical University of Kosice,
Slovakia

Valerio Pascucci

Scientific Computing and Imaging Institute,
University of Utah, USA

Gabriela Pasi

Laboratorio di Information Retrieval,
Università di Milano Bicocca, Milan, Italy

Armando J. Pinho

Departamento de Electrónica,
Telecomunicações e Informática,
Universidade de Aveiro, Portugal

Pavel Pilarczyk

Centre of Mathematics, University of Minho,
Braga, Portugal

Margit Pohl

Human-Computer Interaction Group, Vienna
University of Technology, Vienna, Austria

Paul Rabadan

Biomedical Informatics, Columbia University
College of Physicians and Surgeons,
New York, USA

Heri Ramampiaro

Data and Information Management Group,
Norwegian University of Science and
Technology, Trondheim, Norway

Dietrich Rebholz

European Bioinformatics Institute, Cambridge,
UK

Chandan Reddy

Data Mining and Knowledge Discovery Lab,
Wayne State University, USA

Gerhard Rigoll

Lehrstuhl für Mensch-Maschine
Kommunikation, Technische Universität
München, Germany

Jianhua Ruan

Computational Biology, Department of
Computer Science, University of Texas,
San Antonio, USA

Lior Rokach

Department of Information Systems
Engineering, Ben-Gurion University of the
Negev, Beer-Sheva, Israel

| | |
|---|---|
| Carsten Roecker | e-Health Group, RWTH Aachen University, Germany |
| Timo Ropinski | Scientific Visualization Group, Linköping University, Sweden |
| Giuseppe Santucci | Dipartimento di Informatica e Sistemistica, La Sapienza, University of Rome, Italy |
| Reinhold Scherer | Graz BCI Lab, Institute of Knowledge Discovery, Graz University of Technology, Austria |
| Monica M.C. Schraefel | Agents, Interaction and Complexity Group, Electronics and Computer Science, University of Southampton, UK |
| Paola Sebastiani | Department of Biostatistics, School of Public Health, Boston University, USA |
| Christin Seifert | Media Computer Science, University Passau, Germany |
| Tanja Schultz | Cognitive Systems Lab, Karlsruhe Institute of Technology, Germany |
| Andrzej Skowron | Group of Mathematical Logic, Institute of Mathematics, University of Warszaw, Poland |
| Neil R. Smalheiser | College of Medicine, University of Illinois at Chicago, USA |
| Rainer Spang | Statistical Bioinformatics Department, Institute of Functional Genomics, University of Regensburg, Germany |
| Irena Spasic | Health Informatics, School of Computer Science and Informatics, Cardiff University, UK |
| Jerzy Stefanowski | Institute of Computing Science, Poznan University of Technology, Poland |
| Gregor Stiglic | Stanford Center for Biomedical Informatics, Stanford School of Medicine, Stanford, USA |
| Marc Streit | Institute of Computer Graphics, Johannes Kepler University Linz, Austria |
| Dimitar Trajanov | Department of Computer Science, Cyril and Methodius University, Skopje, Macedonia |
| Catagaj Turkay | Department of Computer Science, City University London, UK |
| A Min Tjoa | Information and Software Engineering Group, Vienna University of Technology, Austria |
| Olof Torgersson | Applied Information Technology, Chalmers University of Technology, Göteborg, Sweden |

Berndt Urlesberger             Neonatalogist, Department of Pediatrics and
                               Adolescent Medicine, Division Neonatology,
                               Graz University Hospital, Austria
Nikolaus Veit-Rubin            Operative Gynaecology and Obstetrics,
                               Department of Gynaecology and Obstetrics,
                               University Hospitals Geneva, Switzerland

## International Industrial Application and Business Committee

Rakesh Agrawal                 Microsoft Search Labs, Mountain View
                               California, USA
Peter Bak                      IBM Haifa Research Lab, Mount Carmel, Israel
Robert Baumgartner             Lixto Web Information Extraction, Vienna,
                               Austria
Andreas Bender                 Unilever Centre for Molecular Science
                               Informatics, Cambridge, UK
Alberto Brabenetz              IBM Vienna Austria, Austria
Anni R. Coden                  IBM T.J. Watson Research Center New York,
                               USA
Hugo Gamboa                    PLUX Wireless Biosensors, Portugal
Leo Grady                      Heart Flow Inc., Redwood, California, USA
Stefan Jaschke                 IBM Vienna Austria, Austria
Homa Javahery                  IBM Centers for Solution Innovation, Canada
Igor Jurisica                  IBM Life Sciences Discovery Centre, Canada
Mei Kobayashi                  IBM Tokyo Laboratory, Tokyo, Japan
Alek Kolcz                     Twitter Inc., USA
Jie Lu                         IBM T.J. Watson Research Center, Hawthorne,
                               New York, USA
Helmut Ludwar                  IBM Vienna Austria, Austria
Sriganesh Madhvanath           Hewlett-Packard Laboratories Bangalore,
                               Republic of India
Roberto Mirizzi                Hewlett-Packard Laboratories Palo Alto,
                               USA
Laxmi Parida                   IBM T.J. Watson Research Center. Yorktown
                               Heights, New York, USA
Gottfried Prohaska             IBM Vienna Austria, Austria
Hugo Silva                     PLUX Wireless Biosensors, Lisbon, Portugal
Gurjeet Singh                  AYASDI, USA
Hong Sun                       Advanced Clinical Applications Research, Agfa
                               HealthCare, Ghent, Belgium
Dan T. Tecuci                  SIEMENS Corporate Research Princeton, USA
Ulli Waltinger                 SIEMENS Business Analytics, Germany

Martin Weigl              AIMC, Vienna, Austria
Raffael Wiemker           Philips Research Hamburg, Germany
Minlu Zhang               NEXTBIO, USA

## International Student Committee

Andre Calero-Valdez        RWTH Aachen, Germany
Pavel Dlotko               Jagiellonian University, Poland
Markus Fassold             hci4all Team Graz, Austria
Fleur Jeanquartier         hci4all Team Graz, Austria
Peter Koncz                Technical University of Kosice, Slovakia
Bernd Malle                hci4all Team Graz, Austria
Emanuele Panzeri           University of Milano Bicocca, Italy
Igor Pernek                University of Maribor, Slovenia
Vito Claudio Ostuni        Politecnico di Bari, Italy
David Rogers               Health Informatics, School of Computer Science
                           and Informatics, Cardiff University, UK
Antonia Saravanou          Knowledge Discovery in Database Laboratory,
                           University of Athens, Greece
Jasmina Smailović          Jožef Stefan Institute, Ljubljana, Slovenia
Christof Stocker           hci4all Team Graz, Austria
Hubert Wagner              Jagiellonian University, Poland

# Table of Contents

Knowledge Discovery and Data Mining in Biomedical Informatics:
The Future Is in Integrative, Interactive Machine Learning Solutions ...   1
  *Andreas Holzinger and Igor Jurisica*

Visual Data Mining: Effective Exploration of the Biological Universe ...   19
  *David Otasek, Chiara Pastrello, Andreas Holzinger, and Igor Jurisica*

Darwin or Lamarck? Future Challenges in Evolutionary Algorithms for
Knowledge Discovery and Data Mining ...........................   35
  *Katharina Holzinger, Vasile Palade, Raul Rabadan, and
  Andreas Holzinger*

On the Generation of Point Cloud Data Sets: Step One in the
Knowledge Discovery Process....................................   57
  *Andreas Holzinger, Bernd Malle, Marcus Bloice, Marco Wiltgen,
  Massimo Ferri, Ignazio Stanganelli, and Rainer Hofmann-Wellenhof*

Adapted Features and Instance Selection for Improving Co-training ....   81
  *Gilad Katz, Asaf Shabtai, and Lior Rokach*

Knowledge Discovery and Visualization of Clusters for Erythromycin
Related Adverse Events in the FDA Drug Adverse Event Reporting
System .......................................................   101
  *Pinar Yildirim, Marcus Bloice, and Andreas Holzinger*

On Computationally-Enhanced Visual Analysis of Heterogeneous Data
and Its Application in Biomedical Informatics .....................   117
  *Cagatay Turkay, Fleur Jeanquartier, Andreas Holzinger, and
  Helwig Hauser*

A Policy-Based Cleansing and Integration Framework for Labour and
Healthcare Data ..............................................   141
  *Roberto Boselli, Mirko Cesarini, Fabio Mercorio, and
  Mario Mezzanzanica*

Interactive Data Exploration Using Pattern Mining .................   169
  *Matthijs van Leeuwen*

Resources for Studying Statistical Analysis of Biomedical Data
and R .......................................................   183
  *Mei Kobayashi*

A Kernel-Based Framework for Medical Big-Data Analytics ...........  197
    *David Windridge and Miroslaw Bober*

On Entropy-Based Data Mining ..................................  209
    *Andreas Holzinger, Matthias Hörtenhuber, Christopher Mayer,*
    *Martin Bachler, Siegfried Wassertheurer, Armando J. Pinho, and*
    *David Koslicki*

Sparse Inverse Covariance Estimation for Graph Representation of
Feature Structure ...............................................  227
    *Sangkyun Lee*

Multi-touch Graph-Based Interaction for Knowledge Discovery on
Mobile Devices: State-of-the-Art and Future Challenges ..............  241
    *Andreas Holzinger, Bernhard Ofner, and Matthias Dehmer*

Intelligent Integrative Knowledge Bases: Bridging Genomics, Integrative
Biology and Translational Medicine .............................  255
    *Hoan Nguyen, Julie D. Thompson, Patrick Schutz, and Olivier Poch*

Biomedical Text Mining: State-of-the-Art, Open Problems and Future
Challenges .....................................................  271
    *Andreas Holzinger, Johannes Schantl, Miriam Schroettner,*
    *Christin Seifert, and Karin Verspoor*

Protecting Anonymity in Data-Driven Biomedical Science ............  301
    *Peter Kieseberg, Heidelinde Hobel, Sebastian Schrittwieser,*
    *Edgar Weippl, and Andreas Holzinger*

Biobanks – A Source of Large Biological Data Sets: Open Problems
and Future Challenges ...........................................  317
    *Berthold Huppertz and Andreas Holzinger*

On Topological Data Mining ....................................  331
    *Andreas Holzinger*

**Author Index** .................................................  357

# Knowledge Discovery and Data Mining in Biomedical Informatics: The Future Is in Integrative, Interactive Machine Learning Solutions

Andreas Holzinger[1] and Igor Jurisica[2]

[1] Medical University Graz, Institute for Medical Informatics, Statistics and Documentation
Research Unit HCI, Austrian IBM Watson Think Group,
Auenbruggerplatz 2/V, A-8036 Graz, Austria
a.holzinger@hci4all.at
[2] Princess Margaret Cancer Centre, University Health Network, IBM Life Sciences Discovery
Centre, and TECHNA Institute for the Advancement of Technology for Health,
TMDT 11-314, 101 College Street, Toronto, ON M5G 1L7, Canada
juris@ai.utoronto.ca

**Abstract.** Biomedical research is drowning in data, yet starving for knowledge. Current challenges in biomedical research and clinical practice include information overload – the need to combine vast amounts of structured, semi-structured, weakly structured data and vast amounts of unstructured information – and the need to optimize workflows, processes and guidelines, to increase capacity while reducing costs and improving efficiencies. In this paper we provide a very short overview on interactive and integrative solutions for knowledge discovery and data mining. In particular, we emphasize the benefits of including the end user into the "interactive" knowledge discovery process. We describe some of the most important challenges, including the need to develop and apply novel methods, algorithms and tools for the integration, fusion, pre-processing, mapping, analysis and interpretation of complex biomedical data with the aim to identify testable hypotheses, and build realistic models. The HCI-KDD approach, which is a synergistic combination of methodologies and approaches of two areas, Human–Computer Interaction (HCI) and Knowledge Discovery & Data Mining (KDD), offer ideal conditions towards solving these challenges: with the goal of supporting human intelligence with machine intelligence. There is an urgent need for integrative and interactive machine learning solutions, because no medical doctor or biomedical researcher can keep pace today with the increasingly large and complex data sets – often called "Big Data".

**Keywords:** Knowledge Discovery, Data Mining, Machine Learning, Biomedical Informatics, Integration, Interaction, HCI-KDD, Big Data.

A. Holzinger, I. Jurisica (Eds.): Knowledge Discovery and Data Mining, LNCS 8401, pp. 1–18, 2014.
© Springer-Verlag Berlin Heidelberg 2014

# 1     Introduction and Motivation

Cinical practice, healthcare and biomedical research of today is drowning in data, yet starving for knowledge as Herbert A. Simon (1916–2001) pointed it out 40 years ago: *"A wealth of information creates a poverty of attention and a need to allocate that attention efficiently among the overabundance of information sources that might consume it* [1]."

The central problem is that biomedical data models are characterized by significant **complexity** [2-5] making manual analysis by the end users difficult, yet often impossible. Hence, current challenges in clinical practice and biomedical research include **information overload** – an often debated phenomenon in medicine for a long time [6-10].

There is the pressing need to combine vast amounts of diverse data, including structured, semi-structured and weakly structured data and unstructured information [11]. Interestingly, many powerful computational tools advancing in recent years have been developed by separate communities following different philosophies: Data mining and machine learning researchers tend to believe in the power of their statistical methods to identify relevant patterns – mostly automatic, without human intervention. There is, however, the danger of modelling artefacts when end user comprehension and control are diminished [12-15]. Additionally, mobile, ubiquitous computing and automatic medical sensors everywhere, together with low cost storage, will even accelerate this avalanche of data [16].

Another aspect is that, faced with unsustainable health care costs worldwide and enormous amounts of under-utilized data, medicine and health care needs more efficient practices; experts consider health information technology as key to increasing efficiency and quality of health care, whilst decreasing the costs [17].

Moreover, we need more research on methods, algorithms and tools to harness the full benefits towards the concept of **personalized medicine** [18]. Yet, we also need to substantially expand automated data capture to further **precision medicine** [19] and truly enable evidence-based medicine [20].

To capture data and task diversity, we continue to expand and improve individual knowledge discovery and data mining approaches and frameworks that let the end users gain insight into the nature of massive data sets [21-23].

The trend is to move individual systems to integrated, ensemble and interactive systems (see Figure 1).

Each type of data requires different, optimized approach; yet, we cannot interpret data fully without linking to other types. Ensemble systems and integrative KDD are part of the answer. Graph-based methods enable linking typed and annotated data further. Rich ontologies [24-26] and aspects from the Semantic Web [27-29] provide additional abilities to further characterize and annotate the discoveries.

## 2     Glossary and Key Terms

*Biomedical Informatics:* similar to medical informatics (see below) but including the optimal use of *biomedical data,* e.g. from the "–omics world" [30];

*Data Mining:* methods, algorithms and tools to extract patterns from data by combining methods from computational statistics [31] and machine learning: *"Data mining is about solving problems by analyzing data present in databases* [32]";

*Deep Learning:* is a machine learning method which models high-level abstractions in data by use of architectures composed of multiple non-linear transformations [33].

*Ensemble Machine Learning:* uses multiple learning algorithms to obtain better predictive performance as could be obtained from any standard learning algorithms [34]; A tutorial on ensemble-based classifiers can be found in [35].

*Human–Computer Interaction:* involves the study, design and development of the interaction between end users and computers (data); the classic definition goes back to Card, Moran & Newell [36], [37]. Interactive user-interfaces shall, for example, empower the user to carry out visual data mining;

*Interactome:* is the whole set of molecular interactions in a cell, i.e. genetic interactions, described as biological networks and displayed as graphs. The term goes back to the work of [38].

*Information Overload:* is an often debated, not clearly defined term from decision making research, when having to many alternatives to make a satisfying decision [39]; based on, e.g. the theory of cognitive load during problem solving [40-42].

*Knowledge Discovery (KDD):* Exploratory analysis and modeling of data and the organized process of identifying valid, novel, useful and understandable patterns from these data sets [21].

*Machine Learning:* the classic definition is "A computer program is said to learn from experience E with respect to some class of tasks T and performance measure P, if its performance at tasks in T, as measured by P, improves with experience E" [43].

*Medical Informatics:* in the classical definition: "... scientific field that deals with the storage, retrieval, and optimal use of medical information, data, and knowledge for problem solving and decision making" [44];

*Usability Engineering:* includes methods that shall ensure that integrated and interactive solutions are useable and useful for the end users [45].

*Visual Data Mining:* An interactive combination of visualization and analysis with the goal to implement workflow that enables integration of user's expertise [46].

# 3     State-of-the-Art of Interactive and Integrative Solutions

Gotz et al. (2014) [47] present in a very recent work an interesting methodology for interactive mining and visual analysis of clinical event patterns using electronic health record data. They start with the evidence that the medical conditions of patients often evolve in *complex* and *unpredictable* ways and that variations between patients in both their progression and eventual outcome can be dramatic. Consequently, they state that understanding the patterns of events observed within a population that most correlate with differences in outcome is an important task. Their approach for **interactive pattern mining** supports ad hoc visual exploration of patterns mined from retrospective clinical patient data and combines three issues: visual query capabilities to interactively specify episode definitions; pattern mining techniques to help discover important intermediate events within an episode; and interactive visualization techniques that help uncover event patterns that most impact outcome and how those associations change over time.

Pastrello et al. (2014) [48] emphasize that first and foremost it is important to integrate the large volumes of heterogeneous and distributed data sets and that interactive data visualization is essential to obtain meaningful hypotheses from the diversity of various data (see Figure 1). They see **network analysis** (see e.g. [49]) as a key technique to integrate, visualize and extrapolate relevant information from diverse data sets and emphasize the huge challenge in integrating different types of data and then focus on systematically exploring network properties to gain insight into network functions. They also accentuate the role of the *interactome* in connecting data derived from different experiments, and they emphasize the importance of network analysis for the recognition of interaction context-specific features.

A previous work of Pastrello et al. (2013) [50] states that, whilst high-throughput technologies produce massive amounts of data, individual methods yield data, specific to the technique and the specific biological setup used. They also emphasize that at first the **integration of diverse data sets** is necessary for the qualitative analysis of information relevant to build hypotheses or to discover knowledge. Moreover, Pastrello et al. are of the opinion that it is useful to integrate these data sets by use of pathways and protein interaction networks; the resulting network needs to be able to focus on either a large-scale view or on more detailed small-scale views, depending on the research question and experimental goals. In their paper, the authors illustrate a workflow, which is useful to integrate, analyze, and visualize data from different sources, and they highlight important features of tools to support such analyses.

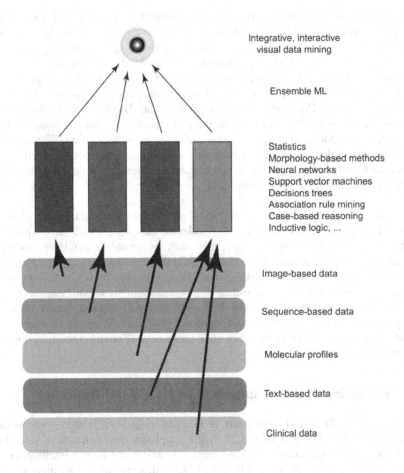

Integrative, interactive
visual data mining

Ensemble ML

Statistics
Morphology-based methods
Neural networks
Support vector machines
Decisions trees
Association rule mining
Case-based reasoning
Inductive logic, ...

Image-based data

Sequence-based data

Molecular profiles

Text-based data

Clinical data

**Fig. 1.** Integrative analysis requires systematically combining various data sets and diverse algorithms. To support multiple user needs and enable integration of user's expertise, it is essential to support visual data mining.

An example from Neuroimaging provided by Bowman et al. (2012) [51], shows that electronic data capture methods will significantly advance the populating of large-scale neuroimaging databases: As these archives grow in size, a particular challenge is in the examination of and interaction with the information that these resources contain through the development of user-driven approaches for data exploration and data mining. In their paper they introduce the visualization for neuroimaging (INVIZIAN) framework for the graphical rendering of, and the dynamic interaction with the contents of large-scale neuroimaging data sets. Their system graphically displays brain surfaces as points in a coordinate space, thereby enabling the classification of clusters of neuroanatomically similar MRI-images and data mining.

Koelling et al. (2012) [52] present a web-based tool for visual data mining colocation patterns in multivariate bioimages, the so-called Web-based Hyperbolic Image Data Explorer (WHIDE). The authors emphasize that bioimaging techniques rapidly develop toward higher resolution and higher dimension; the increase in dimension is achieved by different techniques, which record for each pixel an $n$-dimensional intensity array, representing local abundances of molecules, residues or interaction patterns. The analysis of such Multivariate Bio-Images (MBIs) calls for new approaches to support end users in the analysis of both feature domains: space (i.e. sample morphology) and molecular colocation or interaction. The approach combines principles from computational learning, dimension reduction and visualization within, freely available via: http://ani.cebitec.uni-bielefeld.de/BioIMAX (login: whidetestuser; Password: whidetest).

An earlier work by Wegman (2003) [53], emphasizes that data mining strategies are usually applied to "opportunistically" collected data sets, which are frequently in the focus of the discovery of structures such as clusters, trends, periodicities, associations, correlations, etc., for which a visual data analysis is very appropriate and quite likely to yield insight. On the other hand, Wegman argues that data mining strategies are often applied to large data sets where standard visualization techniques may not be appropriate, due to the limits of screen resolution, limits of human perception and limits of available computational resources. Wegman thus envisioned Visual Data Mining (VDM) as a possible successful approach for attacking high-dimensional and large data sets.

# 4    Towards Finding Solutions: The HCI-KDD Approach

The idea of the HCI-KDD approach is in combining the "best of two worlds": Human–Computer Interaction (HCI), with emphasis on perception, cognition, interaction, reasoning, decision making, human learning and human intelligence, and Knowledge Discovery & Data Mining (KDD), dealing with data-preprocessing, computational statistics, machine learning and artificial intelligence [54].

In Figure 2 it can be seen how the concerted HCI-KDD approach may provide contributions to research and development for finding solutions to some challenges mentioned before. However, before looking at further details, one question may arise: What is the difference between Knowledge Discovery and Data Mining? The paradigm "Data Mining (DM)" has an established tradition, dating back to the early days of databases, and with varied naming conventions, e.g., "data grubbing", "data fishing" [55]; the term "Information Retrieval (IR)" was coined even earlier in 1950 [56, 57], whereas the term "Knowledge Discovery (KD)" is relatively young, having its roots in the classical work of Piatetsky-Shapiro (1991) [58], and gaining much popularity with the paper by Fayyad et al. (1996) [59]. Considering these definitions, we need to explain the difference between Knowledge Discovery and Data Mining itself: Some researchers argue that there is *no* difference, and to emphasize this it is often called "Knowledge Discovery and Data Mining (KDD)", whereas the original definition by Fayyad was "Knowledge Discovery from Data (KDD)", which makes also sense but separates it from Data Mining (DM). Although it makes sense to differentiate between these two terms, we prefer the first notion: "Knowledge

Discovery and Data Mining (KDD)" to emphasize that *both* are of equal importance and necessary in combination. This orchestrated interplay is graphically illustrated in Figure 2: Whilst KDD encompasses the whole *process* workflow ranging from the very physical data representation (left) to the human aspects of information processing (right), data mining goes *in depth* and includes the algorithms for particularly finding patterns in the data. Interaction is prominently represented by HCI in the left side.

Within this "big picture" seven research areas can be identified, numbered from area 1 to area 7:

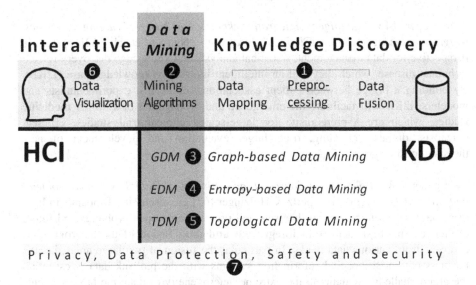

**Fig. 2.** The big picture of the HCI-KDD approach: KDD encompasses the whole **horizontal** process chain from data to information and knowledge; actually from physical aspects of raw data, to human aspects including attention, memory, vision, interaction etc. as core topics in HCI, whilst DM as a **vertical** subject focuses on the development of methods, algorithms and tools for data mining (Image taken from the hci4all.at website, as of March, 2014).

## 4.1 Area 1: Data Integration, Data Pre-processing and Data Mapping

In this volume three papers (#4, #8 and #15) are addressing research area 1:

In paper #4 *"On the Generation of Point Cloud Data Sets: Step one in the Knowledge Discovery Process"* Holzinger et al. [60] provide some answers to the question "How do you get a graph out of your data?" or more specific "How to get **point cloud data sets** from natural images?". The authors present some solutions, open problems and a future outlook when mapping continuous data, such as natural images, into discrete point cloud data sets (PCD). Their work is based on the assumption that geometry, topology and graph theory have much potential for the analysis of arbitrarily high-dimensional data.

In paper #8 *"A Policy-based Cleansing and Integration Framework for Labour and Healthcare Data"* Boselli et al. [61] report on a **holistic data integration strategy** for large amounts of health data. The authors describe how a model based cleansing framework is extended to address such integration activities. Their combined approach facilitates the rapid prototyping, development, and evaluation of data preprocessing activities. They found, that a combined use of formal methods and visualization techniques strongly empower the data analyst, which can effectively evaluate how cleansing and integration activities can affect the data analysis. The authors show also an example focusing on labour and healthcare data integration.

In paper #15 *"Intelligent integrative knowledge bases: bridging genomics, integrative biology and translational medicine"*, Nguyen et al. [62] present a perspective for data management, statistical analysis and knowledge discovery related to human disease, which they call an intelligent integrative knowledge base (I2KB). By building a bridge between patient associations, clinicians, experimentalists and modelers, I2KB will facilitate the emergence and propagation of **systems medicine** studies, which are a prerequisite for large-scaled clinical trial studies, efficient diagnosis, disease screening, drug target evaluation and development of new therapeutic strategies.

In paper #18 *"Biobanks – A Source of large Biological Data Sets: Open Problems and Future Challenges"*, Huppertz & Holzinger [63] are discussing Biobanks in light of a source of large biological data sets and present some open problems and future challenges, amongst them **data integration and data fusion** of the heterogeneous data sets from various data banks. In particular the fusion of two large areas, i.e. the business enterprise hospital information systems with the biobank data is essential, the grand challenge remains in the extreme heterogeneity of data, the large amounts of weakly structured data, in data complexity, and the massive amount of unstructured information and the associated lack of data quality.

## 4.2    Area 2: Data Mining Algorithms

Most of the papers in this volume are dealing with data mining algorithms, in particular:

In paper #3 *"Darwin or Lamarck? Future Challenges in Evolutionary Algorithms for Knowledge Discovery and Data Mining"* Katharina Holzinger et al. [64] are discussing the differences between evolutionary algorithms, beginning with some background on the **theory of evolution** by contrasting the original ideas of Charles Darwin and Jean-Baptiste de Lamarck; the authors provide a discussion on the analogy between biological and computational sciences, and briefly describe some fundamentals of various algorithms, including Genetic Algorithms, but also new and promising ones, including Invasive Weed Optimization, Memetic Search, Differential Evolution Search, Artificial Immune Systems, and Intelligent Water Drops.

In paper #5 *"Adapted Features and Instance Selection for Improving Co-Training"*, Katz et al. [65] report on the importance of high quality, labeled data as it is essential for successfully applying machine learning to real-world problems. Because often the amount of labeled data is insufficient and labeling that data is time consuming, Katz et al. propose co-training algorithms, which use unlabeled data in order to improve classification. The authors propose simple and effective strategies for improving the basic co-training framework, i.e.: the manner in which the features set is partitioned and the method of selecting additional instances. Moreover, they present a study over 25 datasets, and prove that their proposed strategies are especially effective for **imbalanced datasets.**

In paper #6 *"Knowledge Discovery & Visualization of Clusters for Erythromycin Related Adverse Events in the FDA Drug Adverse Event Reporting System"*, Yildirim et al. [66] present a study to discover hidden knowledge in the reports of the public release of the Food and Drug Administration (FDA)'s Adverse Event Reporting System (FAERS) for the antibiotic Erythromycin. This is highly relevant, due to the fact that bacterial infections can cause significant morbidity, mortality and high costs of treatment and are known as a significant health problem in the world. The authors used **cluster analysis** and the DBSCAN algorithm. Medical researchers and pharmaceutical companies may utilize these results and test these relationships along with their clinical studies.

In paper #10 *"Resources for Studying Statistical Analysis of Biomedical Data and R"*, Kobayashi [67] introduces some online resources to help medical practitioners with little or no background in **predictive statistics**, to learn basic statistical concepts and to implement data analysis methods on their personal computers by using R, a high-level open source computer language that requires relatively little training. This offers medical practitioners an opportunity to identify effectiveness of treatments for patients using summary statistics, so to offer patients more personalized medical treatments based on predictive analytics. Some open problems emphasized by Kobayashi include Privacy Preserving Data Mining (PPDM) algorithms and High Speed Medical Data Analysis.

In paper #11 *"A Kernel-based Framework for Medical Big-Data Analytics"*, Windridge & Bober [68] point out that issues of incompleteness and heterogeneity are problematic and that data in the biomedical domain can be as diverse as handwritten notes, blood pressure readings, and MR scans, etc., and typically very little of this data will be co-present for each patient at any given time interval. Windridge & Bober therefore advocate a **kernel-based framework** as being most appropriate for handling these issues, using the neutral point substitution method to accommodate missing inter-modal data, and advocates for the pre-processing of image based MR data a **deep learning** solution for contextual areal segmentation, with edit-distance based kernel measurement, used to characterize relevant morphology. Moreover, the authors promote the use of **Boltzmann machines.**

In paper #16 *"Biomedical Text Mining: Open Problems and Future Challenges"* Holzinger et al. [69] provide a short, concise overview of some selected text mining methods, focusing on **statistical methods** (Latent Semantic Analysis, Probabilistic Latent Semantic Analysis, Latent Dirichlet Allocation, Hierarchical Latent Dirichlet Allocation, Hierarchical Latent Dirichlet Allocation, Principal Component Analysis), but also introduces relatively new and promising text mining methods including **graph-based** approaches and **topological text mining.** Although in our modern graphic-driven multimedia world, the importance of text is often debated, it should not be underestimated, as particularly in the medical domain "free text" is a very important type of data for medical communication; however, the increasing volumes of this unstructured information makes manual analysis nearly impossible, and calls for machine learning approaches for text mining.

### 4.2.1    Area 3: Graph Based Data Mining

In paper #14 *"Multi-touch Graph-Based Interaction for Knowledge Discovery on Mobile Devices: State-of-the-Art and Future Challenges"* Holzinger et al. [70] provide an overview on **graph-based knowledge representation:** Graphs are most powerful tools to map structures within a given data set and to recognize relationships between specific data objects. Many advantages of graph-based data structures can be found in the applicability of methods from network analysis, topology and data mining (e.g. small world phenomenon, cluster analysis). Moreover, Holzinger et al. present graph-based approaches for multi-touch interaction on mobile devices (tablets, smartphones), which is particularly important in the medical domain, as a conceptual graph analysis may provide novel insights on hidden patterns in data, hence support interactive knowledge discovery. Amongst the open problems the authors list the question "Which structural properties possess the multi-touch interaction graphs?", which calls for investigating graph classes beyond small world and random networks.

In paper #13 *"Sparse Inverse Covariance Estimation for Graph Representation of Feature Structure"*, Lee [71] states that higher dimensionality makes it challenging to understand complex systems. The author reports on structure learning with the Gaussian Markov random field, by identifying conditional independence structure of features in a form that is easy to visualize and understand. The learning is based on a convex optimization problem, called the sparse inverse covariance estimation, for which many efficient algorithms have been developed in the past. When dimensions are much larger than sample sizes, **structure learning** requires to consider statistical stability, in which connections to data mining arise in terms of discovering common or rare sub-graphs as patterns. Lee discusses the outcome of structure learning, which can be visualized as graphs provide a perceivable way to investigate complex feature spaces. He identifies two major open challenges for solving the sparse inverse covariance estimation problem in high-dimensions: development of efficient optimization algorithms and consideration of statistical stability of solutions.

### 4.2.2 Area 4: Entropy Based Data Mining

In paper #12 *"On Entropy-based Data Mining"*, Holzinger et al. [72], start with some basics on information entropy as **measure for the uncertainty of data.** Then the authors provide a taxonomy of various entropy methods, whereby describing in more detail: Approximate Entropy, Sample Entropy, Fuzzy Entropy, and particularly **Topological Entropy** for finite sequences. Holzinger et al. state that entropy measures have successfully been tested for analysing short, sparse and noisy time series data, but that they have not yet been applied to weakly structured data in combination with techniques from computational topology, which is a hot and promising research route.

### 4.2.3 Area 5: Topological Data Mining

In paper #19 *"Topological Data Mining in a Nutshell"* [73] Holzinger presents a nutshell-like overview on some basics of **topology and data** and discusses some issues on why this is important for knowledge discovery and data mining: Humans are very good at pattern recognition in dimensions of lower or equal than 3, this suggests that computer science should develop methods for exploring this capacity, whereas computational geometry and topology have much potential for the analysis of arbitrarily high-dimensional data sets. Again, both together could be powerful beyond imagination.

### 4.3 Area 6: Data Visualization

In paper #2 *"Visual Data Mining: Effective Exploration of the Biological Universe"*, Otasek et al. [74] present their experiences with Visual Data Mining (VDM), supported by interactive and scalable network visualization and analysis, which enables effective exploration within multiple biological and biomedical fields. The authors discuss large networks, such as the protein interactome and transcriptional regulatory networks, which contain hundreds of thousands of objects and millions of relationships. The authors report on the involved workflows and their experiences with biological researchers on how they can discover knowledge and new theories from their complex data sets.

In paper #7 *"On Computationally-enhanced Visual Analysis of Heterogeneous Data and its Application in Biomedical Informatics"*, Turkay et al. [75] present a concise overview on the state-of-the-art in interactive data visualization, relevant for knowledge discovery, and particularly focus on the issue of integrating computational tools into the workplace for the analysis of heterogeneous data. Turkay et al. emphasize that seamlessly integrated concepts are rare, although there are several solutions that involve a tight integration between computational methods and visualization. Amongst the open problems, the most pressing one is the application of sophisticated visualization techniques, seamlessly integrated into the (bio)-medical workplace, useable and useable to the medical professional.

In paper #9 *"Interactive Data Exploration using Pattern Mining"* van Leeuwen [76] reports on challenges in exploratory data mining to provide insight in data, i.e. to develop principled methods that allow both user-specific and task-specific information to be taken into account, by directly involving the user into the discovery process. The author states that pattern mining algorithms will need to be combined with techniques from visualization and human-computer interaction. As ultimate goal van Leeuwen states to make pattern mining practically more useful, by enabling the user to interactively explore the data and identify interesting structures.

### 4.4    Area 7: Privacy, Data Protection, Safety and Security

In the biomedical domain it is mandatory to consider aspects of privacy, data protection, safety and security, and a fair use of data sets, and one paper is particularly dealing with these topics:

In paper #17 Kieseberg et al. [77] discuss concerns of the disclosure of research data, which raises considerable privacy concerns, as researchers have the responsibility to protect their (volunteer) subjects and must adhere to respective policies. The authors provide an overview on the most important and well-researched approaches to deal with such concerns and discuss open research problems to stimulate further investigation: One solution for this problem lies in the protection of sensitive information in medical data sets by applying appropriate anonymization techniques, due to the fact that the underlying data set should always be made available to ensure the quality of the research done and to prevent fraud or errors.

## 5    Conclusion and Future Outlook

Some of the most important challenges in clinical practice and biomedical research include the need to develop and apply novel tools for the effective integration, analysis and interpretation of complex biomedical data with the aim to identify testable hypothesis, and build realistic models. A big issue is the limited time to make a decision, e.g. a medical doctor has in average five minutes to make a decision [78], [79].

Data and requirements also evolve over time – we need approaches that seamlessly and robustly handle *change*.

The algorithms must also handle incomplete, noisy, even contradictory/ambiguous information, and they have to support multiple viewpoints and contexts.

Solutions need to be interactive, seamlessly integrating diverse data sources, and able to scale to ultra-high dimensions, support multimodal and rapidly evolving representations.

Major future research areas in HCI-KDD in the biomedical field include graph-based analysis and pattern discovery, streaming data mining, integrative and interactive visual data mining. Thus, solutions will need to use heuristics, probabilistic and data-driven methods, with rigorous train-test-validate steps. Especially the last point highlights the need for **open data.**

It is paramount importance that the data is broadly available in usable formats – without relevant reliable and clean data there is no data mining; without accessible data we cannot assure correctness; without data, we cannot train and validate machine learning systems. It is alarming to see an exponential trend in number of retracted papers per year, and especially since the majority of them are fraud – 21.3% being attributed to error and 67.4% to (suspected) fraud [80]: A detailed review of over 2,000 biomedical research articles indexed by PubMed as retracted by May, 2012 revealed that only 21.3% of retractions were attributable to error [80]. In contrast, 67.4% of retractions were attributable to misconduct, including fraud or suspected fraud (43.4%), or duplicate publication (14.2%), and even plagiarism (9.8%) [80]. Incomplete, uninformative or misleading retraction announcements have led to a previous underestimation of the role of fraud in the ongoing retraction epidemic. Machine learning and data mining also plays a significant role in identifying outliers, errors, and thus could contribute to 'cleaning up' science from fraud and errors.

Concluding, there are a lot of open problems and future challenges in dealing with massive amounts of heterogeneous, distributed, diverse, highly dynamic data sets, complex, high-dimensional and weakly structured data and increasingly large amounts of unstructured and non-standardized information. The limits of our human capacities makes it impossible to deal manually with such data, hence, efficient machine learning approaches becomes indispensable.

**Acknowledgements.** We would like to thank the HCI-KDD network of excellence for valuable comments and our institutional colleagues for appreciated discussions.

# References

1. Simon, H.A.: Designing Organizations for an Information-Rich World. In: Greenberger, M. (ed.) Computers, Communication, and the Public Interest, pp. 37–72. The Johns Hopkins Press, Baltimore (1971)
2. Dugas, M., Hoffmann, E., Janko, S., Hahnewald, S., Matis, T., Miller, J., Bary, C.V., Farnbacher, A., Vogler, V., Überla, K.: Complexity of biomedical data models in cardiology: the Intranet-based AF registry. Computer Methods and Programs in Biomedicine 68(1), 49–61 (2002)
3. Akil, H., Martone, M.E., Van Essen, D.C.: Challenges and opportunities in mining neuroscience data. Science 331(6018), 708–712 (2011)
4. Holzinger, A.: Biomedical Informatics: Computational Sciences meets Life Sciences. BoD, Norderstedt (2012)
5. Holzinger, A.: Biomedical Informatics: Discovering Knowledge in Big Data. Springer, New York (2014)
6. Berghel, H.: Cyberspace 2000: Dealing with Information Overload. Communications of the ACM 40(2), 19–24 (1997)
7. Noone, J., Warren, J., Brittain, M.: Information overload: opportunities and challenges for the GP's desktop. Medinfo 9(2), 1287–1291 (1998)

8. Holzinger, A., Geierhofer, R., Errath, M.: Semantic Information in Medical Information Systems - from Data and Information to Knowledge: Facing Information Overload. In: Procedings of I-MEDIA 2007 and I-SEMANTICS 2007, pp. 323–330 (2007)
9. Holzinger, A., Simonic, K.-M., Steyrer, J.: Information Overload - stößt die Medizin an ihre Grenzen? Wissensmanagement 13(1), 10–12 (2011)
10. Holzinger, A., Scherer, R., Ziefle, M.: Navigational User Interface Elements on the Left Side: Intuition of Designers or Experimental Evidence? In: Campos, P., Graham, N., Jorge, J., Nunes, N., Palanque, P., Winckler, M. (eds.) INTERACT 2011, Part II. LNCS, vol. 6947, pp. 162–177. Springer, Heidelberg (2011)
11. Holzinger, A., Dehmer, M., Jurisica, I.: Knowledge Discovery and interactive Data Mining in Bioinformatics - State-of-the-Art, future challenges and research directions. BMC Bioinformatics 15(suppl. 6), I1 (2014)
12. Shneiderman, B.: Inventing Discovery Tools: Combining Information Visualization with Data Mining. In: Jantke, K.P., Shinohara, A. (eds.) DS 2001. LNCS (LNAI), vol. 2226, pp. 17–28. Springer, Heidelberg (2001)
13. Shneiderman, B.: Inventing Discovery Tools: Combining Information Visualization with Data Mining. Information Visualization 1(1), 5–12 (2002)
14. Shneiderman, B.: Creativity support tools. Communications of the ACM 45(10), 116–120 (2002)
15. Shneiderman, B.: Creativity support tools: accelerating discovery and innovation. Communications of the ACM 50(12), 20–32 (2007)
16. Butler, D.: 2020 computing: Everything, everywhere. Nature 440(7083), 402–405 (2006)
17. Chaudhry, B., Wang, J., Wu, S.Y., Maglione, M., Mojica, W., Roth, E., Morton, S.C., Shekelle, P.G.: Systematic review: Impact of health information technology on quality, efficiency, and costs of medical care. Ann. Intern. Med. 144(10), 742–752 (2006)
18. Chawla, N.V., Davis, D.A.: Bringing Big Data to Personalized Healthcare: A Patient-Centered Framework. J. Gen. Intern. Med. 28, S660–S665 (2013)
19. Mirnezami, R., Nicholson, J., Darzi, A.: Preparing for Precision Medicine. N. Engl. J. Med. 366(6), 489–491 (2012)
20. Sackett, D.L., Rosenberg, W.M., Gray, J., Haynes, R.B., Richardson, W.S.: Evidence based medicine: what it is and what it isn't. BMJ: British Medical Journal 312(7023), 71 (1996)
21. Fayyad, U., Piatetsky-Shapiro, G., Smyth, P.: The KDD process for extracting useful knowledge from volumes of data. Communications of the ACM 39(11), 27–34 (1996)
22. Jurisica, I., Mylopoulos, J., Glasgow, J., Shapiro, H., Casper, R.F.: Case-based reasoning in IVF: prediction and knowledge mining. Artificial Intelligence in Medicine 12(1), 1–24 (1998)
23. Yildirim, P., Ekmekci, I.O., Holzinger, A.: On Knowledge Discovery in Open Medical Data on the Example of the FDA Drug Adverse Event Reporting System for Alendronate (Fosamax). In: Holzinger, A., Pasi, G. (eds.) HCI-KDD 2013. LNCS, vol. 7947, pp. 195–206. Springer, Heidelberg (2013)
24. Gruber, T.R.: Toward principles for the design of ontologies used for knowledge sharing. International Journal of Human-Computer Studies 43(5-6), 907–928 (1995)
25. Pinciroli, F., Pisanelli, D.M.: The unexpected high practical value of medical ontologies. Computers in Biology and Medicine 36(7-8), 669–673 (2006)
26. Eiter, T., Ianni, G., Polleres, A., Schindlauer, R., Tompits, H.: Reasoning with rules and ontologies. In: Barahona, P., Bry, F., Franconi, E., Henze, N., Sattler, U. (eds.) Reasoning Web 2006. LNCS, vol. 4126, pp. 93–127. Springer, Heidelberg (2006)

27. Tjoa, A.M., Andjomshoaa, A., Shayeganfar, F., Wagner, R.: Semantic Web challenges and new requirements. In: Database and Expert Systems Applications (DEXA), pp. 1160–1163. IEEE (2005)
28. d'Aquin, M., Noy, N.F.: Where to publish and find ontologies? A survey of ontology libraries. Web Semantics: Science, Services and Agents on the World Wide Web 11, 96–111 (2012)
29. Ruttenberg, A., Clark, T., Bug, W., Samwald, M., Bodenreider, O., Chen, H., Doherty, D., Forsberg, K., Gao, Y., Kashyap, V., Kinoshita, J., Luciano, J., Marshall, M.S., Ogbuji, C., Rees, J., Stephens, S., Wong, G.T., Wu, E., Zaccagnini, D., Hongsermeier, T., Neumann, E., Herman, I., Cheung, K.H.: Methodology - Advancing translational research with the Semantic Web. BMC Bioinformatics 8 (2007)
30. Shortliffe, E.H., Barnett, G.O.: Biomedical data: Their acquisition, storage, and use. Biomedical informatics, pp. 39–66. Springer, London (2014)
31. Hastie, T., Tibshirani, R., Friedman, J.: The Elements of Statistical Learning: Data Mining, Inference, and Prediction, 2nd edn. Springer, New York (2009)
32. Witten, I.H., Frank, E., Hall, M.A.: Data Mining: Practical machine learning tools and techniques. Morgan Kaufmann, San Francisco (2011)
33. Arel, I., Rose, D.C., Karnowski, T.P.: Deep Machine Learning - A New Frontier in Artificial Intelligence Research [Research Frontier]. IEEE Computational Intelligence Magazine 5(4), 13–18 (2010)
34. Dietterich, T.G.: Ensemble methods in machine learning. Multiple classifier systems, pp. 1–15. Springer (2000)
35. Rokach, L.: Ensemble-based classifiers. Artif. Intell. Rev. 33(1-2), 1–39 (2010)
36. Card, S.K., Moran, T.P., Newell, A.: The keystroke-level model for user performance time with interactive systems. Communications of the ACM 23(7), 396–410 (1980)
37. Card, S.K., Moran, T.P., Newell, A.: The psychology of Human-Computer Interaction. Erlbaum, Hillsdale (1983)
38. Sanchez, C., Lachaize, C., Janody, F., Bellon, B., Roder, L., Euzenat, J., Rechenmann, F., Jacq, B.: Grasping at molecular interactions and genetic networks in Drosophila melanogaster using FlyNets, an Internet database. Nucleic Acids Res. 27(1), 89–94 (1999)
39. McNeil, B.J., Keeler, E., Adelstein, S.J.: Primer on Certain Elements of Medical Decision Making. N. Engl. J. Med. 293(5), 211–215 (1975)
40. Sweller, J.: Cognitive load during problem solving: Effects on learning. Cognitive Science 12(2), 257–285 (1988)
41. Stickel, C., Ebner, M., Holzinger, A.: Useful Oblivion Versus Information Overload in e-Learning Examples in the Context of Wiki Systems. Journal of Computing and Information Technology (CIT) 16(4), 271–277 (2008)
42. Workman, M.: Cognitive Load Research and Semantic Apprehension of Graphical Linguistics. In: Holzinger, A. (ed.) USAB 2007. LNCS, vol. 4799, pp. 375–388. Springer, Heidelberg (2007)
43. Mitchell, T.M.: Machine learning, p. 267. McGraw-Hill, Boston (1997)
44. Shortliffe, E.H., Perrault, L.E., Wiederhold, G., Fagan, L.M.: Medical Informatics: Computer Applications in Health Care and Biomedicine. Springer, New York (1990)
45. Holzinger, A.: Usability engineering methods for software developers. Communications of the ACM 48(1), 71–74 (2005)
46. Keim, D.A.: Information visualization and visual data mining. IEEE Transactions on Visualization and Computer Graphics 8(1), 1–8 (2002)

47. Gotz, D., Wang, F., Perer, A.: A methodology for interactive mining and visual analysis of clinical event patterns using electronic health record data. J. Biomed. Inform. (in print, 2014)
48. Pastrello, C., Pasini, E., Kotlyar, M., Otasek, D., Wong, S., Sangrar, W., Rahmati, S., Jurisica, I.: Integration, visualization and analysis of human interactome. Biochemical and Biophysical Research Communications 445(4), 757–773 (2014)
49. Dehmer, M.: Information-theoretic concepts for the analysis of complex networks. Applied Artificial Intelligence 22(7-8), 684–706 (2008)
50. Pastrello, C., Otasek, D., Fortney, K., Agapito, G., Cannataro, M., Shirdel, E., Jurisica, I.: Visual Data Mining of Biological Networks: One Size Does Not Fit All. PLoS Computational Biology 9(1), e1002833 (2013)
51. Bowman, I., Joshi, S.H., Van Horn, J.D.: Visual systems for interactive exploration and mining of large-scale neuroimaging data archives. Frontiers in Neuroinformatics 6(11) (2012)
52. Kolling, J., Langenkamper, D., Abouna, S., Khan, M., Nattkemper, T.W.: WHIDE–a web tool for visual data mining colocation patterns in multivariate bioimages. Bioinformatics 28(8), 1143–1150 (2012)
53. Wegman, E.J.: Visual data mining. Stat. Med. 22(9), 1383–1397 (2003)
54. Holzinger, A.: Human-Computer Interaction and Knowledge Discovery (HCI-KDD): What Is the Benefit of Bringing Those Two Fields to Work Together? In: Cuzzocrea, A., Kittl, C., Simos, D.E., Weippl, E., Xu, L. (eds.) CD-ARES 2013. LNCS, vol. 8127, pp. 319–328. Springer, Heidelberg (2013)
55. Lovell, M.C.: Data Mining. Review of Economics and Statistics 65(1), 1–12 (1983)
56. Mooers, C.N.: Information retrieval viewed as temporal signalling. In: Proc. Internatl. Congr. of Mathematicians, August 30-September 6, p. 572 (1950)
57. Mooers, C.N.: The next twenty years in information retrieval; some goals and predictions. American Documentation 11(3), 229–236 (1960)
58. Piatetsky-Shapiro, G.: Knowledge Discovery in Real Databases - A report on the IJCAI-89 Workshop. AI Magazine 11(5), 68–70 (1991)
59. Fayyad, U., Piatetsky-Shapiro, G., Smyth, P.: From data mining to knowledge discovery in databases. Ai Magazine 17(3), 37–54 (1996)
60. Holzinger, A., Malle, B., Bloice, M., Wiltgen, M., Ferri, M., Stanganelli, I., Hofmann-Wellenhof, R.: On the Generation of Point Cloud Data Sets: the first step in the Knowledge Discovery Process. In: Holzinger, A., Jurisica, I. (eds.) Knowledge Discovery and Data Mining. LNCS, vol. 8401, pp. 57–80. Springer, Heidelberg (2014)
61. Boselli, R., Cesarini, M., Mercorio, F., Mezzanzanica, M.: A Policy-based Cleansing and Integration Framework for Labour and Healthcare Data. In: Holzinger, A., Jurisica, I. (eds.) Knowledge Discovery and Data Mining. LNCS, vol. 8401, pp. 141–168. Springer, Heidelberg (2014)
62. Nguyen, H., Thompson, J.D., Schutz, P., Poch, O.: Intelligent integrative knowledge bases: bridging genomics, integrative biology and translational medicine. In: Holzinger, A., Jurisica, I. (eds.) Knowledge Discovery and Data Mining. LNCS, vol. 8401, pp. 255–270. Springer, Heidelberg (2014)
63. Huppertz, B., Holzinger, A.: Biobanks – A Source of large Biological Data Sets: Open Problems and Future Challenges. In: Holzinger, A., Jurisica, I. (eds.) Knowledge Discovery and Data Mining, vol. 8401, pp. 317–330. Springer, Heidelberg (2014)

64. Holzinger, K., Palade, V., Rabadan, R., Holzinger, A.: Darwin or Lamarck? Future Challenges in Evolutionary Algorithms for Knowledge Discovery and Data Mining. In: Holzinger, A., Jurisica, I. (eds.) Knowledge Discovery and Data Mining. LNCS, vol. 8401, pp. 35–56. Springer, Heidelberg (2014)
65. Katz, G., Shabtai, A., Rokach, L.: Adapted Features and Instance Selection for Improving Co-Training. In: Holzinger, A., Jurisica, I. (eds.) Knowledge Discovery and Data Mining. LNCS, vol. 8401, pp. 81–100. Springer, Heidelberg (2014)
66. Yildirim, P., Bloice, M., Holzinger, A.: Knowledge Discovery & Visualization of Clusters for Erythromycin Related Adverse Events in the FDA Drug Adverse Event Reporting System. In: Holzinger, A., Jurisica, I. (eds.) Knowledge Discovery and Data Mining. LNCS, vol. 8401, pp. 101–116. Springer, Heidelberg (2014)
67. Kobayashi, M.: Resources for Studying Statistical Analysis of Biomedical Data and R. In: Holzinger, A., Jurisica, I. (eds.) Knowledge Discovery and Data Mining. LNCS, vol. 8401, pp. 183–195. Springer, Heidelberg (2014)
68. Windridge, D., Bober, M.: A Kernel-based Framework for Medical Big-Data Analytics. In: Holzinger, A., Jurisica, I. (eds.) Knowledge Discovery and Data Mining. LNCS, vol. 8401, pp. 197–208. Springer, Heidelberg (2014)
69. Holzinger, A., Schantl, J., Schroettner, M., Seifert, C., Verspoor, K.: Biomedical Text Mining: Open Problems and Future Challenges. In: Holzinger, A., Jurisica, I. (eds.) Knowledge Discovery and Data Mining. LNCS, vol. 8401, pp. 271–300. Springer, Heidelberg (2014)
70. Holzinger, A., Ofner, B., Dehmer, M.: Multi-touch Graph-Based Interaction for Knowledge Discovery on Mobile Devices: State-of-the-Art and Future Challenges. In: Holzinger, A., Jurisica, I. (eds.) Knowledge Discovery and Data Mining. LNCS, vol. 8401, pp. 241–254. Springer, Heidelberg (2014)
71. Lee, S.: Sparse Inverse Covariance Estimation for Graph Representation of Feature Structure. In: Holzinger, A., Jurisica, I. (eds.) Knowledge Discovery and Data Mining. LNCS, vol. 8401, pp. 227–240. Springer, Heidelberg (2014)
72. Holzinger, A., Hortenhuber, M., Mayer, C., Bachler, M., Wassertheurer, S., Pinho, A., Koslicki, D.: On Entropy-based Data Mining. In: Holzinger, A., Jurisica, I. (eds.) Knowledge Discovery and Data Mining. LNCS, vol. 8401, pp. 209–226. Springer, Heidelberg (2014)
73. Holzinger, A.: Topological Data Mining in a Nutshell. In: Holzinger, A., Jurisica, I. (eds.) Knowledge Discovery and Data Mining. LNCS, vol. 8401, pp. 331–356. Springer, Heidelberg (2014)
74. Otasek, D., Pastrello, C., Holzinger, A., Jurisica, I.: Visual Data Mining: Effective Exploration ofthe Biological Universe. In: Holzinger, A., Jurisica, I. (eds.) Knowledge Discovery and Data Mining. LNCS, vol. 8401, pp. 19–33. Springer, Heidelberg (2014)
75. Turkay, C., Jeanquartier, F., Holzinger, A., Hauser, H.: On Computationally-enhanced Visual Analysis of Heterogeneous Data and its Application in Biomedical Informatics. In: Holzinger, A., Jurisica, I. (eds.) Knowledge Discovery and Data Mining. LNCS, vol. 8401, pp. 117–140. Springer, Heidelberg (2014)
76. van Leeuwen, M.: Interactive Data Exploration using Pattern Mining. In: Holzinger, A., Jurisica, I. (eds.) Knowledge Discovery and Data Mining. LNCS, vol. 8401, pp. 169–182. Springer, Heidelberg (2014)
77. Kieseberg, P., Hobel, H., Schrittwieser, S., Weippl, E., Holzinger, A.: Protecting Anonymity in the Data-Driven Medical Sciences. In: Holzinger, A., Jurisica, I. (eds.) Knowledge Discovery and Data Mining. LNCS, vol. 8401, pp. 301–316. Springer, Heidelberg (2014)

78. Gigerenzer, G.: Gut Feelings: Short Cuts to Better Decision Making. Penguin, London (2008)
79. Gigerenzer, G., Gaissmaier, W.: Heuristic Decision Making. In: Fiske, S.T., Schacter, D.L., Taylor, S.E. (eds.) Annual Review of Psychology, vol. 62, pp. 451–482. Annual Reviews, Palo Alto (2011)
80. Fang, F.C., Steen, R.G., Casadevall, A.: Misconduct accounts for the majority of retracted scientific publications. Proc. Natl. Acad. Sci. U.S.A 109(42), 17028–17033 (2012)

# Visual Data Mining:
# Effective Exploration of the Biological Universe

David Otasek[1], Chiara Pastrello[1], Andreas Holzinger[2], and Igor Jurisica[1,3,*]

[1] Princess Margaret Cancer Centre, University Health Network, IBM Life Sciences Discovery Centre, and TECHNA for the Advancement of Technology for Health, TMDT Room 11-314, 101 College Street, Toronto, ON M5G 1L7, Canada
juris@ai.utoronto.ca
[2] Medical University Graz, Institute for Medical Informatics, Statistics and Documentation Research Unit HCI, IBM Watson Think Group, Auenbruggerplatz 2/V, A-8036 Graz, Austria
a.holzinger@hci4all.at
[3] Departments of Medical Biophysics and Computer Science, University of Toronto

**Abstract.** Visual Data Mining (VDM) is supported by interactive and scalable network visualization and analysis, which in turn enables effective exploration and communication of ideas within multiple biological and biomedical fields. Large networks, such as the protein interactome or transcriptional regulatory networks, contain hundreds of thousands of objects and millions of relationships. These networks are continuously evolving as new knowledge becomes available, and their content is richly annotated and can be presented in many different ways. Attempting to discover knowledge and new theories within this complex data sets can involve many workflows, such as accurately representing many formats of source data, merging heterogeneous and distributed data sources, complex database searching, integrating results from multiple computational and mathematical analyses, and effectively visualizing properties and results. Our experience with biology researchers has required us to address their needs and requirements in the design and development of a scalable and interactive network visualization and analysis platform, NAViGaTOR, now in its third major release.

**Keywords:** Visual Data Mining, Interactive Data Mining, Knowledge Discovery, Scalable Network Visualization, Biological Graphs, Networks.

# 1 Introduction and Motivation

## 1.1 The Need for Visual Data Mining

One of the grand challenges in our "networked 21st century" is in dealing with large, complex, and often weakly structured data sets [1], [2], and in big volumes of unstructured information [3].

This "big data" challenge is most evident in the biomedical domain [4]: the emergence of new biotechnologies that can measure many molecular species at once,

---

\* Corresponding author.

A. Holzinger, I. Jurisica (Eds.): Knowledge Discovery and Data Mining, LNCS 8401, pp. 19–33, 2014.

large scale sequencing, high-throughput facilities and individual laboratories worldwide produce vast amounts of data sets including nucleotide and protein sequences, protein crystal structures, gene-expression measurements, protein and genetic interactions, phenotype studies etc. [5]. The increasing trend towards personalized medicine brings together data from very different sources [6].

The problem is that these data sets are characterized by heterogeneous and diverse features. Individual data collectors prefer their own different schema or protocols for data recording, and the diverse nature of the applications used results in various data representations. For example, patient information may include simple demographic information such as gender, age, disease history, and so on as non-standardized text [7]; results of X-ray examination and CT/MR scan as image or video data, and genomic or proteomic-related tests could include microarray expression data, DNA sequence, or identified mutations or peptides. In this context, heterogeneous features refer to the varied ways in which similar features can be represented. Diverse features refer to the variety of features involved in each distinct observation. Consider that different organizations (or health practitioners) have their own schemata representing each patient. Data heterogeneity and diverse dimensionality issues then become major challenges if we are trying to enable data aggregation by combining data from all sources [8], [9].

This increasingly large amount of data requires not only new, but efficient and most of all end-user friendly solutions for handling it, which poses a number of challenges [10]. With the growing expectations of end-users, traditional approaches for data interpretation often cannot keep pace with demand, so there is the risk of modelling artefacts or delivering unsatisfactory results. Consequently, to cope with this flood of data, *interactive* data mining approaches are vital. However, exploration of large data sets is a difficult problem and techniques from interactive visualization and visual analytics may help to assist the knowledge discovery process generally and data mining in particular [11], [12], leading to the approach of Visual Data Mining (VDM).

### 1.2    A Short History of Visual Data Mining

One of the first VDM approaches was in a telecommunications application. This application involved a graph-based representation and a user interface to manipulate this representation in search of unusual calling patterns. This approach proved extremely effective for fraud detection [13].

A further work by Alfred Inselberg (1998) [14] proposed the use of parallel coordinates for VDM, which transforms the search for relations into a 2-D pattern recognition problem. Parallel coordinates are a splendid idea for visualizing multi-dimensional geometry [15]; a good overview on parallel coordinates can be found in [16], however, to date they are still rarely used in biomedical applications.

The field of VDM started to expand to diverse domains, as highlighted in a special issue in issue 5 of the 1999 volume of IEEE Computer Graphics and Applications [17] including a work on visual mining of high-dimensional data [18]. A state-of-the art analysis was provided by Keim et al. at the EUROGRAPHICS 2002 [19]. A good overview of VDM can be found in [20]. A recent overview on VDM for knowledge discovery, with a focus on the chemical process industry can be found in [21] and a recent work on VDM of biological networks is [12]. A very recent medical example for interactive pattern visualization in $n$-dimensional data sets by application of supervised self- organizing maps is [22]. A general overview on the integration of computational tools in visualization for interactive analysis of heterogeneous data in biomedical informatics can be found in [23].

### 1.3    Interactivity and Decision Support

For data mining to be effective, it is important to include the human expert in the data exploration process, and combine the flexibility, creativity, and general knowledge of the human with the enormous computational capacity and analytical power of novel algorithms and systems. VDM integrates the human in the data exploration process; it aims to effectively represent data visually to benefit from human perceptual abilities, allowing the expert to get insight into the data by direct interaction with the data. VDM can be particularly helpful when little is known about the data and the exploration goals are ill-defined or evolve over time. The VDM process can be seen as a hypothesis generation process: the visualizations of the data enable the user to gain insight into the data, and generate new hypotheses to support data mining and interpretation [24], [25].

VDM often provides better results, especially in cases where automatic algorithms fail [11]. However, it is indispensable to combine interactive VDM with automatic exploration techniques; hence we need machine learning approaches due to the complexity and the largeness of data, which humans alone cannot systematically and comprehensively explore. Consequently, a central goal is to work towards enabling effective human control over powerful machine intelligence by the integration of both machine learning methods and manual VDM to enable human insight and decision support [26], the latter is still the core discipline in biomedical informatics [27].

## 2    Glossary and Key Terms

*Biological Pathway Exchange (BioPAX):* is a RDF/OWL-based language to represent biological pathways at the molecular and cellular level to facilitate the exchange of pathway data. It makes explicit use of relations between concepts and is defined as an ontology of concepts with attributes [28].

*CellML:* is an open standard XML, for describing mathematical models, originally created out of the Physiome Project, and hence used primarily to describe models relevant to the field of biology [29, 30].

*Graph dRawing with Intelligent Placement (GRIP):* is based on the algorithm of Gajer, Goodrich & Kobourov [31] and written in C++ and OpenGL, and uses an adaptive Tcl/Tk interface. Given an abstract graph, GRIP produces drawings in 2D and 3D either directly or by projecting higher dimensional drawings into 2D or 3D space [32].

*KEGG Markup Language (KGML):* is an exchange format of the KEGG pathway maps, which is converted from the KGML+ (KGML+SVG) format. KGML enables automatic drawing of KEGG pathways and provides facilities for computational analysis and modeling of gene/protein networks and chemical networks [33].

*Proteomics Standards Initiative Molecular Interaction XML format (PSI MI):* was developed by the Proteomics Standards Initiative (PSI) as part of the Human Proteome Organization (HUPO) [34]. PSI-MI is the standard for protein–protein interaction (PPI), intended as a data exchange format for molecular interactions, not a database structure [35].

*Protein-Protein Interactions (PPIs):* are fundamental for many biological functions [36], [37]. Being able to visualize the structure of a protein and analyze its shape is of great importance in biomedicine: Looking at the protein structure means to locate amino acids, visualize specific regions of the protein, visualize secondary structure elements, determine residues in the score or solvent accessible residues on the surface of the protein, determine binding sites, etc. [38], [39].

*Systems Biology Markup Language (SBML):* is a language intended as future standard for information exchange in computational biology and especially within molecular pathways. The aim of SBML is to model biochemical reaction networks, including cell signaling, metabolic pathways and gene regulation [40].

*Visual Data Mining (VDM):* is an approach for exploring large data sets by combining traditional data mining methods with advanced visual analytics methods and can be seen as a hypothesis generation process [14], [11], [41].

# 3    Representing Biological Graphs

## 3.1    A Constantly Changing Understanding

The functions of life on a sub-cellular level rely on multiple interactions between different types of molecules. Proteins, genes, metabolites, all interact to produce either healthy or diseased cellular processes. Our understanding of this network of interactions, and the interacting objects themselves, is continuously changing; and the network itself is evolving as we age or as disease progresses. Our methods for discovering new relationships and pathways change as well.

NAViGaTOR 3 addresses these realities by having a very basic core rooted in graph theory, with the flexibility of a modular plugin architecture that provides data input and output, analysis, layout and visualization capabilities. NAViGaTOR 3 implements this architecture by following the OSGi standard (http://www.osgi.org/Main/HomePage). Available API enables developers to expand standard distribution by integrating new features and extending the functionality of the program to suit their specific needs.

## 3.2    Data Formats

The ability to share data effectively and efficiently is the starting point for successful analysis, and thus several attempts have been made to standardize formats for such data exchange: PSI-MI [35], BioPAX [42], KGML, SBML [40], GML, CML, and CellML [30].

Each of these formats has a different focus and thus uniquely affects the way a particular network can be described. Some formats, like PSI, focus on describing binary interactions. Others, such as BioPAX, can describe more complex topology, allowing for many-to-many interactions and concepts such as meta-graphs. However, the majority of biological data remains represented in tabular format, which can vary wildly in content and descriptiveness.

NAViGaTOR 3 was designed with the knowledge that a researcher may need to combine heterogeneous and distributed data sources. The standard distribution supports the loading, manipulation, and storage of multiple XML formats and tabular data. XML data is handled using a suite of file loaders, including XGMML, PSI-MI, SBML, KGML, and BioPAX, which store richly-annotated data and provide links to corresponding objects in the graph. Tabular data is stored using DEX [43], a dedicated graph database from Sparsity Technologies (http://www.sparsity-technologies.com/dex).

## 3.3    Biological Scale

A sense of the scale biologists might contend with in attempting to model protein behavior can be seen in UniProt (http://www.uniprot.org), a database that documents protein sequences. In its 2013_10 release, UniProt contained 20,277 sequences for human proteins, while I2D (http://ophid.utoronto.ca/i2d) [44], a database that includes interactions between these proteins, in its 2.3 version contains 241,305 experimental or predicted interactions among 18,078 human proteins. If the protein interaction network is integrated with other data of similar size, such as transcriptome regulatory network, microRNA:gene regulation network, or drug:protein target network, the visualization can become challenging, not only because of the size of the graph, but due to rich annotation and underlying topology of these 'interactomes'.

Often, even the best case layouts produce a gigantic 'hairball' in which a user is unable to trace paths between different objects in the network. It is important to keep in mind that such a network is still limited in scope; it doesn't take into account genetic, metabolite or drug interactions. In a true 'systems biology' view, we need to integrate multiple layers of these individual networks into a larger, comprehensive, typed graph. Tools that attempt to analyse this data must take this scale into account. To be useful, visualization tools, and particularly interactive visualization tools must effectively handle networks of this size. In the case of NAViGaTOR, DEX can handle networks of up to 1 Billion objects. Visualizing networks is handled through JOGL (http://jogamp.org/jogl/www/), a library that speeds up large network rendering by taking advantage of the acceleration provided by GPU hardware whenever it is available.

# 4    Visualization, Layout and Analysis

Exploring data is often a combination of analysis, layout and visualization. We have found that being able to utilize and combine all three of these aspects quickly and efficiently simplifies and in turn enables effective research.

A central idea to NAViGaTOR 3's architecture is providing multiple views of the data. While the structure of the network and its annotations remains constant, NAViGaTOR 3 allows the user to view and manipulate it as a spreadsheet of nodes or edges, a matrix, or an OpenGL rendered graph. Individual views allow a user to make a selection of objects, which can then be transferred to another view. For example, a user can select the top 10 rows of a spreadsheet that sorts the network's nodes by a measurement such as gene expression, and then transfer that selection to the OpenGL view, allowing them to see those nodes in the context of their neighbors.

The most basic level of analysis supports access, search and data organization. The tabular data associated with a network can be searched using DEX queries, allowing for basic numeric searches (equals, greater than, less than, etc.) and text (exact match, regular expression, etc.). The spreadsheet view supports effective searching, data sorting and selecting. XML data benefits from rich data annotation, and can be searched using XPath, a dedicated XML query language.

XPath is extremely versatile, mixing logical, numeric and text queries in a single language. It also handles translation of XML data into tabular data.

Network structure provides additional insights, as it relates to the function of proteins that form it [45], [46]. Examining the network structure can range from searches for node neighbors and nodes of high degree to more mathematically complex operations such as all pairs shortest path calculations, flow analysis, or graphlets [47].

A key part of NAViGaTOR's tool set is the subset system, which enables the storage of selections from various graph views. Once they are stored, they can be manipulated with set arithmetic operations (union, difference, intersection). This allows the user to intelligently combine the results of searches and selections from other views.

Further strengthening the link between visualization and data is the concept of filters. Filters are visualization plugins for the OpenGL view that allow a user to map node or edge feature to a visual attribute, i.e., enabling interactive exploration of typed graphs by seamlessly combining analysis and human insight. For example, a confidence value for an edge can be translated into its width, color, shape or transparency. Similarly, node height, width, color, transparency, outline color, and outline size can be used to visualize gene, protein or drug characteristics and measurements. Thus, layout and presentation of rich, annotated networks can be easily modified, enabling new insight into complex data.

Graph layout is essential for effective visual analysis of complex graphs. NAViGaTOR 3 uses a combination of manual and automated layout tools. The standard distribution includes several versions of the GRIP (Graph dRawing with Intelligent Placement) [48], [49], [50] layout algorithm, which enables fast layouts of tens of thousands of nodes and edges. For example, visualizing protein interaction network topology changes in the presence or absence of specific receptors [51].

Besides GRIP, the user also has a selection of circular, arc and linear layouts, as well as moving, scaling and rotating tools to manually place nodes in a desired topology.

Usually, combinations of these layouts are necessary to effectively visualize the network [12]. Large and complex biological networks, even with the benefit of the GRIP layout, are usually tangled and poorly interpretable graphs. Analyzing network topology (hubs, graphlets, cliques, shortest path, flow, etc.) provides rich topological features that may aid in discovery and visualization of important insights. Researchers may have to map a data attribute to transparency to make areas of interest visible, or use an overlap of searches to color a selection of nodes or edges. Being able to use different analysis and layout methods combined with user's insight provides the flexibility to highlight desired results in the network, or discover novel insights and form hypotheses. Thus, NAViGaTOR extends the basic concept of network visualization to visual data mining.

To demonstrate the versatility of NAViGaTOR 3 we created an integrated network by combining metabolic pathways, protein-protein interactions, and drug-target data. We first built a network using metabolic data collected and curated in our lab, combining several steroid hormone metabolism pathways: androgen, glutathione, N-nitrosamine and benzo(a)pyrene pathway, the ornithine-spermine biosynthesis pathway, the retinol metabolism pathway and the TCA cycle aerobic respiration pathway. The reactions in the dataset are in the following format: metabolite A → enzyme → metabolite B. As shown in Figure 1, the different pathways are integrated and highlighted with different edge colours. The edge directionality highlights reactions and flow between the individual pathways.

As the dataset is centred on steroid hormone metabolism, we decided to include data from hormone-related cancers [52]. In particular, we retrieved the list of FDA-approved drugs used for breast, ovarian and prostate cancer from the National Cancer Institute website (http://www.cancer.gov/). We then searched in the DrugBank (http://www.drugbank.ca [53]) for targets for each drug and integrated them in the network.

Three targets are enzymes that are part of the original network (HSD11B1, CYP19A1, CYP17A1). Polymorphisms in CYP19 have been associated with increased risk of breast cancer [54], while polymorphisms in CYP17 have been linked to increased risk of prostate cancer [55].

CYP17 inhibitors are considered key drugs for castration resistant prostate tumours, due to their ability to block the signaling of androgen receptors even when the receptor expression is increased [56].

Thanks to the ability of NAViGaTOR to include various types of nodes, we can also see how frequently DNA is a target. In fact, many of the drugs used for breast and ovarian cancer treatment are DNA intercalating agents [57].

To further investigate whether drug targets are directly connected to the metabolic network we searched for direct interactions between the two types of nodes using protein interactions from I2D and identified three such targets (TUBA1, TOP1 and EGFR).

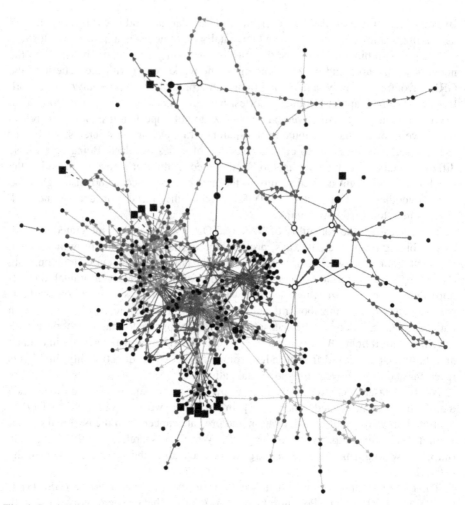

**Fig. 1.** Partially explored network – connecting drugs and metabolism. A network comprising metabolites, enzymes, and drugs in the early stages of exploration, colored according to the pathway (see complete overview in Figure 2).

EGFR overexpression appears in breast cancer, especially in triple-negative and in inflammatory breast cancer, and is associated with large tumor size, poor differentiation, and poor clinical outcomes [58]. EGFR inhibitor treatments (e.g., Erlotinib or Cetuximab) have been suggested for triple-negative breast cancer patients, and a few clinical trials showed promising results [59].

It would be interesting to study the effect of EGFR mutations in this network, to evaluate if they can have an effect on the patient's response to inhibitors similar to response to Erlotinib in non-small-cell-lung cancer patients [60].

Interestingly, several CYP and UGT proteins are key connectors of different metabolic pathways (highlighted in green in Figure 2), and have a biologically important role in the network. Both families of proteins have important roles in metabolic pathways (CYP450 are ubiquitously expressed in the body as they catalyze the fundamental carbon–oxidation reaction used for unnumbered metabolic reactions, while UGTs are used in reactions that form lipophilic glucuronides from a high variety of non–membrane-associated substrates, either endogenous or xenobiotics and has evolved as a highly specialized function in higher organisms) but they have mainly been associated with drug metabolism, in their wild-type or polymorphic forms [61], [62], [63].

This example shows only one of the several possible integrated networks that can be built using NAViGaTOR 3, and highlights the role of the analysis of the network structure in pointing out major biological players.

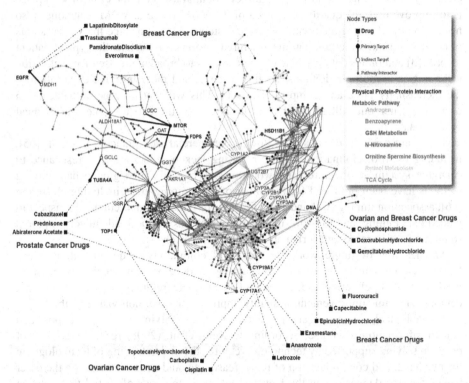

**Fig. 2.** Completed network – the same network as in Figure 1 with drugs and biologically relevant components emphasized

Biological networks will continue becoming larger and more complex thanks to the higher throughput of novel technologies and increased data integration. This highlights the need for tools that scale up to large and complex networks. Moreover, and maybe more importantly, this highlights the necessity for tools with the ability to integrate different -omics data collections, to discover cross-talk and to build an increasingly more complete representation of the real cell or an organism. NAViGaTOR fits perfectly in this context and provides the researcher with the functionality needed to advance data discovery at the same speed of high-throughput data production.

# 5    Open Problems and Future Work

The deployment of VDM techniques in commercial products remains sparse – and in today's traditional hospital information systems such approaches are completely missing. Future work must involve the tight integration of sophisticated interactive visualization techniques with traditional techniques from machine learning with the aim to combine fast automatic data mining algorithms with the intuitive power and creativity of the human mind [64]. A further essential aspect at the clinical workplace is to improve both the quality and speed of the VDM process. VDM techniques also need to be tightly integrated with available systems used to manage the vast amounts of relational, semi-structured and unstructured information such as the typical patient records [3] and omics data [9]. The ultimate goal is to broaden the use of visualization technologies in multiple domains, leading to faster and more intuitive exploration of the increasingly large and complex data sets. This will not only be valuable in an economic sense but will also enhance the power of the end user, i.e. the medical professional.

There are several reasons for slower commercial acceptance of VDM [65], including multi-disciplinarity and the resulting lack of expertise, and resistance to changing system architectures and workflows. While so-called guided data mining methods have been produced for a number of data mining areas including clustering [66], association mining [67] and classification [68], there is an architectural aspect to guided data mining, and to VDM in general, which has not been adequately explored so far, and which represents a rich area for future research.

Another area of future work for the VDM community is quantification. Since VDM methods can be more time-consuming to develop and special expertise is needed for their effective use, successful deployment requires proper metrics that demonstrates time improvement or quality improvement over non-visual methods.

Technological challenges are present in problem solving, decision support and human information discourse; according to Keim et al. (2008) [65], the process of problem solving supported by technology requires the understanding of technology on the one hand, and comprehension of logic, reasoning, and common sense on the other hand. Here the danger lies in the fact that automatic methods often fail to recognize the context, if not explicitly trained.

A grand challenge is to find the most appropriate visualization methodology and/or metaphor to communicate analytical results in an appropriate manner. A recent example on Glyph-based visualizations can be seen in [69], while noting that most often such approaches are limited to a certain domain.

User acceptability, which is also on Keim's 2008 list is an additional grand challenge: many sophisticated visualization techniques have been introduced, but they are not yet integrated in the clinical workplace, mainly due to end users' refusal to change their routine – this is most apparent in the medical domain [70]; an often ignored aspect in that respect is the previous exposure to technology [71]; in particular elderly end users are not so enthusiastic in adopting new technologies to their daily routine. Consequently, it is very important that advantages of VDM tools are presented and communicated to future users to overcome such usage barriers, taking usability engineering into full account [72].

Faced with unsustainable costs and enormous amounts of under-utilized data, health care needs more efficient practices, research, and tools to harness the full benefits towards the concept of personalized medicine [73].

A major challenge lies in the development of new machine learning methods for knowledge discovery in protein-protein interaction sites, e.g. to study gene regulatory networks and functions. However, when applied to such big data, the computational complexities of these methods become a major drawback. To overcome such limitations Extreme Learning Machines provide a trade-off between computational time and generalization performance [74].

**Acknowledgements.** We would like to thank Dr. M. Kotlyar and G. Morrison for their help on data retrieval.

# References

1. Holzinger, A.: On Knowledge Discovery and Interactive Intelligent Visualization of Biomedical Data - Challenges in Human–Computer Interaction & Biomedical Informatics. In: DATA 2012, Rome, Italy, pp. 9–20. INSTICC (2012)
2. Holzinger, A.: Weakly Structured Data in Health-Informatics: The Challenge for Human-Computer Interaction. In: Proceedings of INTERACT 2011 Workshop: Promoting and Supporting Healthy Living by Design. IFIP, pp. 5–7 (2011)
3. Holzinger, A., Stocker, C., Ofner, B., Prohaska, G., Brabenetz, A., Hofmann-Wellenhof, R.: Combining HCI, Natural Language Processing, and Knowledge Discovery - Potential of IBM Content Analytics as an assistive technology in the biomedical domain. In: Holzinger, A., Pasi, G. (eds.) HCI-KDD 2013. LNCS, vol. 7947, pp. 13–24. Springer, Heidelberg (2013)
4. Holzinger, A.: Biomedical Informatics: Discovering Knowledge in Big Data. Springer, New York (2014)
5. Howe, D., Costanzo, M., Fey, P., Gojobori, T., Hannick, L., Hide, W., Hill, D.P., Kania, R., Schaeffer, M., St Pierre, S., Twigger, S., White, O., Rhee, S.Y.: Big data: The future of biocuration. Nature 455(7209), 47–50 (2008)
6. Holzinger, A., Dehmer, M., Jurisica, I.: Knowledge Discovery and interactive Data Mining in Bioinformatics - State-of-the-Art, future challenges and research directions. BMC Bioinformatics 15(suppl. 6), I1 (2014)
7. Kreuzthaler, M., Bloice, M.D., Faulstich, L., Simonic, K.M., Holzinger, A.: A Comparison of Different Retrieval Strategies Working on Medical Free Texts. J. Univers. Comput. Sci. 17(7), 1109–1133 (2011)
8. Wu, X.D., Zhu, X.Q., Wu, G.Q., Ding, W.: Data Mining with Big Data. IEEE Transactions on Knowledge and Data Engineering 26(1), 97–107 (2014)

9.  Huppertz, B., Holzinger, A.: Biobanks – A Source of large Biological Data Sets: Open Problems and Future Challenges. In: Holzinger, A., Jurisica, I. (eds.) Interactive Knowledge Discovery and Data Mining: State-of-the-Art and Future Challenges in Biomedical Informatics. LNCS, vol. 8401, pp. 317–330. Springer, Heidelberg (2014)

10. Jeanquartier, F., Holzinger, A.: On Visual Analytics And Evaluation In Cell Physiology: A Case Study. In: Cuzzocrea, A., Kittl, C., Simos, D.E., Weippl, E., Xu, L. (eds.) CD-ARES 2013. LNCS, vol. 8127, pp. 495–502. Springer, Heidelberg (2013)

11. Keim, D.A.: Information visualization and visual data mining. IEEE Transactions on Visualization and Computer Graphics 8(1), 1–8 (2002)

12. Pastrello, C., Otasek, D., Fortney, K., Agapito, G., Cannataro, M., Shirdel, E., Jurisica, I.: Visual Data Mining of Biological Networks: One Size Does Not Fit All. PLoS Computational Biology 9(1), e1002833 (2013)

13. Cox, K., Eick, S., Wills, G., Brachman, R.: Brief Application Description; Visual Data Mining: Recognizing Telephone Calling Fraud. Data Min. Knowl. Discov. 1(2), 225–231 (1997)

14. Inselberg, A.: Visual data mining with parallel coordinates. Computational Statistics 13(1), 47–63 (1998)

15. Inselberg, A., Dimsdale, B.: Parallel coordinates: A tool for visualizing multi-dimensional geometry, pp. 361–378. IEEE Computer Society Press (1990)

16. Heinrich, J., Weiskopf, D.: State of the Art of Parallel Coordinates. In: Eurographics 2013-State of the Art Reports, pp. 95–116. The Eurographics Association (2012)

17. Wong, P.C.: Visual data mining. IEEE Computer Graphics and Applications 19(5), 20–21 (1999)

18. Hinneburg, A., Keim, D.A., Wawryniuk, M.: HD-eye: Visual mining of high-dimensional data. IEEE Computer Graphics and Applications 19(5), 22–31 (1999)

19. Keim, D., Müller, W., Schumann, H.: Information Visualization and Visual Data Mining; State of the art report. In: Eurographics (2002)

20. de Oliveira, M.C.F., Levkowitz, H.: From visual data exploration to visual data mining: A survey. IEEE Transactions on Visualization and Computer Graphics 9(3), 378–394 (2003)

21. Stahl, F., Gabrys, B., Gaber, M.M., Berendsen, M.: An overview of interactive visual data mining techniques for knowledge discovery. Wiley Interdisciplinary Reviews-Data Mining and Knowledge Discovery 3(4), 239–256 (2013)

22. Rosado-Munoz, A., Martinez-Martinez, J.M., Escandell-Montero, P., Soria-Olivas, E.: Visual data mining with self-organising maps for ventricular fibrillation analysis. Computer Methods and Programs in Biomedicine 111(2), 269–279 (2013)

23. Turkay, C., Jeanquartier, F., Holzinger, A., Hauser, H.: On computationally-enhanced visual analysis of heterogeneous data and its application in biomedical informatics. In: Holzinger, A., Jurisica, I. (eds.) Interactive Knowledge Discovery and Data Mining in Biomedical Informatics. LNCS, vol. 8401, pp. 117–140. Springer, Heidelberg (2014)

24. Blandford, A., Attfield, S.: Interacting with Information. Synthesis Lectures on Human-Centered Informatics 3(1), 1–99 (2010)

25. Holzinger, A., Scherer, R., Seeber, M., Wagner, J., Müller-Putz, G.: Computational Sensemaking on Examples of Knowledge Discovery from Neuroscience Data: Towards Enhancing Stroke Rehabilitation. In: Böhm, C., Khuri, S., Lhotská, L., Renda, M.E. (eds.) ITBAM 2012. LNCS, vol. 7451, pp. 166–168. Springer, Heidelberg (2012)

26. Holzinger, A.: Interacting with Information: Challenges in Human-Computer Interaction and Information Retrieval (HCI-IR). In: IADIS Multiconference on Computer Science and Information Systems (MCCSIS), Interfaces and Human-Computer Interaction, pp. 13–17. IADIS, Rome (2011)

27. Holzinger, A.: Biomedical Informatics: Computational Sciences meets Life Sciences. BoD, Norderstedt (2012)
28. Strömbäck, L., Lambrix, P.: Representations of molecular pathways: an evaluation of SBML, PSI MI and BioPAX. Bioinformatics 21(24), 4401–4407 (2005)
29. Lloyd, C.M., Halstead, M.D., Nielsen, P.F.: CellML: Its future, present and past. Progress in biophysics and molecular biology 85(2), 433–450 (2004)
30. Miller, A.K., Marsh, J., Reeve, A., Garny, A., Britten, R., Halstead, M., Cooper, J., Nickerson, D.P., Nielsen, P.F.: An overview of the CellML API and its implementation. BMC Bioinformatics 11(1), 178 (2010)
31. Gajer, P., Goodrich, M.T., Kobourov, S.G.: A multi-dimensional approach to force-directed layouts of large graphs. In: Marks, J. (ed.) GD 2000. LNCS, vol. 1984, pp. 211–221. Springer, Heidelberg (2001)
32. Gajer, P., Kobourov, S.G.: GRIP: Graph dRawing with Intelligent Placement. In: Marks, J. (ed.) GD 2000. LNCS, vol. 1984, pp. 222–228. Springer, Heidelberg (2001)
33. http://www.kegg.jp/kegg/xml/
34. Hermjakob, H., Montecchi-Palazzi, L., Bader, G., Wojcik, J., Salwinski, L., Ceol, A., Moore, S., Orchard, S., Sarkans, U., von Mering, C.: The HUPO PSI's molecular interaction format—a community standard for the representation of protein interaction data. Nature Biotechnology 22(2), 177–183 (2004)
35. Kerrien, S., Orchard, S., Montecchi-Palazzi, L., Aranda, B., Quinn, A., Vinod, N., Bader, G., Xenarios, I., Wojcik, J., Sherman, D.: Broadening the horizon–level 2.5 of the HUPO-PSI format for molecular interactions. BMC Biology 5(1), 44 (2007)
36. Jones, S., Thornton, J.M.: Principles of protein-protein interactions. Proceedings of the National Academy of Sciences 93(1), 13–20 (1996)
37. Zhang, A.: Protein Interaction Networks: Computational Analysis. Cambridge University Press, Cambridge (2009)
38. Wiltgen, M., Holzinger, A.: Visualization in Bioinformatics: Protein Structures with Physicochemical and Biological Annotations. In: Zara, J., Sloup, J. (eds.) Central European Multimedia and Virtual Reality Conference (available in EG Eurographics Library), pp. 69–74. Czech Technical University (CTU), Prague (2005)
39. Wiltgen, M., Holzinger, A., Tilz, G.P.: Interactive Analysis and Visualization of Macromolecular Interfaces Between Proteins. In: Holzinger, A. (ed.) USAB 2007. LNCS, vol. 4799, pp. 199–212. Springer, Heidelberg (2007)
40. Hucka, M., Finney, A., Sauro, H.M., Bolouri, H., Doyle, J.C., Kitano, H., Arkin, A.P., Bornstein, B.J., Bray, D., Cornish-Bowden, A.: The systems biology markup language (SBML): A medium for representation and exchange of biochemical network models. Bioinformatics 19(4), 524–531 (2003)
41. Wong, B.L.W., Xu, K., Holzinger, A.: Interactive Visualization for Information Analysis in Medical Diagnosis. In: Holzinger, A., Simonic, K.-M. (eds.) USAB 2011. LNCS, vol. 7058, pp. 109–120. Springer, Heidelberg (2011)
42. Demir, E., Cary, M.P., Paley, S., Fukuda, K., Lemer, C., Vastrik, I., Wu, G., D'Eustachio, P., Schaefer, C., Luciano, J.: The BioPAX community standard for pathway data sharing. Nature Biotechnology 28(9), 935–942 (2010)
43. Martinez-Bazan, N., Gomez-Villamor, S., Escale-Claveras, F.: DEX: A high-performance graph database management system. In: IEEE 27th International Conference on Data Engineering (ICDEW), pp. 124–127 (2011)
44. Brown, K.R., Jurisica, I.: Online predicted human interaction database. Bioinformatics 21(9), 2076–2082 (2005)

45. Pržulj, N., Wigle, D.A., Jurisica, I.: Functional topology in a network of protein interactions. Bioinformatics 20(3), 340–348 (2004)
46. Ghersi, D., Singh, M.: Disentangling function from topology to infer the network properties of disease genes. BMC Systems Biology 7(1), 1–12 (2013)
47. Memišević, V., Pržulj, N.: C-GRAAL: Common-neighbors-based global GRAph ALignment of biological networks. Integrative Biology 4(7), 734–743 (2012)
48. Gajer, P., Kobourov, S.G.: GRIP: Graph drawing with intelligent placement. J. Graph Algorithms Appl. 6(3), 203–224 (2002)
49. Gajer, P., Goodrich, M.T., Kobourov, S.G.: A multi-dimensional approach to force-directed layouts of large graphs. Computational Geometry 29(1), 3–18 (2004)
50. Ma, K.-L., Muelder, C.W.: Large-Scale Graph Visualization and Analytics. Computer 46(7), 39–46 (2013)
51. Lissanu Deribe, Y., Wild, P., Chandrashaker, A., Curak, J., Schmidt, M.H., Kalaidzidis, Y., Milutinovic, N., Kratchmarova, I., Buerkle, L., Fetchko, M.J.: Regulation of epidermal growth factor receptor trafficking by lysine deacetylase HDAC6. Science Signaling 2(102), ra84 (2009)
52. Henderson, B.E., Feigelson, H.S.: Hormonal carcinogenesis. Carcinogenesis 21(3), 427–433 (2000)
53. Knox, C., Law, V., Jewison, T., Liu, P., Ly, S., Frolkis, A., Pon, A., Banco, K., Mak, C., Neveu, V.: DrugBank 3.0: A comprehensive resource for 'omics' research on drugs. Nucleic Acids Research 39(suppl. 1), D1035–D1041 (2011)
54. Ma, X., Qi, X., Chen, C., Lin, H., Xiong, H., Li, Y., Jiang, J.: Association between CYP19 polymorphisms and breast cancer risk: Results from 10,592 cases and 11,720 controls. Breast Cancer Research and Treatment 122(2), 495–501 (2010)
55. Douglas, J.A., Zuhlke, K.A., Beebe-Dimmer, J., Levin, A.M., Gruber, S.B., Wood, D.P., Cooney, K.A.: Identifying susceptibility genes for prostate cancer—a family-based association study of polymorphisms in CYP17, CYP19, CYP11A1, and LH-$\beta$. Cancer Epidemiology Biomarkers & Prevention 14(8), 2035–2039 (2005)
56. Reid, A.H., Attard, G., Barrie, E., de Bono, J.S.: CYP17 inhibition as a hormonal strategy for prostate cancer. Nature Clinical Practice Urology 5(11), 610–620 (2008)
57. Brana, M., Cacho, M., Gradillas, A., de Pascual-Teresa, B., Ramos, A.: Intercalators as anticancer drugs. Current Pharmaceutical Design 7(17), 1745–1780 (2001)
58. Masuda, H., Zhang, D., Bartholomeusz, C., Doihara, H., Hortobagyi, G.N., Ueno, N.T.: Role of epidermal growth factor receptor in breast cancer. Breast Cancer Research and Treatment 136(2), 331–345 (2012)
59. Gelmon, K., Dent, R., Mackey, J., Laing, K., McLeod, D., Verma, S.: Targeting triple-negative breast cancer: Optimising therapeutic outcomes. Annals of Oncology 23(9), 2223–2234 (2012)
60. Tsao, M.-S., Sakurada, A., Cutz, J.-C., Zhu, C.-Q., Kamel-Reid, S., Squire, J., Lorimer, I., Zhang, T., Liu, N., Daneshmand, M.: Erlotinib in lung cancer—molecular and clinical predictors of outcome. N. Engl. J. Med. 353(2), 133–144 (2005)
61. Tukey, R.H., Strassburg, C.P.: Human UDP-glucuronosyltransferases: Metabolism, expression, and disease. Annual Review of Pharmacology and Toxicology 40(1), 581–616 (2000)
62. Haining, R.L., Nichols-Haining, M.: Cytochrome P450-catalyzed pathways in human brain: Metabolism meets pharmacology or old drugs with new mechanism of action? Pharmacology & Therapeutics 113(3), 537–545 (2007)

63. Kilford, P.J., Stringer, R., Sohal, B., Houston, J.B., Galetin, A.: Prediction of drug clearance by glucuronidation from in vitro data: Use of combined cytochrome P450 and UDP-glucuronosyltransferase cofactors in alamethicin-activated human liver microsomes. Drug Metabolism and Disposition 37(1), 82–89 (2009)
64. Holzinger, A.: Human–Computer Interaction & Knowledge Discovery (HCI-KDD): What is the benefit of bringing those two fields to work together? In: Cuzzocrea, A., Kittl, C., Simos, D.E., Weippl, E., Xu, L. (eds.) CD-ARES 2013. LNCS, vol. 8127, pp. 319–328. Springer, Heidelberg (2013)
65. Keim, D.A., Mansmann, F., Schneidewind, J., Thomas, J., Ziegler, H.: Visual Analytics: Scope and Challenges. In: Simoff, S.J., Böhlen, M.H., Mazeika, A. (eds.) Visual Data Mining. LNCS, vol. 4404, pp. 76–90. Springer, Heidelberg (2008)
66. Anderson, D., Anderson, E., Lesh, N., Marks, J., Perlin, K., Ratajczak, D., Ryall, K.: Human-guided simple search: Combining information visualization and heuristic search. In: Proceedings of the 1999 Workshop on New Paradigms in Information Visualization and Manipulation in Conjunction with the Eighth ACM Internation Conference on Information and Knowledge Management, pp. 21–25. ACM (1999)
67. Ng, R.T., Lakshmanan, L.V., Han, J., Pang, A.: Exploratory mining and pruning optimizations of constrained associations rules. In: ACM SIGMOD Record, pp. 13–24. ACM (1998)
68. Ankerst, M., Ester, M., Kriegel, H.-P.: Towards an effective cooperation of the user and the computer for classification. In: Proceedings of the Sixth ACM SIGKDD International Conference on Knowledge Discovery and Data Mining, pp. 179–188. ACM (2000)
69. Mueller, H., Reihs, R., Zatloukal, K., Holzinger, A.: Analysis of biomedical data with multilevel glyphs. BMC Bioinformatics 15(suppl. 6), S5 (2014)
70. Holzinger, A., Leitner, H.: Lessons from Real-Life Usability Engineering in Hospital: From Software Usability to Total Workplace Usability. In: Holzinger, A., Weidmann, K.-H. (eds.) Empowering Software Quality: How can Usability Engineering Reach These Goals?, pp. 153–160. Austrian Computer Society, Vienna (2005)
71. Holzinger, A., Searle, G., Wernbacher, M.: The effect of Previous Exposure to Technology (PET) on Acceptance and its importance in Usability Engineering. Universal Access in the Information Society International Journal 10(3), 245–260 (2011)
72. Holzinger, A.: Usability engineering methods for software developers. Communications of the ACM 48(1), 71–74 (2005)
73. Chawla, N.V., Davis, D.A.: Bringing Big Data to Personalized Healthcare: A Patient-Centered Framework. J. Gen. Intern. Med. 28, S660–S665 (2013)
74. Wang, D.A., Wang, R., Yan, H.: Fast prediction of protein-protein interaction sites based on Extreme Learning Machines. Neurocomputing 128, 258–266 (2014)

# Darwin or Lamarck?
# Future Challenges in Evolutionary Algorithms
# for Knowledge Discovery and Data Mining

Katharina Holzinger[1], Vasile Palade[2,3], Raul Rabadan[4], and Andreas Holzinger[1]

[1] Medical University Graz, Institute for Medical Informatics, Statistics and Documentation
Research Unit HCI, Graz, Austria
{k.holzinger,a.holzinger}@hci4all.at
[2] Coventry University, Faculty of Engineering and Computing, Coventry, UK
vasile.palade@coventry.ac.uk
[3] Oxford University, Department of Computer Science, Oxford, UK
[4] Columbia University, Department of Systems Biology and
Department of Biomedical Informatics, New York, US
rabadan@dbmi.columbia.edu

**Abstract.** Evolutionary Algorithms (EAs) are a fascinating branch of computational intelligence with much potential for use in many application areas. The fundamental principle of EAs is to use ideas inspired by the biological mechanisms observed in nature, such as selection and genetic changes, to find the best solution for a given optimization problem. Generally, EAs use iterative processes, by growing a population of solutions selected in a guided random search and using parallel processing, in order to achieve a desired result. Such population based approaches, for example particle swarm and ant colony optimization (inspired from biology), are among the most popular metaheuristic methods being used in machine learning, along with others such as the simulated annealing (inspired from thermodynamics). In this paper, we provide a short survey on the state-of-the-art of EAs, beginning with some background on the theory of evolution and contrasting the original ideas of Darwin and Lamarck; we then continue with a discussion on the analogy between biological and computational sciences, and briefly describe some fundamentals of EAs, including the Genetic Algorithms, Genetic Programming, Evolution Strategies, Swarm Intelligence Algorithms (i.e., Particle Swarm Optimization, Ant Colony Optimization, Bacteria Foraging Algorithms, Bees Algorithm, Invasive Weed Optimization), Memetic Search, Differential Evolution Search, Artificial Immune Systems, Gravitational Search Algorithm, Intelligent Water Drops Algorithm. We conclude with a short description of the usefulness of EAs for Knowledge Discovery and Data Mining tasks and present some open problems and challenges to further stimulate research.

**Keywords:** Evolutionary Algorithms, Optimization, Nature inspired computing, Knowledge Discovery, Data Mining.

A. Holzinger, I. Jurisica (Eds.): Knowledge Discovery and Data Mining, LNCS 8401, pp. 35–56, 2014.
© Springer-Verlag Berlin Heidelberg 2014

# 1    Introduction

The original idea behind the EAs goes back to the early days of computer science [1] and started with some initial thoughts on **adaptive systems** introduced by John H. Holland [2]. Since the 1980ies, EAs have been used to address optimization problems due to their robustness and flexibility, especially in fields where traditional greedy algorithms did not provide satisfactory results. A typical example can be found in [3] in finding near-minimal phylogenetic trees from protein sequence data; a good Web-based tool for the display, manipulation and annotation of such phylogenetic trees is described in [4].

Traditional evolutionary paradigms are usually divided into two groups according to the principle invoked to explain the biological change: While Lamarck (see section 3.3) proposed the inheritance of acquired characteristics; Darwin (see section 3.2) underlines the role of selection on *random genetic variation*. A Lamarckian Algorithm, for example, would have nothing to do with selection.

Rather than referring to Darwin's original work [5], computer scientists use terms like "natural selection theory", "natural genetics", "the genetic theory of natural selection", etc., because EAs are inspired from the **selection** and **genetic principles observed in nature.** However, EAs do not prove anything with respect to the evolution in nature presumed in the original work by Darwin. So, a good question is why are we speaking then of "evolutionary algorithms"?

One aim of this paper is to shortly introduce to computer scientists the original work of Darwin, and to contrast these ideas to an earlier evolution theory of Lamarck, which might be even less familiar to the computer science community, but which has started to gain some popularity among researchers in evolutionary computing in recent years. For example, a search in the Web of Science repository, with the words "evolutionary algorithms" in the title, returns 1,886 results (as of February, 19, 2014). The oldest contribution is a paper in Lecture Notes in Economics and Mathematical Systems dating back to 1991 [6], which, interestingly, got no citation so far; the newest is a contribution in the April 2014 issue of the Journal of Industrial Management Optimization [7]; and the paper with the highest number of citations is in the Nov. 1999 issue of the IEEE Transactions on Evolutionary Computation [8].

This paper is organized as follows: First, we define the key terms to ensure mutual understanding. Then, we contrast the work of Darwin and Lamarck and focus on some computational aspects, because it will be necessary to define a new terminology for the Lamarckian version of an evolutionary algorithm. In the central part of the paper, we describe the state-of-the-art in EAs, where we shortly describe the main classes of current EA approaches. We finally stimulate a discussion on the use of EAs for Knowledge Discovery and Data Mining tasks, by presenting current challenges in the area and some new "hot ideas" that may inspire future research.

# 2    Glossary and Key Terms

*Classification:* Computational learning process to identify the class or category (from a set of possible classes) to which a new observation belongs, on basis of a training set containing observations whose category memberships are known.

*Clustering:* Grouping a set of objects in such a way that objects in the same group (or cluster) are more similar to each other than to those in other groups (clusters).

*Epigenetics:* is the study of heritable changes in genes, not caused by changes in the DNA. Whereas genetics is based on changes to the DNA sequence (the genotype), the changes in gene expression or cellular phenotype of epigenetics have other causes, therefore the prefix epi- (Greek: επί- outside) [9], [10].

*Evolution:* The change of inherited characteristics of biological populations over successive generations.

*Evolutionary Computation (EC):* Subfield of computational intelligence that involves mainly optimization with a metaheuristic or stochastic character inspired from biological processes observed in nature.

*Evolutionary Algorithm (EA):* An algorithm that uses mechanisms inspired by biological evolution, such as reproduction, mutation, recombination, and selection.

*Genetic Algorithm (GA):* Search heuristic that mimics the processes from natural genetics to generate useful solutions in optimization and search problems.

*Genetic Programming (GP):* Set of genetic operations and a fitness function to measure how well a computer program has performed a task, and used to optimize a population of computer programs.

*Knowledge Discovery (KDD):* Exploratory analysis and modeling of data and the organized process of identifying valid, novel, useful and understandable patterns from data sets.

*Machine Learning:* The discipline concerned with methods and systems that can built and used to learn from data; a subfield of computer science.

*Multi-Objective Optimization:* aka Pareto optimization, involves more objective functions to be optimized simultaneously.

*Optimization:* is the selection of a best solution to a given problem (with regard to some criteria) from a set of available alternatives.

*Phylogenetic tree:* is a branching tree diagram displaying the evolutionary relationships among biological species [11], [12].

# 3     Background

## 3.1     Basic Principles

The fundamental principle of evolutionary algorithms is to use ideas inspired by selection and genetic mechanisms observed in nature to find the best solution for a given optimization problem. Consequently, EAs include a class of optimization techniques that imitate natural selection principles and social behavior in nature, and embrace genetic algorithms, swarm optimization algorithms, ant colony algorithms, bacteria foraging algorithms, to name only a few.

Today, EAs field has grown to represent a big branch of computational intelligence and machine learning research [13]. Evolutionary methods are used in many different research fields such as medicine [14], genetics [15], or engineering [16], and there are nearly countless application areas of EAs, due to their **adaptive nature** and ability in solving difficult optimization problems [17], [18], [19].

EAs scale well into high dimensions, are robust to noise and are in general a good choice for problems where traditional methods do not provide a solid foundation. However, due to the global search process of evolutionary methods, an optimal solution within finite time cannot be guaranteed. Before we continue with recent state-of-the-art on EAs, we will shortly look back into history first.

## 3.2    Darwin's Theory

The theory of evolution, which Charles Darwin (1809–1882) presented in 1859 in his book "On the origin of species" [5] can be summarized with a simple algorithm: Mutation – variability – competition – selection – inheritance.

*Fitness:* A key concept in Darwinian evolution is the idea of fitness, or the capability of organisms to survive and reproduce. Genomic variations in the form of mutation or recombination could cause changes in fitness. Fitter organisms are positively selected and their genomic information is inherited by their descendants. The descendants inherit the selected variations and the phenotypic traits associated with them. The phenotypic variability is then caused by inherited mutations in the DNA sequence. Similar to individuals, there is also a competition among the alleles, for the presence in the DNA of the population. Alleles are the possible genetic variations of a gene that are present in the population. Depending on how successful the carriers of this specific allele are, after several generations it will either be fixed or die out – therefore, disappear from the gene pool. However, the success of an allele carrier only depends on the allele, if it occurs phenotypically in morphological, physiological or ethological terms, therefore, has an influence on appearance, body function or behavior of the organism in question. Consequently, in Darwinism, the evolution is only a secondary process. The organisms do not actively adapt to their environment, but out of a variety of different characteristics and manifestations, the ones that are selected are those that give their bearers an advantage in survival or reproduction. As has already been emphasized above, what a central role the selection plays in Darwinism, it is essential to look at the different types of selection:

*Natural Selection:* This is the selection by biotic or abiotic environmental factors. Abiotic factors for example include climate, biotic factors include pressure from predators. Darwin used the term as opposed to artificial selection and emphasized that natural selection must end with the death or incapacity of reproduction of the organism. *"(…) for of the many individuals of any species which are periodically born, but a small number can survive. I have called this principle, by which each slight variation, if useful, is preserved, by the term of Natural selection (…)"* [5].

*Sexual Selection:* In modern evolutionary biology, sexual selection is counted among natural selection. Darwin himself described sexual selection as "less rigorous" than natural selection because it does not decide over life and death, but on the number of offspring, which is only indirectly crucial for the survival or success of a species. Sexual selection is the competition within a species to reproduce, hence, the efforts of the males to impress the females and the males fighting each other for the right to mate. The structures and trades resulting from these processes do not always coincide with natural selection, but often are even contradictory to it. Well known examples of such structures are the tail feathers of a male peacock and the antlers of a male deer. As for the survival of a species, however natural selection is the stronger force.

*Artificial Selection:* Artificial selection occurs when humans select animals with desired characteristics and breed them. The many breeds of dogs and horses are a result of artificial selection.

*Gene Selection:* It is of great importance in modern evolutionary research, as individual alleles compete for the maximum frequency in the population. In modern evolutionary biology, gene selection has replaced the selection of individuals as postulated in the theory of classical Darwinism, where individuals are selected because of phenotypic characteristics.

*Stabilizing selection:* eliminates individuals with an extreme value of a specific characteristic, for example size. A possible scenario would be a pond with fish in different sizes, where the small fish are prayed on by birds and the large fish get caught by fishermen. Therefore medium sized fish will become a majority within the pond.

*Distributive Selection:* This is the exact opposite of stabilizing selection, because it eliminates individuals with mediocre value of a certain characteristic. If we return to our exemplary pond of fish, this time the medium sized fish will get prayed on by bigger birds. On the other hand the extreme fish – the small and the big – will survive.

*Directional Selection:* This type of selection is particularly interesting and aimed at one side of the extremes and the mediocre; e.g., in our exemplary pond directional selection, if an otter preyed on small and medium sized fish. Thus, the chances of survival increase for the fish with their size. The bigger the safer. Under such a kind of selective pressure this species of fish will gradually increase in size.

*Hard selection:* This refers to selective pressure at which an individual is eliminated if it does not reach a certain value, such as size or color. For example, all fish bigger than 30 cm will be caught in the nets of fishermen.

*Soft selection:* This does not use an absolute value, but a ratio. In our fish example soft selection would mean the biggest fish will be caught, no matter how big they are exactly.

## 3.3    Lamarck's Theory

However, Darwinism was not the only theory of evolution of the time. In addition to the catastrophism of Georges Cuvier (1769–1832), there is also Lamarckism, which states, unlike Darwinism, that selection is **not** the driving force of evolution, but the inheritance of acquired characteristics or inherited **"effort"** of the organisms themselves. Jean-Baptiste de Lamarck (1744–1829) assumed that appropriate characteristics arise from the desire of the organisms to achieve them (strive for perfection).

Unlike Darwinism, where evolution is only a result of competition and selection, in Lamarckism the organisms themselves control evolution. This is accomplished through practice, training, and the frequent use of specific organs. Lesser used organs, however, wither with time. The most popular example to illustrate the idea

Lamarckism is the evolution of the giraffe's neck: The giraffe is striving to reach the highest leaves, and stretched her neck. This acquired trait is inherited by her descendants, who again stretch their necks. However, this very simple explanation of a deliberate adaptation results in some questions from modern biological perspective: Why should organisms have the desire to change? Can new structures be build trough training? By what means is it decided which adaptions will be passed on? Why does not an amputated leg get inherited? In biology, Lamarckism would be possible if there was a mechanism that translates phenotypic changes into the sequence of the responsible gene. However, Lamarckism should not be entirely rejected, as it can provide some answers, especially in modern genetics and medicine. In epigenetics – which very early dealt with questions of evolution [20],[21], it was found that there are special traits which can be inherited without being part of the genetic code; That would, for example, explain a possible higher function of the thumb in the upcoming post-millennial younger generations ("Net Gen" [22]) due to frequent use of text messaging on mobile phones, which is being allegedly claimed by some people, but still to be confirmed. The possibility that acquired behavior or marks can be passed from parents to children is in serious debate and the advent of epigenetics is hailed as a profound shift in our understanding of inheritance, i.e. that genes also have a kind of "memory" [23], [24], epigenetics being an upcoming hype in medical research [25], with a very recent example in cancer research found here [26].

# 4     Brief Survey on Evolutionary Algorithms

## 4.1     Why Evolutionary Algorithms?

Due to the adaptive and robust nature of performing a global instead of a local search for solutions in the search space, which improves their handling of interactions between attributes [27], methods based on evolutionary algorithms are being used in a wide array of different research fields. They are mostly used for traditional KDD tasks, such as clustering and classification as well as for optimization. Another benefit of evolutionary methods is the possibility of using them for multi-objective optimization, making them well suited for many real-world use-cases where simultaneous optimization of several objectives is of importance [28]. There are many different algorithms in the universe of evolutionary methods, but the most prevalent are genetic algorithms and genetic programming which we describe in section 4.4.

## 4.2     Biological Sciences versus Computational Sciences

Darwin explains in his book *"The Origin of Species by Means of Natural Selection, or the Preservation of Favoured Races in the Struggle for Life"* [5] the diversity and complexity of living organisms: Beneficial traits resulting from random variation are favored by natural selection, i.e. individuals with beneficial traits have better chances to survive, procreate and multiply, which may also be captured by the expression differential reproduction. In order to understand evolutionary algorithms, some basic notions are important, which will highlight the applicability of biological principles to computer science. Good resources for further details are: [13], which is also available in German [29], and [30], [31], [32], [33].

Evolutionary algorithms operate on a search space $S$, where $S$ denotes a given set. Points are assigned via an objective function $f$. In the context of evolutionary algorithms, this is usually called **fitness function** $f: S \to R$, where $R$ is the set of arbitrary possible fitness values, and the evolutionary algorithm operates on a collection of points from $S$, called a population $P$. Each member of the population (points in the search space) is called individual. A number $\mu \in \mathbb{N}$ is used to denote the size of the population, i.e. $\mu = |P|$.

A population is a multiset over $S$, i.e., it may contain multiple copies of individuals. Since the population changes from generation to generation, we denote the population at the $t$-th generation as $P_t$. Choosing the first population, $P_0$, at the beginning is called initialization.

**Table 1.** Biology vs Computing: basic evolutionary notions in the biological vs. computational sciences; compare with Kruse et al. (2013) [13]

| NOTION | BIOLOGICAL UNIVERSE | COMPUTATIONAL UNIVERSE |
|---|---|---|
| Allele | "Value" of a gene | Value of a information object |
| Chromosome | DNA, protein, and RNA sequence in cells (describes the "construction plan" and traits of an individual) | Sequence of information objects (describes the "construction plan" and "traits of an individual") |
| Fitness | Aptitude/conformity of a living organism, determines chances of survival and reproduction | Aptitude/quality of a solution candidate, determines chances of survival and reproduction |
| Gene | Part of a Chromosome, as a fundamental unit of inheritance, which determines a (partial) characteristic of an individual | Information object, e.g. a bit, a character, number etc., fundamental unit of inheritance, which determines a (partial) characteristic of an individual |
| Generation | Population at a point in time | Population at a point in time |
| Genotype | Genetic constitution of a living organism | Encoding of a solution candidate |
| Individual | Living organism | Solution candidate |
| Locus | position of a gene, at each position in a Chromosome there is exactly one gene | position of an information object, at each position in a Chromosome there is exactly one gene |
| Phenotype | Physical appearance of a living organism | Implementation or application of a solution candidate |
| Population | Set of living organisms | Bag or multi-set of Chromosomes |
| Reproduction | Creating offspring of one or multiple (usually two) parent organisms | Creating (child) chromosomes from one or multiple (parent) chromosomes |

For each member $x$ of the population, its fitness $f(x)$ is computed and stored. The first step in each generation is to select some individuals from the population that will be used to create new points in the search space. These individuals are referred to as parents. This process is called selection for reproduction. Often this selection is done fitness-based, i.e., the chances of individuals to become parents increase with their fitness. Then some random variation is applied to the parents, where small changes are more likely than large changes [30].

## 4.3    Foundations of Evolutionary Algorithms

As already mentioned, the basic idea of an evolutionary algorithm is to apply evolutionary principles to generate increasingly better solution candidates in order to solve an optimization problem. This may be achieved by evolving a population of solution candidates by random variation and fitness-based selection of the next generation. According to [13], an EA requires the following building blocks:

- an encoding for the solution candidates,
- a method to create an initial population,
- a fitness function to evaluate the individual solutions (chromosomes),
- a selection method on the basis of the fitness function,
- a set of genetic operators to modify chromosomes,
- a termination criterion for the search, and
- values for various parameters.

The (natural) selection process of biological evolution can be simulated by a method for selecting candidate solutions according to their fitness, i.e., to select the parents of offspring that are transferred to the next generation. Such a selection method may simply transform the fitness values into a selection probability, such that better individuals have higher chances of getting chosen for the next generation. The random variation of chromosomes can be simulated by so-called genetic operators that modify and recombine chromosomes, for example, mutation, which randomly changes individual genes, and crossover, which exchanges parts of the chromosomes of parent individuals to produce offspring. While biological evolution is unbounded, we need a criterion to decide when to stop the process in order to retrieve a final solution. Such a criterion may be, for example, that the algorithm is terminated (1) after a user-specified number of generations have been created, (2) there has been no improvement (of the best solution candidate) for a user-specified number of generations, or (3) a user-specified minimum solution quality has been obtained. To complete the specification of an evolutionary algorithm, we have to choose the values of several parameters, which include, for example, the size of the population to evolve, the fraction of individuals that is chosen from each population to produce offsprings, the probability of a mutation occurring in an individual etc. [13]. The general procedure of such an evolutionary algorithm may look as presented in table 2:

**Table 2.** General Scheme of an Evolutionary Algorithm

```
procedure evolutionary algorithm;
begin
    t ← 0; (* initialize the generation counter *)
    initialize pop(t);(* create the initial population *)
    evaluate pop(t); (* and evaluate it (compute fitness) *)
    while not termination criterion do (* loop until termination *)
            t ← t+1;  (* count the created generation *)
                    select pop(t)from pop(t-1);(*select individuals
                    based on fitness*)
            alter pop(t);  (* apply genetic operators *)
            evaluate pop(t); (* evaluate the new population *)
    end
end
```

## 4.4    Types of Evolutionary Algorithms

### 4.4.1    Genetic Algorithms (GA)

Genetic algorithms (GAs) are a machine learning method inspired from genetic and selection mechanisms found in nature [34], which conduct a randomized and parallel search for solutions that optimize a predefined fitness function [35].

In nature, the genetic information is defined in a quaternary code, based on the four nucleotides **A**denine, **C**ytosine, **G**uanine and **T**hymine, stringed together in a DNA sequence, which forms the basis of the genetic code [36]. In transferring this structure to computer science, it seems natural to base all encodings on the ultimately binary structure of information in a computer. That is, we use chromosomes that are bit strings, to encode problem solutions, and exactly this is the distinctive feature of genetic algorithms [37]. The algorithm performs a global search in the space of solution candidates, where the space consists of data vectors. The first step is to initialize the solution candidate space with randomly generated individual solutions. At each iteration, the available candidates are mutated or crossed with other solutions in order to create new candidates. At the end of each iteration, every individual solution candidate is evaluated using a predefined fitness function. Consequently, the fitness function is the core part of every evolutionary algorithm, and designed to find out which solutions are the best fits for the problem. Once each individual has been evaluated, the least fit candidates get dismissed, leaving only the best available solutions in the population. This is Darwin's principle of survival of the fittest in solving computing problems. The loop of iterations is repeated until a predefined stopping criterion has been reached. Stopping criteria can vary in their definition from just the number of iterations to go through to a certain threshold of fitness value that has to be reached within the solution space. For more details on GAs refer to [38], [39], [40].

### 4.4.2   Genetic Programming (GP)

Genetic programming (GP) differs from genetic algorithms mainly in the form of the input and output values the algorithm needs and produces [41]. In the case of GP, the values are not simple data points, but parts of functions or programs. The goal is to find a procedure which solves the given problem in the most efficient way. The algorithm itself works in the same way as described in the section above, where initially there is a randomly generated space of candidate solutions (random programs in this case), which are evolved using mutation and crossover processes, generating new program trees. The end result is supposed to be a function or a program, which can be used to solve a specific type of problem. An example of linear genetic programming applied to medical classification problems from a benchmark database compared with results obtained by neural networks can be found in [42].

### 4.4.3   Evolution Strategies (ES)

Evolution Strategies (ES) are a stochastic approach to numerical optimization that shows good optimization performance in general and which goes attempt to imitate principles of organic evolution in the field of parameter optimization [43]. In order to improve the "self-adaptive" property of strategy parameters, Ohkura et al. (2001) [44] proposed an extended ES called **Robust Evolution Strategy (RES),** which has redundant neutral strategy parameters and which adopts new mutation mechanisms in order to utilize selectively neutral mutations to improve the adaptability of strategy parameters, a similar approach was proposed in [45] and more details can be found in [46], [47], [48].

### 4.4.4   Swarm Intelligence (SI)

Swarm intelligence (SI) studies the collective behavior of self-organized systems composed of many individuals interacting locally with each other and with their environment, using decentralized control to achieve their goals. Swarm-based systems have been developed in response to the observed success and efficiency of such swarms in nature [49].

Approaches that came out as a result of studying the **collective behavior** of populations of "simple agents", i.e. individuals with limited abilities without central control, can be employed in many different areas. They have been inspired by the behavior of certain species of animals, especially social insects (ants, bees) and animals that live and search for food in swarms, flocks, herds or packs (fish, birds, deer, wolves, rabbits etc.) and also bacteria. Such swarms can find the shortest paths to food sources, they can build complex nests like bee hives, hunt for prey (for example, packs of wolves), and protect themselves against predators [13]. In joint efforts, these animals are often able to solve complex problems – demonstrating collective intelligence [50]. This is a recent and important research area in computer science [51] which can be applied for many purposes, a prominent example being the NASA crater finding [52] using human collective intelligence [53], [54].

### Particle Swarm Optimization (PSO)

Particle swarm optimization (PSO) is an evolutionary computation technique developed by Eberhart & Kennedy in 1995 [55], the concept being originated from the simulation of a simplified social system, i.e. to graphically simulate the graceful but unpredictable choreography of a bird flock.

Initial simulations were modified to incorporate nearest-neighbor velocity matching, eliminate ancillary variables, and incorporate multidimensional search and acceleration by distance. At some point in the evolution of this algorithm, it was realized that the conceptual model was **an optimizer.** Through a process of trial and error, a number of parameters extraneous to optimization were eliminated from the algorithm, resulting in a very simple implementation [56], similar to a genetic algorithm, where the system is initialized with a population of random solutions.

Unlike GAs, there is no mutation operator, although each potential solution is also assigned a randomized velocity, and the potential solutions, called particles, are then "flown" through the problem space. Each particle keeps track of its personal best position in the problem space, which is associated with the best fitness value of the particle found so far. Another "best" value that is tracked by the particle swarm optimizer is the overall best value, and its location, obtained by any particle in the population [57], [58] – the so-called "global best".

### Ant Colony Optimization (ACO)

Ants do not possess a great deal of intelligence by themselves, but collectively a colony of ants performs sophisticated tasks such as finding the shortest path to food sources and sharing this information with other ants by depositing *pheromone.* Ant Colony Optimization (ACO) models the collective intelligence of ants, which are transformed into optimization techniques [59]. ACO was introduced by Dorigo et al. (1991) [60], [61] as a novel nature-inspired metaheuristic for the solution of hard combinatorial optimization (CO) problems. Such metaheuristics are approximate algorithms used to obtain satisfactory solutions to hard CO problems in a reasonable amount of computational time. Other examples of such metaheuristics are tabu search, simulated annealing, and evolutionary computation [62]. More details can be found in [63], [64] and a recent example can be found in [65]. A prominent example as a data mining algorithm is the Ant-Miner (Ant-colony-based data miner), aiming at extracting classification rules from data. This algorithm was inspired by both research on the behavior of real ant colonies and known data mining concepts [66].

### Bacteria Foraging Algorithms (BFA)

Foraging theory is based on the assumption that animals search for and obtain nutrients in a way that maximizes their energy intake $E$ per unit time $T$ spent foraging. The Escherichia coli bacterium is probably the best understood microorganism and much what is known cytokinesis in bacteria has come from studies with E. coli, and efforts to understand fundamental processes in this organism continue to intensify [67]. When E. coli grows, it gets longer, then divides in the middle into two so-called "daughters." Given sufficient food and held at the temperature of the human gut (one place where they live) of 37° C, this bacterium can synthesize and replicate everything it needs to make a copy of itself in about 20 minutes. Hence, the growth of a population of bacteria is exponential, with a relatively short time to double [68]. The foraging behavior of E. coli can be used by analogy in the Bacteria Foraging Algorithms (BFA) to solve global optimization problems [69]. An example of an electrical engineering application of the BFA can be found in [70]. An approach applied in human psychology is the Information Foraging Theory by Pirolli & Card (1999) [71]; this assumes that people try to modify their information seeking strategies to maximize their rate in gaining valuable information. The adaptation analysis develops information patch models, which deal with *time allocation* and *information filtering*; *information scent* models, which address the identification of information value from proximal cues; and *information diet models*, which address decisions about the selection and pursuit of information items. The theory has been used to study e.g. the "surf behaviour" on the Web [72], but has also been used for data mining [73], and for knowledge discovery in the biomedical domain [74].

*Bees Algorithm (BA)*

The population-based search algorithm called the Bees Algorithm (BA) mimics the food foraging behaviour of a swarm of honey bees and was proposed by Pham et al. (2006) [75]. In its basic version, the algorithm performs a kind of neighbourhood search combined with random search, and can be used for combinatorial optimisation as well as functional optimisation [76]. BAs are also meta-heuristics, which try to model the natural behavior of bees in food foraging, such as mechanisms like waggle dance to optimally locate food sources and to search for new ones [77]. Basturk & Karaboga (2007), [78] proposed the Artificial Bee Colony (ABC) algorithm for constrained optimization problems. The idea is that the collective intelligence of bee swarms consists of three components: food sources, employed bees, and unemployed bees; the latter further segregated into onlookers and scouts. This results into three main phases of ABC: employed phase, onlooker phase, and scout phase.A recent work described the integration of Artificial Bee Colony (ABC) and Bees Algorithm (BA) to an ABC–BA algorithm which performs better than each single one [79].

*Invasive Weed Optimization (IWO)*

The Invasive Weed Optimization Algorithm (IWO) was proposed by Mehrabian & Lucas (2006) [80], as an ecologically inspired metaheuristic that mimics the process of weeds colonization and distribution, which is capable of solving multi-dimensional, linear and nonlinear optimization problems with appreciable efficiency. Moreover, the IWO can also be used in the validation of reached optima and in the development of regularization terms and non-conventional transfer functions that do not necessarily provide gradient information [81]. A recent example of IWO for knowledge discovery purposes can be found in [82], .

### 4.4.5    Memetic Algorithms (MA)

Memetic algorithms (MA) are amongst the growing areas in evolutionary computation and were inspired by Richard Dawkins' meme [83]; an implementation of an "selfish gene algorithm" can be found here [84]. The term MA is widely used as a synergy of evolutionary or any other population-based approach with separate individual learning or local improvement procedures for search problems [85]. MAs are often also referred to as Baldwinian evolutionary algorithms (see [86] about the Baldwin effect), Lamarckian EAs, cultural algorithms, or genetic local search.

A novel correlation based memetic framework (MA-C), which is a combination of a genetic algorithm (GA) and local search (LS) using correlation based filter ranking has been proposed in [87]: The local filter method fine-tunes the population of GA solutions by adding or deleting features based on Symmetrical Uncertainty (SU) measures. Such approaches have many possibilities for the use in real-world problems, particularly in bio-computing and data mining for high-dimensional problems [88]. Amongst a very recent meta-heuristic is the Grey Wolf Optimizer (GWO), which mimics the leadership hierarchy and hunting mechanism of grey wolves (canis lupus) in nature [89].

### 4.4.6    Differential Evolution Search

An example of Differential Evolution (DE) search is the Artificial Bee Colony (ABC) algorithm, mentioned in section 4.3.4. Its main idea is that the algorithm makes use of differential evolution operators to update the information on the food source in order to enhance the local search ability at the stage of onlooker bees, and a chaotic sequence is introduced to the differential mutation operator for this purpose. Simulation results show that this algorithm, introducing *chaotic differential evolution search*, is a promising one in terms of convergence rate and solution accuracy, compared to the ABC algorithm [90]. A memetic DE algorithm, that utilizes a chaotic local search (CLS) with a shrinking strategy, in order to improve the optimizing performance of the canonical DE by exploring a huge search space in the early run phase to avoid premature convergence can be found in [91].

### 4.4.7    Artificial Immune Systems (AIS)

Artificial immune systems (AIS) developed by Farmer et al. (1986) [92], can be defined as adaptive computational systems inspired from immunology, i.e. by the observed immune functions, principles and mechanisms. The idea was that the immune system as highly evolved biological system, is able to identify (and eliminate) foreign substances [93]. Consequently, it must be able to determine between gens and antigens, which requires a powerful capability of learning, memory and pattern recognition. The development and application domains of AIS follow those of soft computing paradigms [94], such as artificial neural networks (ANN) and fuzzy systems (FS). A framework which discusses the suitability of AIS as a soft computing paradigm that integrate AIS with other approaches, focusing on ANN, EA and FS has been proposed by [95].

### 4.4.8    Gravitational Search Algorithm (GSA)

Gravitational Search Algorithms (GSA) are based on the analogy with the law of gravity and mass interactions: the search agents are a collection of masses which interact with each other based on the Newtonian gravity and the laws of motion [96].

GSA falls also under the category of metaheuristics as general search strategies that, at the exploitation stage, exploit areas of the solution space with high quality solutions and, at the exploration stage, move to unexplored areas of the solution space [97]. GSA is a stochastic population-based metaheuristic that was originally designed for solving *continuous* optimization problems.

The Binary Gravitational Search Algorithm (BGSA) is a new variant for discrete optimization problems, and experimental results confirm its efficiency in solving various nonlinear benchmark problems [98].

A recent work on a Discrete Gravitational Search Algorithm (DGSA) to solve combinatorial optimization problems [99] can be found in [97].

### 4.4.9    Intelligent Water Drops Algorithm (IWD)

A natural river often finds optimal paths among a number of different possible paths in its ways from the source to destination. These near optimal or optimal (natural) paths are obtained by the actions and reactions that occur among the water drops and between the water drops and the riverbeds.

The Intelligent Water Drops (IWD) algorithm is a new population-based optimisation algorithm inspired from observing natural water drops flowing in rivers. The authors of [100] tested this algorithm to find solutions of the *n*-queen puzzle with a simple local heuristic, solved the travelling salesman problem (TSP) and tested it with multiple knapsack problems (MKP) in which near-optimal or optimal solutions were obtained [101].

There are various application areas for IWD thinkable, e.g. Agarwal et al. (2012) [102], propose the use of IWD as an optimised code coverage algorithm by using dynamic parameters for finding all the optimal paths using basic properties of natural water drops. A recent example application is in using IWD for solving multi-objective job-shop scheduling: Niu et al. (2013) customized it to find the best compromising solutions (Pareto non-dominance set) considering multiple criteria, namely make-span, tardiness and mean flow time of schedules, and proved that the customized IWD algorithm can identify the Pareto non-dominance schedules efficiently.

## 5    Evolutionary Algorithms for Knowledge Discovery and Data Mining

### 5.1    Classification and Clustering with EAs

In traditional data mining tasks, evolutionary algorithms can easily be used for both classification and clustering as well as for data preparation in the form of attribute generation and selection [27].

**Classification** is a central application for EAs, where they can be used for classification *rule mining*. These rules can be of different complexity and forms. In some cases, a whole set of rules is the goal, where interactions between the rules play an important role, whereas it is also possible to mine independent rules for classification. For details on the topic of *classification rule mining,* please refer to [27] and [103]. A very recent work, which shows that the implementation of evolutionary algorithms in machine learning can be achieved without extensive effort, meaning much experimentation can be performed quickly in order to discover novel areas where genetic algorithms can complement machine learning algorithms to achieve better classification results [104].

**Clustering** analysis is another application area for EAs to knowledge discovery tasks. There are different approaches to this problem, which are discussed in detail in [103]. The most important criteria when performing clustering analysis using EAs is the representation of solution candidates as well as the fitness evaluation, which can be a problematic issue considering the complexity of evaluating unsupervised knowledge discovery methods in general.

## 5.2    Advantages and Disadvantages

EAs have certain pros and cons as general optimization methods, including when they are used for knowledge discovery and data mining tasks, as shown in Table 3.

**Table 3.** Advantages and Disadvantages of EAs

| Advantages | Disadvantages |
|---|---|
| Robust to noise | EA methods do not guarantee finding of an optimal solution in finite time |
| Deals well with attribute interaction | Domain specific knowledge has to be explicitly added using external processes |
| Comparatively easy to implement | Optimization runtime not constant, variance between best- and worst-case can differ greatly |
| Well suited for multi-objective optimization | Computational complexity can be an issue |
| Good scalability due to parallelization | Fitness-function needs to be specified, otherwise EAs do not work |
| Very flexible (widely usable) | Slower than greedy algorithms in many cases |
| Good option for problems without a traditional best practice method | Not the first choice if a traditional method already solves the problem in an efficient way |
| Good amount of programming libraries available | |
| Small amount of specific mathematical knowledge necessary for using EAs | |
| Suitable for efficiently solving NP-hard problems | |

## 5.3    Available Software and Programming Libraries

There is a broad range of different software packages and libraries available for using EAs in KDD and DM tasks, The list below contains only the most well-known examples:

WEKA - http://www.cs.waikato.ac.nz/ml/weka
KEEL - http://www.keel.es
SolveIT - http://www.solveitsoftware.com
MCMLL - http://mcmll.sourceforge.net
Jenetics - http://jenetics.sourceforge.net
Jenes - http://jenes.intelligentia.it

jMetal - `http://jmetal.sourceforge.net`
JGAP - `http://jgap.sourceforge.net`
epochX - `http://www.epochx.org`
SAS - `https://www.sas.com`
Discipulus - `http://www.rmltech.com`
XpertRule - `http://www.attar.com`
MATLAB GA-Toolbox `http://www.mathworks.com/discovery/genetic-algorithm`

## 6     Open Problems and Challenges

Evolutionary algorithms, by default, are so called "blind" methods, which means that the used operators do not use or depend on domain specific knowledge. While this feature enriches their generality, it is in most cases a negative factor compared to methods making use of existing relevant knowledge within the domain [103]. This aspect can however be remedied by introducing mechanisms such as a preceding local search into the execution of evolutionary algorithms, and enriching the fitness function with domain specific data.

Another shortcoming of evolutionary approaches for knowledge discovery tasks is that they do not guarantee an optimal solution in finite time. They also do not guarantee constant optimization runtimes and the differences between the best and worst case scenarios are usually larger than for most traditional optimization methods, making EAs a suboptimal choice for real-time systems [105].

Computational complexity can, as with all other KDD methods, also be an issue. However with the increase of processing power as well as the possibility to easily parallelize evolutionary methods, especially in combination with cloud services and the island model [105], the issue should be, at most, of a temporary nature.

## 7     Future Work

A specific area of future research, according to [103], should be the application of genetic programming for data mining tasks. There have been attempts to create generic rule induction algorithms using GP [106], [107], but they are still comparatively under-discovered and under-used within the domain of knowledge discovery.

Biology has traditionally been a source of inspiration for evolutionary algorithms. In most organisms, evolution proceeds in small steps by random mutations and in large steps by horizontal events (recombination, reassortments, gene transfer and hybridizations). Horizontal events combine the genetic information from two or more organisms to generate a new one that incorporate alleles from parental strains. Whilst mutations allow efficient local searches in the fitness landscape, horizontal events combine information from fit individuals exploring larger regions of search space. Humans and eukaryotes in general recombine during meiosis, retroviruses during retrotranscription, each presenting different ways of combining genetic information. Segmented viruses, viruses with more than one chromosome as influenza, combine genetic information through reassortments, a process where a new individual is created by exchange of chromosomes between two or more parental strains. This is the very effective process behind **influenza pandemics** that could allow viruses to jump from one host to another and rapidly propagate in the new population. Such mechanisms, and others, are found in nature and represent different strategies to go beyond mutations with distinct advantages. Each of these evolutionary strategies can be used to address different problems – but it needs much further research, testing and experimenting.

# References

1. Box, G.E.: Evolutionary operation: A method for increasing industrial productivity. Applied Statistics 6(2), 81–101 (1957)
2. Holland, J.H.: Outline for a Logical Theory of Adaptive Systems. J. ACM 9(3), 297–314 (1962)
3. Hendy, M.D., Penny, D.: Branch an Bound Algorithms to determine minimal Evolutionary Trees. Mathematical Biosciences 59(2), 277–290 (1982)
4. Letunic, I., Bork, P.: Interactive Tree Of Life (iTOL): An online tool for phylogenetic tree display and annotation. Bioinformatics 23(1), 127–128 (2007)
5. Darwin, C.: On the origin of species by means of natural selection, or the preservation of favoured races in the struggle for life. John Murray, London (1859)
6. Hoffmeister, F.: Scalable Parallelism by Evolutionary Algorithms. Lecture Notes in Economics and Mathematical Systems 367, 177–198 (1991)
7. Cheng, A., Lim, C.C.: Optimizing System-On-Chip verifications with multi-objective genetic evolutionary algorithms. Journal of Industrial and Management Optimization 10(2), 383–396 (2014)
8. Zitzler, E., Thiele, L.: Multiobjective evolutionary algorithms: A comparative case study and the Strength Pareto approach. IEEE Transactions on Evolutionary Computation 3(4), 257–271 (1999)
9. Waddington, C.H.: Canalization of development and the inheritance of acquired characters. Nature 150(3811), 563–565 (1942)
10. Trygve, T.: Handbook of Epigenetics. Academic Press, San Diego (2011)
11. Fitch, W.M., Margoliash, E.: Construction of phylogenetic trees. Science 155(760), 279–284 (1967)
12. Saitou, N., Nei, M.: The neighbor-joining method: A new method for reconstructing phylogenetic trees. Molecular Biology and Evolution 4(4), 406–425 (1987)
13. Kruse, R., Borgelt, C., Klawonn, F., Moewes, C., Steinbrecher, M., Held, P.: Computational Intelligence: A Methodological Introduction. Springer, Heidelberg (2013)
14. Lollini, P.-L., Motta, S., Pappalardo, F.: Discovery of cancer vaccination protocols with a genetic algorithm driving an agent based simulator. BMC Bioinformatics 7(1), 352 (2006)
15. Ritchie, M.D., Motsinger, A.A., Bush, W.S., Coffey, C.S., Moore, J.H.: Genetic programming neural networks: A powerful bioinformatics tool for human genetics. Applied Soft Computing 7(1), 471–479 (2007)
16. Winstein, K., Balakrishnan, H.: TCP ex Machina: Computer-Generated Congestion Control. In: ACM SIGCOMM, pp. 123–134. ACM (2013)
17. Gen, M., Cheng, R.: Genetic algorithms and engineering optimization. John Wiley & Sons (2000)
18. Rafael, B., Oertl, S., Affenzeller, M., Wagner, S.: Music segmentation with genetic algorithms. In: 20th International Workshop on Database and Expert Systems Application, DEXA 2009, pp. 256–260. IEEE (2009)

19. Soupios, P., Akca, I., Mpogiatzis, P., Basokur, A., Papazachos, C.: Application of Genetic Algorithms in Seismic Tomography. In: EGU General Assembly Conference Abstracts, p. 1555 (2010)
20. Waddington, C.H.: Epigenetics and Evolution. Symposia of the Society for Experimental Biology 7, 186–199 (1953)
21. Jablonka, E.: Epigenetic inheritance and evolution: The Lamarckian dimension. Oxford University Press, Oxford (1999)
22. Tapscott, D.: Grown Up Digital: How the Net Generation is Changing Your World HC. Mcgraw-Hill (2008)
23. Bird, A.: Perceptions of epigenetics. Nature 447(7143), 396–398 (2007)
24. Handel, A., Ramagopalan, S.: Is Lamarckian evolution relevant to medicine? BMC Medical Genetics 11(1), 73 (2010)
25. Kiberstis, P.A.: All Eyes on Epigenetics. Science 335(6069), 637 (2012)
26. Emmert-Streib, F., de Matos Simoes, R., Glazko, G., McDade, S., Haibe-Kains, B., Holzinger, A., Dehmer, M., Campbell, F.: Functional and genetic analysis of the colon cancer network. BMC Bioinformatics 15(suppl. 6), S6 (2014)
27. Freitas, A.A.: A survey of evolutionary algorithms for data mining and knowledge discovery. In: Advances in Evolutionary Computing, pp. 819–845. Springer (2003)
28. Coello Coello, C.A., Lechuga, M.S.: MOPSO: A proposal for multiple objective particle swarm optimization. In: Proceedings of the 2002 Congress on Evolutionary Computation (CEC 2002), pp. 1051–1056. IEEE (2002)
29. Kruse, R., Borgelt, C., Klawonn, F., Moewes, C., Ruß, G., Steinbrecher, M.: Computational Intelligence: Eine methodische Einführung in Künstliche Neuronale Netze, Evolutionäre Algorithmen, Fuzzy-Systeme und Bayes-Netze Vieweg+Teubner, Wiesbaden (2011)
30. Jansen, T.: Analyzing evolutionary algorithms: The computer science perspective. Springer Publishing Company (2013) (incorporated)
31. Yu, X., Gen, M.: Introduction to evolutionary algorithms. Springer, Heidelberg (2010)
32. Eiben, A.E., Smith, J.E.: Introduction to evolutionary computing. Springer, Berlin (2010)
33. De Jong, K.A.: Evolutionary computation: A unified approach. MIT press, Cambridge (2006)
34. Goldberg, D.E., Holland, J.H.: Genetic algorithms and machine learning. Mach. Learn. 3(2), 95–99 (1988)
35. Mitchell, T.M.: Machine learning, p. 267. McGraw-Hill, Boston (1997)
36. Forrest, S.: Genetic algorithms: Principles of natural selection applied to computation. Science 261(5123), 872–878 (1993)
37. Grefenstette, J.J.: Optimization of control parameters for genetic algorithms. IEEE Transactions on Systems Man and Cybernetics 16(1), 122–128 (1986)
38. Goldberg, D.E.: Genetic algorithms in search, optimization, and machine learning. Addison-Wesley Reading, MA (1989)
39. Mitchell, M.: An Introduction to Genetic Algorithms (Complex Adaptive Systems). MIT Press, Cambridge (1998)
40. Coley, D.A.: An introduction to Genetic Algorithms for Scientists and Engineers. World Scientific Publishing, Singapore (1999)
41. Koza, J.R.: Genetic programming as a means for programming computers by natural selection. Statistics and Computing 4(2), 87–112 (1994)
42. Brameier, M., Banzhaf, W.: A comparison of linear genetic programming and neural networks in medical data mining. IEEE Transactions on Evolutionary Computation 5(1), 17–26 (2001)

43. Bäck, T., Hoffmeister, F., Schwefel, H.P.: A survey of evolution strategies. In: Proceedings of the 4th International Conference on Genetic Algorithms, pp. 2-9 (1991)
44. Ohkura, K., Matsumura, Y., Ueda, K.: Robust evolution strategies. Applied Intelligence 15(3), 153–169 (2001)
45. Huhse, J., Zell, A.: Evolution Strategy with Neighborhood Attraction–A Robust Evolution Strategy. In: Proceedings of the Genetic and Evolutionary Computation Conference, GECCO 2001, pp. 1026–1033 (2001)
46. Auger, A., Hansen, N.: Theory of Evolution Strategies: A new perspective. In: Auger, A., Doerr, B. (eds.) Theory of Randomized Search Heuristics: Foundations and Recent Developments, pp. 289–325. World Scientific Publishing, Singapore (2011)
47. Beyer, H.-G., Schwefel, H.-P.: Evolution strategies–A comprehensive introduction. Natural Computing 1(1), 3–52 (2002)
48. Beyer, H.-G.: The theory of evolution strategies. Springer, Heidelberg (2001)
49. Martens, D., Baesens, B., Fawcett, T.: Editorial survey: Swarm intelligence for data mining. Mach. Learn. 82(1), 1–42 (2011)
50. Franks, N.R., Pratt, S.C., Mallon, E.B., Britton, N.F., Sumpter, D.J.T.: Information flow, opinion polling and collective intelligence in house-hunting social insects. Philosophical Transactions of the Royal Society of London Series B-Biological Sciences 357(1427), 1567–1583 (2002)
51. Kennedy, J.F., Eberhart, R.C.: Swarm intelligence. Morgan Kaufmann, San Francisco (2001)
52. van't Woud, J., Sandberg, J., Wielinga, B.J.: The Mars crowdsourcing experiment: Is crowdsourcing in the form of a serious game applicable for annotation in a semantically-rich research domain? In: 2011 16th International Conference on Computer Games (CGAMES), pp. 201–208. IEEE (2011)
53. Woolley, A.W., Chabris, C.F., Pentland, A., Hashmi, N., Malone, T.W.: Evidence for a Collective Intelligence Factor in the Performance of Human Groups. Science 330(6004), 686–688 (2010)
54. Bonabeau, E.: Decisions 2.0: The power of collective intelligence. MIT Sloan Management Review 50(2), 45–52 (2009)
55. Eberhart, R., Kennedy, J.: A new optimizer using particle swarm theory. In: IEEE Proceedings of the Sixth International Symposium on Micro Machine and Human Science, MHS 1995 (1995)
56. Eberhart, R., Simpson, P., Dobbins, R.: Computational intelligence PC tools. Academic Press Professional, Inc. (1996)
57. Kennedy, J., Eberhart, R.C.: A discrete binary version of the particle swarm algorithm. In: 1997 IEEE International Conference on Systems, Man, and Cybernetics, Computational Cybernetics and Simulation, pp. 4104–4108. IEEE (1997)
58. Eberhart, R.C., Shi, Y.H.: Particle swarm optimization: Developments, applications and resources. IEEE, New York (2001)
59. Sim, K.M., Sun, W.H.: Ant colony optimization for routing and load-balancing: Survey and new directions. IEEE Trans. Syst. Man Cybern. Paart A-Syst. Hum. 33(5), 560–572 (2003)
60. Colorni, A., Dorigo, M., Maniezzo, V.: Distributed optimization by ant colonies. In: Proceedings of the First European Conference on Artificial Life, vol. 142, pp. 134–142 (1991)
61. Dorigo, M., Gambardella, L.M.: Ant colony system: A cooperative learning approach to the traveling salesman problem. IEEE Transactions on Evolutionary Computation 1(1), 53–66 (1997)

62. Dorigo, M., Blum, C.: Ant colony optimization theory: A survey. Theoretical Computer Science 344(2-3), 243–278 (2005)
63. Colorni, A., Dorigo, M., Maniezzo, V.: An Investigation of some Properties of an "Ant Algorithm". In: Parallel Problem Solving from Nature Conference (PPSN), pp. 509–520. Elsevier (1992)
64. Dorigo, M., Birattari, M., Stutzle, T.: Ant colony optimization - Artificial ants as a computational intelligence technique. IEEE Computational Intelligence Magazine 1(4), 28–39 (2006)
65. Chen, Y.J., Wong, M.L., Li, H.B.: Applying Ant Colony Optimization to configuring stacking ensembles for data mining. Expert Systems with Applications 41(6), 2688–2702 (2014)
66. Parpinelli, R.S., Lopes, H.S., Freitas, A.A.: Data mining with an ant colony optimization algorithm. IEEE Transactions on Evolutionary Computation 6(4), 321–332 (2002)
67. de Boer, P.A.J.: Advances in understanding E. coli cell fission. Current Opinion in Microbiology 13(6), 730–737 (2010)
68. Passino, K.M.: Biomimicry of bacterial foraging for distributed optimization and control. IEEE Control Systems 22(3), 52–67 (2002)
69. Kim, D.H., Abraham, A., Cho, J.H.: A hybrid genetic algorithm and bacterial foraging approach for global optimization. Inf. Sci. 177(18), 3918–3937 (2007)
70. Tripathy, M., Mishra, S., Lai, L.L., Zhang, Q.P.: Transmission loss reduction based on FACTS and bacteria foraging algorithm. In: Runarsson, T.P., Beyer, H.-G., Burke, E.K., Merelo-Guervós, J.J., Whitley, L.D., Yao, X. (eds.) PPSN 2006. LNCS, vol. 4193, pp. 222–231. Springer, Heidelberg (2006)
71. Pirolli, P., Card, S.: Information foraging. Psychological Review 106(4), 643–675 (1999)
72. Pirolli, P.: Rational analyses of information foraging on the Web. Cognitive Science 29(3), 343–373 (2005)
73. Liu, J.M., Zhang, S.W., Yang, J.: Characterizing Web usage regularities with information foraging agents. IEEE Transactions on Knowledge and Data Engineering 16(5), 566–584 (2004)
74. Goodwin, J.C., Cohen, T., Rindflesch, T.: Discovery by scent: Discovery browsing system based on the Information Foraging Theory. In: Gao, J., Dubitzky, W., Wu, C., Liebman, M., Alhaij, R., Ungar, L., Christianson, A., Hu, X. (eds.) 2012 IEEE International Conference on Bioinformatics and Biomedicine Workshops. IEEE, New York (2012)
75. Pham, D., Ghanbarzadeh, A., Koc, E., Otri, S., Rahim, S., Zaidi, M.: The bees algorithm-a novel tool for complex optimisation problems. In: Proceedings of the 2nd Virtual International Conference on Intelligent Production Machines and Systems (IPROMS 2006), pp. 454–459 (2006)
76. Pham, D.T., Castellani, M.: The Bees Algorithm: Modelling foraging behaviour to solve continuous optimization problems. Proceedings of the Institution of Mechanical Engineers Part C-Journal of Mechanical Engineering Science 223(12), 2919–2938 (2009)
77. Ozbakir, L., Baykasoglu, A., Tapkan, P.: Bees algorithm for generalized assignment problem. Applied Mathematics and Computation 215(11), 3782–3795 (2010)
78. Karaboga, D., Basturk, B.: A powerful and efficient algorithm for numerical function optimization: artificial bee colony (ABC) algorithm. Journal of global optimization 39(3), 459–471 (2007)
79. Tsai, H.C.: Integrating the artificial bee colony and bees algorithm to face constrained optimization problems. Inf. Sci. 258, 80–93 (2014)

80. Mehrabian, A.R., Lucas, C.: A novel numerical optimization algorithm inspired from weed colonization. Ecological Informatics 1(4), 355–366 (2006)
81. Giri, R., Chowdhury, A., Ghosh, A., Das, S., Abraham, A., Snasel, V.: A Modified Invasive Weed Optimization Algorithm for training of feed- forward Neural Networks. In: 2010 IEEE International Conference on Systems, Man and Cybernetics (SMC 2010), pp. 3166–3173 (2010)
82. Huang, H., Ding, S., Zhu, H., Xu, X.: Invasive Weed Optimization Algorithm for Optimizating the Parameters of Mixed Kernel Twin Support Vector Machines. Journal of Computers 8(8) (2013)
83. Dawkins, R.: The selfish gene. Oxford University Press, Oxford (1976)
84. Corno, F., Reorda, M.S., Squillero, G.: The selfish gene algorithm: a new evolutionary optimization strategy. In: Proceedings of the 1998 ACM Symposium on Applied Computing, pp. 349–355. ACM (1998)
85. Ishibuchi, H., Yoshida, T., Murata, T.: Balance between genetic search and local search in memetic algorithms for multiobjective permutation flowshop scheduling. IEEE Transactions on Evolutionary Computation 7(2), 204–223 (2003)
86. Simpson, G.G.: The Baldwin Effect. Evolution 7(2), 110–117 (1953)
87. Kannan, S.S., Ramaraj, N.: A novel hybrid feature selection via Symmetrical Uncertainty ranking based local memetic search algorithm. Knowledge-Based Systems 23(6), 580–585 (2010)
88. Molina, D., Lozano, M., Sanchez, A.M., Herrera, F.: Memetic algorithms based on local search chains for large scale continuous optimisation problems: MA-SSW-Chains. Soft Computing 15(11), 2201–2220 (2011)
89. Mirjalili, S., Mirjalili, S.M., Lewis, A.: Grey Wolf Optimizer. Advances in Engineering Software 69, 46–61 (2014)
90. Yin, J., Meng, H.: Artificial bee colony algorithm with chaotic differential evolution search. Computer Engineering and Applications 47(29), 27–30 (2011)
91. Jia, D.L., Zheng, G.X., Khan, M.K.: An effective memetic differential evolution algorithm based on chaotic local search. Inf. Sci. 181(15), 3175–3187 (2011)
92. Farmer, J.D., Packard, N.H., Perelson, A.S.: The immune system, adaptation, and machine learning. Physica D: Nonlinear Phenomena 22(1), 187–204 (1986)
93. Parham, P.: The Immune System, 3rd edn. Garland Science, Taylor and Francis, New York (2009)
94. Dasgupta, D., Yu, S.H., Nino, F.: Recent Advances in Artificial Immune Systems: Models and Applications. Applied Soft Computing 11(2), 1574–1587 (2011)
95. de Castro, L.N., Timmis, J.I.: Artificial immune systems as a novel soft computing paradigm. Soft Computing 7(8), 526–544 (2003)
96. Rashedi, E., Nezamabadi-Pour, H., Saryazdi, S.: GSA: A Gravitational Search Algorithm. Inf. Sci. 179(13), 2232–2248 (2009)
97. Dowlatshahi, M.B., Nezamabadi-Pour, H., Mashinchi, M.: A discrete gravitational search algorithm for solving combinatorial optimization problems. Inf. Sci. 258, 94–107 (2014)
98. Rashedi, E., Nezamabadi-pour, H., Saryazdi, S.: BGSA: Binary gravitational search algorithm. Natural Computing 9(3), 727–745 (2010)
99. Blum, C., Roli, A.: Metaheuristics in combinatorial optimization: Overview and conceptual comparison. ACM Comput. Surv. 35(3), 268–308 (2003)
100. Shah-Hosseini, H.: The intelligent water drops algorithm: A nature-inspired swarm-based optimization algorithm. International Journal of Bio-Inspired Computation 1(1-2), 71–79 (2009)
101. Shah-Hosseini, H.: Problem solving by intelligent water drops. IEEE, New York (2007)

102. Agarwal, K., Goyal, M., Srivastava, P.R.: Code coverage using intelligent water drop (IWD). International Journal of Bio-Inspired Computation 4(6), 392–402 (2012)
103. Maimon, O., Rokach, L. (eds.): Data Mining and Knowledge Discovery Handbook. Springer, New York (2010)
104. Holzinger, A., Blanchard, D., Bloice, M., Holzinger, K., Palade, V., Rabadan, R.: Darwin, Lamarck, or Baldwin: Applying Evolutionary Algorithms to Machine Learning Techniques. In: World Intelligence Congress (WIC). IEEE (2014) (in print)
105. Whitley, D.: An overview of evolutionary algorithms: Practical issues and common pitfalls. Information and Software Technology 43(14), 817–831 (2001)
106. Pappa, G.L., Freitas, A.A.: Discovering new rule induction algorithms with grammar-based genetic programming. In: Soft Computing for Knowledge Discovery and Data Mining, pp. 133–152. Springer (2008)
107. Pappa, G.L., Freitas, A.A.: Evolving rule induction algorithms with multi-objective grammar-based genetic programming. Knowledge and Information Systems 19(3), 283–309 (2009)

# On the Generation of Point Cloud Data Sets: Step One in the Knowledge Discovery Process

Andreas Holzinger[1], Bernd Malle[1], Marcus Bloice[1], Marco Wiltgen[1],
Massimo Ferri[2], Ignazio Stanganelli[3],
and Rainer Hofmann-Wellenhof[4]

[1] Research Unit Human-Computer Interaction, Institute for Medical Informatics,
Statistics & Documentation,
Medical University Graz, Austria
{a.holzinger,b.malle,m.bloice,m.wiltgen}@hci4all.at
[2] Department of Mathematics, University of Bologna, Italy
massimo.ferri@unibo.it
[3] Skin Cancer Unit IRCCS Istituto Tumori Romagna, Meldola, Italy
[4] Department of Dermatology, Graz University Hospital, Austria

**Abstract.** Computational geometry and topology are areas which have much potential for the analysis of arbitrarily high-dimensional data sets. In order to apply geometric or topological methods one must first generate a representative point cloud data set from the original data source, or at least a metric or distance function, which defines a distance between the elements of a given data set. Consequently, the first question is: How to get point cloud data sets? Or more precise: What is the optimal way of generating such data sets? The solution to these questions is not trivial. If a natural image is taken as an example, we are concerned more with the content, with the shape of the *relevant* data represented by this image than its mere matrix of pixels. Once a point cloud has been generated from a data source, it can be used as input for the application of graph theory and computational topology. In this paper we first describe the case for natural point clouds, i.e. where the data already are represented by points; we then provide some fundamentals of medical images, particularly dermoscopy, confocal laser scanning microscopy, and total-body photography; we describe the use of graph theoretic concepts for image analysis, give some medical background on skin cancer and concentrate on the challenges when dealing with lesion images. We discuss some relevant algorithms, including the watershed algorithm, region splitting (graph cuts), region merging (minimum spanning tree) and finally describe some open problems and future challenges.

**Keywords:** data preprocessing, point cloud data sets, dermoscopy, graphs, image analysis, skin cancer, watershed algorithm, region splitting, graph cuts, region merging, mathematical morphology.

A. Holzinger, I. Jurisica (Eds.): Knowledge Discovery and Data Mining, LNCS 8401, pp. 57–80, 2014.

# 1   Introduction and Motivation

Today we are challenged with complex, high-dimensional, heterogenous, and weakly-structured biomedical data sets and unstructured information from various sources [1]. Within such data, relevant structural or temporal patterns ("knowledge") are often hidden, difficult to extract, and therefore not immediately accessible to the biomedical expert. Consequently, a major challenge is to interactively discover such patterns within large data sets. Computational geometry and algebraic topology may be of great help here [2], however, to apply these methods we need point cloud data sets, or at least distances between data entities. Point cloud data (PCD) sets can be seen as primitive manifold representation for use in algebraic topology [3]. For a rough guide to topology see [4].

A good example of a direct source for point clouds are 3D acquisition devices such as laser scanners, a recent low-cost commercial product being the Kinect device (see section 3). Medical images in nuclear medicine are also usually represented in 3D, where a point cloud is a set of points in the space, with each node of the point cloud characterized by its position and intensity (see section 3 and 5). In dimensions higher than three, point clouds (feature vectors) can be found in the representation of high-dimensional manifolds, where it is usual to work directly with this type of data [5].

Some data sets are naturally available as point clouds, for example protein structures or protein interaction networks, where techniques from graph theory can be directly applied [6].

Despite the fact that naturally occurring point clouds do exist, a concerted effort must focus on how to get representative point cloud data sets from raw data. Before continuing, and for clarification purposes, some key terms are defined in the next section. This is followed by discussing natural point clouds in section 3 as well as the case of text documents in section 4, before examining the case of medical images, and in particular dermatological images, in section 5. We first introduce some dermatological image sources, describe shortly some problems facing the processing of such images, and present some related work, as well as relevant algorithms. Finally, we discuss open problems and provide an outline to future research routes in sections 6 and 7, respectively.

# 2   Glossary and Key Terms

*Point clouds:* are finite sets equipped with a family of *proximity* (or *similarity measure*) functions $sim_q\colon S^{q+1} \to [0,1]$, which measure how "close" or "similar" $(q+1)$-tuples of elements of $S$ are (a value of 0 means totally different objects, while 1 corresponds to essentially equivalent items).

*Space:* a set of points $a_i \in S$ which satisfy some geometric postulate.

*Topology:* the study of shapes and spaces, especially the study of properties of geometric figures that are not changed by continuous deformations such as stretching (but might be by cutting or merging) [7], [8].

*Topological Space:* A pair $(X, T)$ with $X$ denoting a non-empty set and $T$ a collection of subsets of $X$ such that $\emptyset \in T$, $X \in T$ and arbitrary unions and finite intersections of elements of $T$ are also $\in T$.

*Algebraic Topology:* the mathematical field which studies topological spaces by means of algebraic invariants [9].

*Topological Manifold:* A topological space which is locally homeomorphic (has a continuous function with an inverse function) to a real $n$-dimensional space (e.g. Euclidean space) [10].

*Distance:* Given a non-empty set $S$, a function $d : S \times S \rightarrow \mathbb{R}$ such that for all $x, y, z \in S$ (i) $d(x, y) \geq 0$, (ii) $d(x, y) = 0 \iff x = y$, (iii) $d(x, y) = d(y, x)$, and (iv) $d(x, z) \leq d(x, y) + d(y, z)$.

*Metric space:* A pair $(S, d)$ of a set and a distance on it. Every metric space is automatically also a topological space.

*Computational geometry:* A field concerned with algorithms that can be defined in terms of geometry (line segments, polyhedra, etc.) [11].

*Supervised Learning:* Method within Machine Learning that uses labeled training data to develop an accurate prediction algorithm. Let $\{(x_1, y_1), ..., (x_n, y_n)\}$ be n training samples with $x_1...x_n$ being the predictor variables and $y_1...y_n$ the labels, we want a function $g : X \rightarrow Y$ such that a cost function (usually the difference between predicted values $g(x)$ and $y$) is minimized.

*Unsupervised Learning:* Method in machine learning which is used to group similar objects together, e.g. points within geometric groups or objects of similar properties (color, frequency). No labeled training data is used.

*Optimization:* is the selection of cluster a best element (with regard to some criteria) from some set of available alternatives.

*Classification:* Identification to which set of categories (sub-populations) a new observation belongs, on the basis of a training set of data containing observations (or instances) whose category membership is known.

*Clustering:* Grouping a set of objects in such a way that objects in the same group (cluster) are more similar to each other than to those in other groups (clusters).

*Feature:* A measurable property of an object (e.g. the age of a person).

*Feature Vector:* A collection of numerical features interpreted as the dimensional components of a (Euclidean) vector.

*Vector space model:* Approach whose goal is to make objects comparable by establishing a similarity measure between pairs of feature vectors (Euclidean distance, cosine similarity etc.). The space spanned by all possible feature vectors is called the feature space.

*Voronoi region:* Given a set of points in a metric space $p_1, ...p_n$, a Voronoi diagram erects regions around a point $p_i$ such that all points $q$ within its region are closer to $p_i$ than to any other point $p_j$ [12].

*Delaunay triangulation:* Given a set of points in a plane $P = p_1, ...p_n$, a Delaunay triangulation separates the set into triangles with $p's \in P$ as their corners, such that no circumcircle of any triangle contains any other point in its interior.

*Minimum Spanning Tree:* Given a graph $G = (V, E, \omega)$ with $V$ being the set of vertices, $E$ being the set of edges and $\omega$ being the sets of edge weights, a Minimum Spanning tree is the connected acyclic subgraph defined by the subset $E' \subseteq E$ reaching all vertices $v \in V$ with the minimal sum of edge weights possible.

## 3   The Case for Natural Point Clouds

A prototypical example of natural point clouds are the data produced by 3D acquisition devices (Figure 1, Left), such as laser scanners [13]. Methods for the extraction of surfaces from such devices can roughly be divided into two categories: those that segment a point cloud based on criteria such as proximity of points and/or similarity of locally estimated surface normals, and those that directly estimate surface parameters by clustering and locating maxima within a parameter space; the latter is more robust, but can only be used for simple shapes such as planes and cylinders that can be described by only a few parameters [14]. A recent low-cost example is the Kinect (Figure 1, Center) device [15]. This sensor is particularly interesting as such devices will continue to gain popularity as their prices drop while at the same time becoming smaller and more powerful and the open source community will promote its use [16]. Such sensors have the potential to be used for diverse mapping applications; however, the random error of depth measurement increases with increasing distance to the sensor, and ranges from a few millimeters up to about four centimeters at the maximum range of the Kinect device [17]. Some recent examples demonstrate the potential of this sensor for various applications, where high precision is not an issue, e.g. in rehabilitation exercises monitoring [18] or in health games [19].

It seems reasonable to assume the presence of 3D-scanners within mobile devices in the not-so-distant future, which in combination with faster, more powerful algorithms and advances in software engineering could potentially transform each smartphone into a mobile medical laboratory and mobile wellness center [20]. Although applications in this area will likely not be an adequate substitution for the work of trained professionals, it would help reduce data preprocessing time and could make some hospital visits for purely diagnostic purposes a thing of the past, consequently help to tame the worldwide exploding health costs.

Medical images, e.g. in nuclear medicine, are usually also represented in 3D, following the same principle (Figure 1), where a point cloud is a set of points in $\mathbb{R}^3$, whose vertices are characterized by their position and intensity. The density of the point cloud determines the resolution, and the reconstructed volume, which in general could be of any resolution, size, shape, and topology, is represented by a set of non-overlapping tetrahedra defined by the points. The intensity at any point within the volume is defined by linearly interpolating inside a tetrahedron from the values at the four nodes that define such a tetrahedron, see [21] for more details and see [22] for some basic principles.

Some data sets are "naturally" available as point clouds, which is convenient as $n$-dimensional point clouds can easily be mapped into graph data structures by defining some similarity functions to pairs of nodes (e.g. the Euclidean distance, however a multitude of methods are available) and assigning that similarity to edges between them. Examples of this include protein structures or protein interaction networks (Figure 1, Right), where techniques from graph theory can be applied [6].

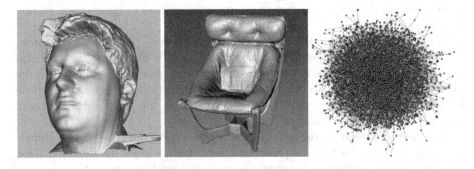

**Fig. 1.** Left: A 3D scan of Bernd Malle taken in 1998 by a stationary device worth around EUR 100,000. Center: 3D scan taken in 2013 by a Microsoft Kinect device worth EUR 200 (Source: http://www.kscan3d.com/). Right: Protein-protein interaction network (Source: http://www.pnas.org/).

## 4   The Case of Text Documents

Based on the vector space model, which is a standard tool in text mining [23], a collection of text documents (aka corpus) can be mapped into a set of points (vectors) in $\mathbb{R}^n$. Each word can also be mapped into vectors, resulting in a very high dimensional vector space. These vectors are the so-called term vectors, with each vector representing a single word. If there, for example, are $n$ keywords extracted from all the documents then each document is mapped to a point (*term vector*) in $\mathbb{R}^n$ with coordinates corresponding to the weights. In this way the whole corpus can be transformed into a point cloud set. Usually, instead of the Euclidean metric, using a specialized similarity (proximity) measure is more convenient. The *cosine similarity measure* is one example which is now a standard tool in text mining, see for example [24]. Namely, the cosine of the angle between two vectors (points in the cloud) reflects how "similar" the underlying weighted combinations of keywords are. By following this approach, methods from computational topology may be applied [25], which offers a lot of interesting research perspectives.

## 5    The Case of Medical Images

### 5.1    Some Fundamentals of Digital Images

**Dermoscopy.** The dermoscopy, aka epiluminescence microscopy (ELM), is a non-invasive diagnostic technique and tool used by dermatologists for the analysis of pigmented skin lesions (PSLs) and hair, that links clinical dermatology and dermatopathology by enabling the visualization of morphological features otherwise not visible to the naked eye [26]. Digital dermoscopy images can be stored and later compared to images obtained during the patient's next visit for melanoma and non-melanoma skin cancer diagnosis. The use of digital dermoscopes permitted the documentation of any examinations in the medical record [27] [28].

Skin and pathology appearance varies with light source, polarization, oil, pressure, and sometimes temperature of the room, so it is important that the examination and documentation be performed in a standardized manner. To do so, some of the most modern spectrometers use an adjustable light source which adjusts according to the room light to try to mimic the "daylight" spectrum from a standardized light source.

Although images produced by polarised light dermoscopes are slightly different from those produced by a traditional skin contact glass dermoscope, they have certain advantages, such as vascular patterns not being potentially missed through compression of the skin by a glass contact plate. Dermoscopy only evaluates the down level of papillary dermis, leaving pathologies in the reticular dermis unseen. Amelanotic melanoma is missed with this method and high pigmented lesions can also hide structures relevant for the diagnosis. A negative surface exam is no guarantee that there is no pathology. In case of doubt a biopsy and experienced clinical judgment is required [29].

**Confocal Laser Scanning Microscopy.** Reflectance confocal microscopy (RCM) allows non-invasive imaging of the epidermis and superficial dermis. Like dermoscopy, RCM acquires images in the horizontal plane (en face), allowing assessment of the tissue pathology and underlying dermoscopic structures of interest at a cellular-level resolution [30].

The confocal image uses a low-power laser and special optics to magnify living cells at approximately 1,000 times zoom. Confocal images are created by the natural refractive difference within and between cells. Melanin is highly refractive and results in brighter images. The confocal microscope captures the images in three dimensions within the top layers of the skin. Imaging each lesion takes between 5 and 10 minutes. A tissue ring is attached with medical adhesive to hold the skin stable and the laser tracks through the lesion in three dimensions to create vertical and horizontal maps of the cell fields. There is no pain or scarring in this non-invasive procedure [29].

The application of a wide array of new synthetic and naturally occurring fluorochromes in confocal microscopy has made it possible to identify cells and sub-microscopic cellular components with a high degree of specificity amid non-fluorescing material. In fact the confocal microscope is often capable of revealing the presence of a single molecule. Confocal microscopy offers several advantages over conventional widefield optical microscopy, including the ability to control depth of field, elimination or reduction of background information away from the focal plane (which leads to image degradation), and the capability to collect serial optical sections from thick specimens, making possible multi-dimensional views of living cells and tissues that include image information in the $x$, $y$, and $z$ dimensions as a function of time and presented in multiple colours (using two or more fluorophores). The temporal data can be collected either from time-lapse experiments conducted over extended periods or through real time image acquisition in smaller frames for shorter periods of time. A concise overview on biological image analysis can be found here [31].

**Total-Body Photography.** Total body photography (TBP) is a diagnostic technique where a series of high resolution digital photographs are taken from head to toe of the patients skin for active skin cancer surveillance [32]. A photographic baseline of the body is important when attempting to detect new lesions or changes in existing lesions in patients with many nevi and create a pigment lesion mapping of the entire body. Changes in moles can be in the form of size, shape and colour change and it can also be useful for other conditions as psoriasis or eczema.

The main advantages of total body photography are that it reduces unnecessary biopsies, and melanomas are often caught at a much earlier stage. A recent approach is Gigapixel Photography (GP), which was used to capture high-res panoramas of landscapes; recent developments in GP hardware have led to the production of consumer devices (see e.g. www.GigaPan.com). GP has a one billion pixel resolution capacity, which is 1000 times higher than TBP, and therefore has a lot of potential for dermatology use [33].

## 5.2   Point Cloud Data Sets

To sum up at this point, let us define in accordance with [34]:

- **Multivariate dataset** is a data set that has *many dependent variables* and they might be correlated to each other to varying degrees. Usually this type of dataset is associated with *discrete data models*.
- **Multidimensional dataset** is a data set that has *many independent variables* clearly identified, and one or more dependent variables associated to them. Usually this type of dataset is associated with *continuous data models*.

In other words, every data item (or object) in a computer is represented (and therefore stored) as a set of features. Instead of the term features we may use the term dimensions, because an object with $n$ features can also be represented as a multidimensional point in an $n$-dimensional space. Dimensionality reduction is the process of mapping an $n$-dimensional point, into a lower $k$-dimensional space, which basically is the main challenge in visualization .

The number of dimensions can sometimes be small, e.g. simple 1D data such as temperature measured at different times, to 3D applications such as medical imaging, where data is captured within a volume. Standard techniques like contouring in 2D, and isosurfacing and volume rendering in 3D, have emerged over the years to handle these types of data. There is no dimension reduction issue in these applications, since the data and display dimensions essentially match.

One fundamental problem in analysing images via graph theoretical methods is when first translating them into a point cloud. While pixels in images naturally have some coordinates in 2D, their colour value as well as relation to pixels around them is not encoded within those coordinates. Thus, some transformation of the 2D image into a higher-dimensional space has to occur as a first step. This, however, entails many problems such as inadvertently modelling artefacts or 'inventing' information that is not contained in the image. The following gives an example of a simple 2D to 3D transform of a melanoma image (Figure 2).

## 5.3   Two Examples of Creating Point Clouds

The functional behaviour of a genome can be studied by determining which genes are induced and which genes are repressed in a cell during a defined snapshot. The behaviour can change in different development phases of the cell (from a stem cell to a specialized cell), in response to a changing environment (triggering of the gene expression by factor proteins with hormonal function) or in response to a drug treatment. The microarray technology makes it possible to explore gene expression patterns of entire genomes (a recent work from cancer research can be found in [35]. Technically, a microarray is usually a small glass slide (approximately 2.0 cm × 2.0 cm) covered with a great number (20,000 or more) of precisely placed spots. Each spot contains a different single stranded DNA sequence fragment: the gene probe. A microarray experiment is done as follows: From reference and test tissue samples, mRNA is isolated and converted into cDNA. The cDNAs are labelled green (reference) and red (test). The cDNA

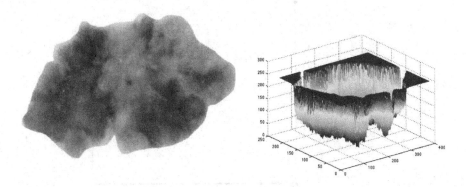

**Fig. 2.** Simple 2D-3D transform using the mesh function built into MATLAB

samples are mixed together and incubated with the probe on the microarray. The location and intensities of the fluorescent dyes are recorded with a scanner. Using the ratios of the dyes, a red spot indicates induced gene activity within the test probe; a green spot shows repressed gene activity in the test probe and a yellow spot indicates that there is no change in the gene activity level in the two probes. The amount of data resulting from microarray experiments is very big and too complex to be interpreted manually by a human observer. Machine learning algorithms extract from a vast amount of data the information that is needed to make the data interpretable. The gene expression pattern of the gene $y_n$ along $P$ experiments is described by a vector:

$$y_n = (x_{n1}, x_{n2}, \ldots, x_{nk}, \ldots, x_{nP})$$

where $x_{nk}$ is the expression value of the gene during the experiment number $k$. The genes can be geometrically interpreted as a point cloud in a $P$-dimensional space (Figure 3).

In the diagnosis of CLSM views of skin lesions, architectural structures at different scales play a crucial role. The images of benign common nevi show pronounced architectural structures, such as arrangements of nevi cells around basal structures and tumour cell nests (Figure 4).

The images of malign melanoma show melanoma cells and connective tissue with few or no architectural structures. Features based on the wavelet transform have been shown to be particularly suitable for the automatic analysis of CLSM images because they enable an exploration of images at different scales. The multi resolution analysis takes scale information into consideration and successively decomposes the original image into approximations (smooth parts) and details. That means, through the wavelet transformation, the two-dimensional image array is split up into several frequency bands (containing various numbers of wavelet coefficients), which represent information at different scales. At each scale the original image is approximated with more or fewer details. The frequency bands, representing information at a large scale, are labelled with

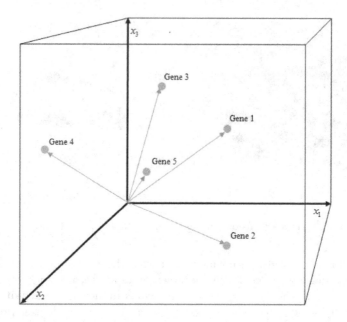

**Fig. 3.** Every gene is represented by a point in a $P$-dimensional space, which is built by the $P$ experiments (for example: $P$ different kinds of tissue). The position of the point is determined by the expression values on each axis of the coordinate system.

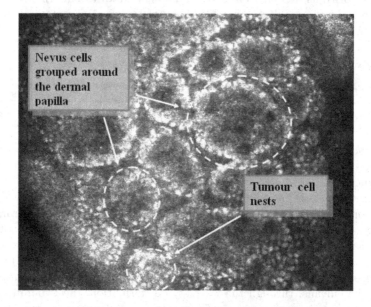

**Fig. 4.** Nevi cell arrangement and tumour cell nests

low indices and the frequency bands representing successively decreasing scales are labelled with higher indices. Then the architectural structure information in the CLSM images is accumulated along the energy bands (from course to fine). Therefore the wavelet transformation allows the analysis of a given texture by its frequency components. In wavelet texture analysis, the features are mostly derived from statistical properties of the resulting wavelet coefficients inside the frequency bands. Then the tissue textures, in the CLSM images, are represented by feature vectors, as for example:

$$\mathbf{x}_n = \left( F_{\mathrm{STD}}^n(i) \right); i = 0, \ldots, N$$

Whereby $N$ is the number of frequency bands. The index $n$ refers to the $n$-th image. $F_{\mathrm{STD}}^n(i)$ represents a statistical property of the wavelet coefficients in the $i$-th frequency band. From an ensemble of images results a point cloud of different feature vectors in the feature space.

**Data Set Example:** A relatively recent development is the creation of the UCI Knowledge Discovery in Databases Archive available at http://kdd.ics.uci.edu. This contains a range of large and complex datasets as a challenge to the data mining research community to scale up its algorithms as the size of stored datasets, especially commercial ones, inexorably rises [36].

## 5.4   Graphs in Image Analysis

The idea of using graph theoretic concepts for image processing and analysis goes back to the early 1970's. Since then, many powerful image processing methods have been formulated on pixel adjacency graphs. These are graphs whose vertex set is the set of image elements (pixels), and whose edge set is determined by an adjacency relation among the image elements.

More recently, image analysis techniques focus on using graph-based methods for segmentation, filtering, clustering and classification. Also, graphs are used to represent the topological relations of image parts.

**Definition 1 (Graph).** A graph $G = (V, E)$ is given by a finite set $V$ of elements called vertices, a finite set $E$ of elements called edges, and a relation of incidence, which associates with each edge $e$ an unordered pair $(v_1, v_2) \in V \times V$. The vertices $v_1$ and $v_2$ are called the end vertices of $e$.

**Definition 2 (Planar Graph, Embedded Graph).** A graph is said to be **planar** if it can be drawn in a plane so that its edges intersect only at its end vertices. A graph already drawn in a surface $S$ is referred to as **embedded in** $S$ [37].

## 5.5   Medical Background

**Skin Cancer** is still the most common and most increasing form of human cancer worldwide. Skin cancer can be classified into melanoma and non-melanoma and although melanomas are much less common than non-melanomas, they account for the majority of skin cancer mortality. Detection of malignant melanoma in its early stages considerably reduces morbidity and mortality and may save hundreds of millions of Euros that otherwise would be spent on the treatment of advanced diseases. If cutaneous malign melanoma can be detected in its early stages and removed, there is a very high likelihood that the patient will survive.

However, melanomas are very complex and a result of accumulated alterations in genetic and molecular pathways among melanocytic cells, generating distinct subsets of melanomas with different biological and clinical behavior. Melanocytes can proliferate to form nevi (common moles), initially in the basal epidermis [38]. A melanoma can also occasionally simply look like a naevus.

Image analysis techniques for measuring these features have indeed been developed. The measurement of image features for the diagnosis of melanoma requires that lesions first be detected and localized in an image. It is essential that lesion boundaries are determined accurately so that measurements, such as maximum diameter, asymmetry, irregularity of the boundary, and color characteristics, can be accurately computed. For delineating lesion boundaries, various image segmentation methods have been developed. These methods use color and texture information in an image to find the lesion boundaries [39].

## 5.6   Challenges

Basic difficulties when dealing with such lesions include:

1. **Morphology is not enough**
   Melanomas can sometimes appear like naevi. This suggests relying on follow-ups and to perhaps prefer sensitivity to specificity.
2. **Detail Level**
   Medical doctors are understandably fond of details, whereas preprocessing often needs to blur images together with noise.
3. **Diversity**
   Especially in dermoscpy there is a great variety of established criteria to describe melanocytic and non melanocytic lesions [40].
4. **Segmentation**
   Segmentation is one of the main hurdles in lesion analysis, as a good segmentation of different skin lesions is crucial for total body imaging. It is also seen as a problem by dermatologists themselves [41]: There has been research on interoperator and *intraoperator* differences in segmentation by hand of one and the same lesion.
5. **Noise**
   Having said that, it is a requirement to split the lesion from the background. This is even more problematic with people of darker complexion. A further

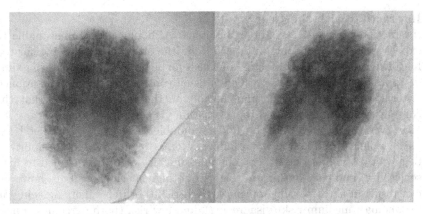

**Fig. 5.** A naevus (left) and a melanoma (right)[42]

problem is hair: the pragmatic solution is to physically remove any hair using a razor. But it is much better to eliminate it (or to "ignore" it) at the image level, for example through the use of the Hough transform [43].

The **Hough transform** is a method for detecting curves by exploiting the duality between points on a curve and the parameters of that curve, hence it is well-suited for the detection of arbitrary shapes, and therefore ideal for removing hair. The method is robust to partial deformation in shape and very tolerant to noise and can detect multiple occurrences of a shape in the same region, however, it requires a lot of memory and computational power [44].

The most optimal segmentations we obtained were through the Mumford-Shah functional, but it requires much processing time [45]. It is therefore better to rely on a cleverly engineered mixture of morphological operations and thresholding. A big issue here is in interactivity, because exactly here the expert end user could come into play, by making her/him either simply to accept or reject a segmentation or even initialize it or modify it (see below Interaction with the user).

6. **Diagnostic Criteria**

Dermatologists trust the following criteria:

- A: Asymmetry
- B: Boundary (border irregularity)
- C: Colour (variegation and uneven distribution)
- D: Diameter (greater than 6 mm)
- E: Elevation (Alternatively: Evolution)

Moreover in patients with many nevi or other skin lesions this simplified algorithm is not sufficient to diagnose such lesions correctly. Experience, comparison of multiple lesions, and follow-up information is crucial to come to a correct diagnosis. At this point one may ask how to make this procedure at least partially automatic, and persistent homology is certainly one approach, as we shall see.

7. **Interaction with the User**

   Interaction in time is an important issue. Although it is unreasonable to expect "real time" outputs, a procedure in the order of minutes is a far too long time for a medical doctor and also for a patient. A processing time of approximately 2 minutes, which is usual considering the aforementioned criteria, requires that something be put on the screen, showing that the computer has not frozen and that something is actually happening.

   Moreover the output must be understandable. Therefore, a trade-off between richness and simplicity of information is required. One possibility is to have two (hidden) classifiers, one "pessimistic" algorithm (tuned to high sensitivity) and one "optimistic" algorithm (high specificity). This, however, can result in three possible outputs: High risk (both classifiers agreeing on melanoma), medium risk (disagreeing), and low risk (both agreeing on naevus). This approach is certainly not satisfactory for the present purposes.

8. **Representation**

   On the strictly technical side, one can simply represent the images as graphs with pixels as vertices, and 4-neighbours as adjacent vertices. Of course, much more elaborate methods have been developed, which shall be discussed further in the following sections.

## 5.7   Related Work

De Mauro, Diligenti, Gori & Maggini [46] in 2003 presented a very relevant piece of work: they proposed an approach based on neural networks by which the retrieval criterion is derived on the basis of learning from examples. De Mauro et al. used a graph-based image representation that denoted the relationships among regions in the image and on recursive neural networks which can process directed ordered acyclic graphs. This graph-based representation combines structural and sub-symbolic features of the image, while recursive neural networks can discover the optimal representation for searching the image database. Their work was presented for the first time at the GBR 2001 conference in Ischia and the authors subsequently expanded it for a journal contribution.

Bianchini (2003) [47] reported on the computationally difficult task of recognizing a particular face in a complex image or in a video sequence, which humans can simply accomplish using contextual information. The face recognition problem is usually solved having assumed that the face was previously localized, often via heuristics based on prototypes of the whole face or significant details. In their paper, they propose a novel approach to the solution of the face localization problem using recursive neural networks. In particular, the proposed approach assumes a **graph-based representation of images** that combines structural and subsymbolic visual features. Such graphs are then processed by recursive neural networks, in order to establish the eventual presence and the position of the faces inside the image.

Chen & Freedman (2011) [48] reported on an alternative method in the preprocessing stage: In cortex surface segmentation, the extracted surface is required to have a particular topology, namely, a two-sphere. The authors presented a novel method for removing topology noise of a curve or surface within the level set framework, and thus produce a cortal surface with the correct topology. They defined a new energy term which quantifies topology noise and showed how to minimize this term by computing its functional derivative with respect to the level set function. This method differs from existing methods in that it is inherently continuous and not digital; and in the way that our energy directly relates to the topology of the underlying curve or surface, versus existing knot-based measures which are related in a more indirect fashion.

## 5.8   Relevant Algorithms

**The Watershed Algorithm** is a popular tool for segmenting objects whose contours appear as crest lines on a gradient image as it is the case with melanomas. It associates to a topographic surface a partition into catchment basins, defined as attraction zones of a drop of water falling on the relief and following a line of steepest descent [49].

Each regional minimum corresponds to such a catchment basin. Points from where several distinct minima may be reached are problematic as it is not clear to which catchment basin they should be assigned. Such points belong to watershed zones, which may be thick. Watershed zones are empty if for each point, there exists a unique steepest path towards a unique minimum. Unfortunately, the classical watershed algorithm accepts too many steep trajectories, as they use neighborhoods which are too small for estimating their steepness. In order to produce a unique partition despite this, they must make arbitrary choices that are out of the control of the user. Finally, their shortsightedness results in imprecise localizations of the contours.

We propose an algorithm without myopia, which considers the total length of a trajectory for estimating its steepness; more precisely, a lexicographic order relation of infinite depth is defined for comparing non ascending paths and choosing the steepest. For the sake of generality, we consider topographic surfaces defined on node weighted graphs. This allows us to easily adapt the algorithms to images defined on any type of grid in any number of dimensions. The graphs are pruned in order to eliminate all downwards trajectories which are not the steepest. An iterative algorithm with simple neighborhood operations performs the pruning and constructs the catchment basins. The algorithm is then adapted to gray tone images. The neighborhood relations of each pixel are determined by the grid structure and are fixed; the directions of the lowest neighbors of each pixel are encoded as a binary number. In that way, the graph may be recorded as an image. A pair of adaptive erosions and dilations prune the graph and extend the catchment basins. As a result, one obtains a precise detection of the catchment basin and a graph of the steepest trajectories [50].

Note: Stable image features, such as SIFT or MSER features, can also be taken to be the nodes of the graph.

The watershed segmentation is a **regionbased technique** making use of image morphology; a classic description can be found in [51]. It requires the selection of markers ("seed" points) interior to each object of the image, including the background as a separate object.

**The markers are chosen by a human expert who takes into account the application-specific knowledge of the objects.** Once the objects are marked, they can be grown using a morphological watershed transformation (Figure 6) [52].

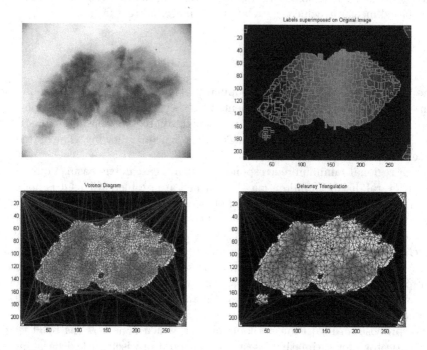

**Fig. 6.** Result of applying a watershed transform to an image of relatively distinguished regions. The resulting segmentation (and thus vertices for the output graph) corresponds well to the overall shape of the image and represents regions of about equal size.

## 5.9    Region Splitting (Graph Cuts)

Understanding the original image as a graph consisting of one large, connected component, the goal of region splitting is to obtain a graph $G(V, E)$ with a number of vertices ($|V|$) significantly smaller than the number of input pixels ($|V| << n$). In order to achieve this we have to group certain areas consisting of varying amounts of pixels together. This can be done via a partition of the image, with a partition being defined as a subgraph ($G'(V, E')$) of the original graph with the set of vertices being the same as in the original and the set of edges being a strict subset of the original set ($E' \subset E$) (one must remove edges in order to separate formerly connected components). This separation occurs recursively until a cutting threshold is obtained for all remaining connected components, which are then interpreted as regions or superpixels (-voxels) represented by some additionally extracted information, stored as a feature vector for the individual partition.

## 5.10  Region Merging (Minimum Spanning Tree)

This is essentially the opposite from the method just mentioned, in that the input image is considered as a set of pixels, each constituting its own region. The goal is to merge regions based on a (dis-)similarity measure. Felzenswalb (2004) [53] proposed an algorithm which in effect defines one numerical figure representing the internal similarity of a region, and a second figure representing the dissimilarity between two adjacent regions. In short, the approach works like this:

$$\text{Int}(C) = \max_{e \in \text{MST}(C,E)} \omega(e)$$

is the internal region similarity figure, given by the maximum edge weight of the regions MST (Minimum Spanning Tree).

$$\text{Dif}(C1, C2) = \min_{v_i \in C1, v_j \in C2, (v_i, v_j) \in E} \omega(v_i, v_j)$$

denotes any two regions' dissimilarity figure, given by the minimum edge weight connecting them.

Finally,

$$\text{D}(C1, C2) = \begin{cases} true & \text{if } \text{Dif}(C1, C2) > \text{MInt}(C1, C2) \\ false & \text{otherwise} \end{cases}$$

determines if two regions should be merged, based on the relation of their inter-region dissimilarity and minimum respective internal similarities.

As per the region splitting approach, once no further regions can be merged, the final image partition is obtained.

# 6  Open Problems

## 6.1  Medical Problems

One of the greatest problems in skin cancer screening is to select the right lesion for further investigation. An adult person has anywhere between 20 and one hundred different lesions. The segmentation and recognition of suspicious lesions, which need further investigation by dermoscopy or RCM or another procedure, is of utmost importance.

Furthermore the differentiation of physiologic changes from malignant changes in a lesion is a great challenge for the dermatologist. The same is true for the validation of benign and malignant criteria in one lesion. The question is, does a small part of the lesion showing criteria of malignancy justify an excision or not?

## 6.2  Graphs from Images

In implementing and testing different techniques for graph extraction out of medical image data several areas of consideration have arisen.

**Is a Graph a Good Representation of an Image?** This is logical as every image consists of pixels that share some form of collocation with one another, may it be geometrical neighborhoods or distances in some feature space. Secondly, image representation through graphs is already used by several segmentation algorithms, as the above sections have sufficiently discussed. The difference between our approach and the aforementioned methods is that the former are treating the raw structure of the image as the input graph to their algorithm, whose output then is a general segmentation. This work however intends to produce a graph representation of the image as its output for further use, while it may or may not use a graph based algorithm to compute it.

**Why Compute another Graph?** One could argue that every image in pixel form (there are other representations like wavelets used in JPG) already contains an implicit graph. While this is certainly true, an image of several megapixels would translate to a graph containing millions of vertices ($n$) and (given a $k$-neighborhood for each pixel) $m = k * n$ edges. This input size is clearly too large for any algorithm of polynomial runtime complexity, especially if it is intended to be used on standard desktop computers or even mobile devices. It is thus imperative to reduce the number of vertices by first applying some form of segmentation or clustering.

**Can a Reliable Graph Be Extracted from One Image Alone?** Another interesting question is how well a (2D) image represents a surface topography at all. Usually the only pieces of information contained in an image are the coordinates of its pixels plus their corresponding color values. The latter (after a transform to an intensity value) is typically interpreted as the height of its pixel, thereby transforming the image to a topographic map. This information however might be imprecise due to light conditions at the time of photography, hardware inaccuracies, angle of the recording device etc., leading to artifacts and thus misrepresentation. The only solution to this problem would be to take several images in a sequence over time, from different angles, or applying a different image taking technology (3D or radar scanning) altogether.

Based on this, a topological analysis of a graph extracted and merged from several images (sources) might reveal information not contained in a single image, while avoiding the incorporation of the same artifacts or inaccuracies that a single input source might contain.

**Is Image Segmentation the Pertinent Approach in Our Case.** In traditional applications the goal of segmenting an image is mostly object recognition or detection, either as an unsupervised grouping of areas belonging together or by matching a template representation to an area within the image, often considering different scales, angles or other deviations. The output segmentation of this class of tasks consists of a small set of image regions, representing either the locations of potential object matches or regions logically belonging together. This approach however does not yield enough differentiated regions in order to constitute a usable graph (a graph of 5 vertices cannot topologically analyzed in any useful way). Thus the major traditional goal of image segmentation is incompatible with the goal of this work.

Nevertheless, segmentation does use techniques that could be adapted to generate hundreds or even thousands of smaller regions representing the different topological elements within an image – this is usually referred to as overseg-mentation, yet it has already been used to generate finer grained partitions [54]. Depending on the algorithm, this can be accomplished by setting some region merging criteria to a higher threshold or adapting the rules for erecting watersheds.

**Supervised or Unsupervised Learning?** Because the final goal of most image processing techniques in medicine is to differentiate between healthy and pathological tissue, they belong to the group of problems known as classification problems, and are therefore supervised learning problems. However, the methods described above presuppose no anterior knowledge about the input images (or parts thereof) in order to group regions of pixels or features together, so the segmentation is done in an unsupervised fashion. This is certainly not the only possibility, as templates of individual features could be provided to the algorithm. Then again, the method would lose its generality, as different templates would be needed for different types of images. A possible solution to this problem is discussed later.

**What Information to Put into a Feature Vector?** Once a satisfying segmentation is obtained, some representative information has to be extracted from the individual regions in order to be stored as the feature vector of the resulting graph node. A whole phalanx of region properties can be chosen, and some will make more sense than others for a particular purpose. Aside from basic geometric information (centroid coordinates, length, or length-to-width ratio) [55] describes common features like histogram-based (mean grey values or grey level entropy distribution), pixel-co-occurrence related (angular moment, correlation, sum variance) as well as frequency-based (such as the wavelet) properties.

## 7   Future Challenges

**Computational Efficiency.** In comparison to extracting point cloud data from text documents, multimedia content such as images or video streams contain a very large amount of data (that might not necessarily contain much information).

As a simple example, in order to represent a 5 megapixel image as an adjacency graph, 25 billion entries would be necessary, while a more efficient representation as an adjacency list would still hold (depending on the neighborhood-definition) on the order of several dozen million list entries. This calls for efficient segmentation and clustering algorithms, as even quadratic runtime complexity would result in unacceptable computing times for interactive data mining in a real-world working environment. Possible solutions comprise downsizing images and the exclusive use of algorithms with near-linear ($O(n * log(n))$ being acceptable) runtime behaviour, as several graph-based algorithms like MST fortunately exhibit. Moreover, depending on the features selected to extract per output node, additional computation will be needed. While this may result in computing times acceptable for professionals depending on that particular information, it might not be to others, which calls for the inclusion of the professional end user into the data mining process.

**User Interaction Pipeline.** Although most algorithms discussed can produce results in a purely unsupervised fashion, in order to achieve excellent and relevant results, we propose designing an interactive data mining work flow. For example, a trained medical professional could identify regions-of-interest in an image which are then utilized by our algorithms to extract templates (feature vectors of those regions) for further use in future classification tasks. While most algorithms proposed today focus on very narrow fields of application (colon images, melanoma samples etc.), this would add to our software the flexibility to include per-user parameters into its machine learning process, solving the problem of what feature vectors to extract, thus significantly widening the applicability of our work.

**Visualizing $n$-Dimensional Point Clouds as Topological Landscapes.** A very promising research route has been opened by [56], [57], [58]: they utilize a landscape metaphor to images, which presents clusters and their nesting as hills whose height, width, and shape reflect cluster coherence, size, and stability. A second local analysis phase utilizes this global structural knowledge to select individual clusters, or point sets, for further, localized data analysis. The big advantage is that the focus on structural entities significantly reduces visual clutter in established geometric visualizations and permits a more efficient data analysis. This analysis complements the global topological perspective and enables the end user to study subspaces or geometric properties, such as shape. This is a very promising research route to follow.

## 8   Conclusion

Much further promising research routes are open for further exploration in the discovery of knowledge from natural images, however, the first question is how to preprocess the raw data as to get relevant data which is applicable for the use of methods from geometry and topology. As this paper only describes methods to extract point cloud data from different weakly structured sources, once a point cloud (or graph) is extracted, it will have to be topologically analysed in order to produce workable results. The quality of those results will not only depend on the quality of the algorithms themselves, but to a large degree also on the quality of the input graphs they receive. In order to determine how well suited our graphs are for further computation, we will have to conduct those experiments, adapting our methods and parameters as needed.

# References

1. Holzinger, A., Dehmer, M., Jurisica, I.: Knowledge discovery and interactive data mining in bioinformatics state-of-the-art, future challenges and research directions. BMC Bioinformatics 15(suppl. 6), S1 (2014)
2. Edelsbrunner, H., Harer, J.L.: Computational Topology: An Introduction. American Mathematical Society, Providence (2010)
3. Memoli, F., Sapiro, G.: A theoretical and computational framework for isometry invariant recognition of point cloud data. Foundations of Computational Mathematics 5(3), 313–347 (2005)
4. Holzinger, A.: Topological Data Mining in a Nutshell. Springer, Heidelberg (2014) (in print)
5. Mmoli, F., Sapiro, G.: A theoretical and computational framework for isometry invariant recognition of point cloud data. Foundations of Computational Mathematics 5(3), 313–347 (2005)
6. Canutescu, A.A., Shelenkov, A.A., Dunbrack, R.L.: A graph-theory algorithm for rapid protein side-chain prediction. Protein Science 12(9), 2001–2014 (2003)
7. Zomorodian, A.: Topology for computing, vol. 16. Cambridge University Press, Cambridge (2005)
8. Vegter, G.: Computational topology, pp. 517–536. CRC Press, Inc., Boca Raton (2004)
9. Hatcher, A.: Algebraic Topology. Cambridge University Press, Cambridge (2002)
10. Cannon, J.W.: The recognition problem: What is a topological manifold? Bulletin of the American Mathematical Society 84(5), 832–866 (1978)
11. De Berg, M., Van Kreveld, M., Overmars, M., Schwarzkopf, O.C.: Computational geometry, 3rd edn. Springer, Heidelberg (2008)
12. Aurenhammer, F.: Voronoi diagrams - a survey of a fundamental geometric data structure. Computing Surveys 23(3), 345–405 (1991)
13. Axelsson, P.E.: Processing of laser scanner data - algorithms and applications. ISPRS Journal of Photogrammetry and Remote Sensing 54(2-3), 138–147 (1999)
14. Vosselman, G., Gorte, B.G., Sithole, G., Rabbani, T.: Recognising structure in laser scanner point clouds. International Archives of Photogrammetry, Remote Sensing and Spatial Information Sciences 46(8), 33–38 (2004)
15. Smisek, J., Jancosek, M., Pajdla, T.: 3D with Kinect, pp. 3–25. Springer (2013)
16. Dal Mutto, C., Zanuttigh, P., Cortelazzo, G.M.: Time-of-Flight Cameras and Microsoft Kinect. Springer, Heidelberg (2012)
17. Khoshelham, K., Elberink, S.O.: Accuracy and resolution of kinect depth data for indoor mapping applications. Sensors 12(2), 1437–1454 (2012)

18. Kayama, H., Okamoto, K., Nishiguchi, S., Yamada, M., Kuroda, T., Aoyama, T.: Effect of a kinect-based exercise game on improving executive cognitive performance in community-dwelling elderly: Case control study. Journal of Medical Internet Research 16(2) (2014)

19. Gonzalez-Ortega, D., Diaz-Pernas, F.J., Martinez-Zarzuela, M., Anton-Rodriguez, M.: A kinect-based system for cognitive rehabilitation exercises monitoring. Computer Methods and Programs in Biomedicine 113(2), 620–631 (2014)

20. Holzinger, A., Dorner, S., Födinger, M., Valdez, A.C., Ziefle, M.: Chances of Increasing Youth Health Awareness through Mobile Wellness Applications. In: Leitner, G., Hitz, M., Holzinger, A. (eds.) USAB 2010. LNCS, vol. 6389, pp. 71–81. Springer, Heidelberg (2010)

21. Sitek, A., Huesman, R.H., Gullberg, G.T.: Tomographic reconstruction using an adaptive tetrahedral mesh defined by a point cloud. IEEE Transactions on Medical Imaging 25(9), 1172–1179 (2006)

22. Caramella, D., Bartolozzi, C.: 3D image processing: techniques and clinical applications (Medical Radiology / Diagnostic Imaging). Springer, London (2002)

23. Salton, G., Wong, A., Yang, C.S.: A vector space model for automatic indexing. Commun. ACM 18(11), 613–620 (1975)

24. Holzinger, A.: On Knowledge Discovery and Interactive Intelligent Visualization of Biomedical Data - Challenges in Human Computer Interaction & Biomedical Informatics. INSTICC, Rome, pp. 9–20 (2012)

25. Wagner, H., Dlotko, P., Mrozek, M.: Computational topology in text mining, pp. 68–78 (2012)

26. Argenziano, G., Soyer, H.P.: Dermoscopy of pigmented skin lesions–a valuable tool for early diagnosis of melanoma. The Lancet Oncology 2(7) (2001)

27. Eisemann, N., Waldmann, A., Katalinic, A.: Incidence of melanoma and changes in stage-specific incidence after implementation of skin cancer screening in Schleswig-Holstein. Bundesgesundheitsblatt, Gesundheitsforschung, Gesundheitsschutz 57, 77–83 (2014)

28. Argenziano, G., Giacomel, J., Zalaudek, I., Blum, A., Braun, R.P., Cabo, H., Halpern, A., Hofmann-Wellenhof, R., Malvehy, J., Marghoob, A.A., Menzies, S., Moscarella, E., Pellacani, G., Puig, S., Rabinovitz, H., Saida, T., Seidenari, S., Soyer, H.P., Stolz, W., Thomas, L., Kittler, H.: A Clinico-Dermoscopic Approach for Skin Cancer Screening. Recommendations Involving a Survey of the International Dermoscopy Society (2013)

29. Australia, M.I.: Dermoscopy (November 2013)

30. Ahlgrimm-Siess, V., Hofmann-Wellenhof, R., Cao, T., Oliviero, M., Scope, A., Rabinovitz, H.S.: Reflectance confocal microscopy in the daily practice. Semin. Cutan. Med. Surg. 28(3), 180–189 (2009)

31. Meijering, E., van Cappellen, G.: Biological image analysis primer (2006), booklet online available via www.imagescience.org

32. Risser, J., Pressley, Z., Veledar, E., Washington, C., Chen, S.C.: The impact of total body photography on biopsy rate in patients from a pigmented lesion clinic. Journal of the American Academy of Dermatology 57(3), 428–434

33. Mikailov, A., Blechman, A.: Gigapixel photography for skin cancer surveillance: A novel alternative to total-body photography. Cutis 92(5), 241–243 (2013)

34. dos Santos, S., Brodlie, K.: Gaining understanding of multivariate and multidimensional data through visualization. Computers & Graphics 28(3), 311–325 (2004)

35. Emmert-Streib, F., de Matos Simoes, R., Glazko, G., McDade, S., Haibe-Kains, B., Holzinger, A., Dehmer, M., Campbell, F.: Functional and genetic analysis of the colon cancer network. BMC Bioinformatics 15(suppl. 6), S6 (2014)

36. Bramer, M.: Principles of data mining, 2nd edn. Springer, Heidelberg (2013)
37. Kropatsch, W., Burge, M., Glantz, R.: Graphs in Image Analysis, pp. 179–197. Springer, New York (2001)
38. Palmieri, G., Sarantopoulos, P., Barnhill, R., Cochran, A.: 4. Current Clinical Pathology. In: Molecular Pathology of Melanocytic Skin Cancer, pp. 59–74. Springer, New York (2014)
39. Xu, L., Jackowski, M., Goshtasby, A., Roseman, D., Bines, S., Yu, C., Dhawan, A., Huntley, A.: Segmentation of skin cancer images. Image and Vision Computing 17(1), 65–74 (1999)
40. Argenziano, G., Soyer, H.P., Chimenti, S., Talamini, R., Corona, R., Sera, F., Binder, M., Cerroni, L., De Rosa, G., Ferrara, G., Hofmann-Wellenhof, R., Landthaler, M., Menzies, S.W., Pehamberger, H., Piccolo, D., Rabinovitz, H.S., Schiffner, R., Staibano, S., Stolz, W., Bartenjev, I., Blum, A., Braun, R., Cabo, H., Carli, P., De Giorgi, V., Fleming, M.G., Grichnik, J.M., Grin, C.M., Halpern, A.C., Johr, R., Katz, B., Kenet, R.O., Kittler, H., Kreusch, J., Malvehy, J., Mazzocchetti, G., Oliviero, M., Özdemir, F., Peris, K., Perotti, R., Perusquia, A., Pizzichetta, M.A., Puig, S., Rao, B., Rubegni, P., Saida, T., Scalvenzi, M., Seidenari, S., Stanganelli, I., Tanaka, M., Westerhoff, K., Wolf, I.H., Braun-Falco, O., Kerl, H., Nishikawa, T., Wolff, K., Kopf, A.W.: Dermoscopy of pigmented skin lesions: Results of a consensus meeting via the internet. Journal of the American Academy of Dermatology 48, 679–693 (2003)
41. Ferri, M., Stanganelli, I.: Size functions for the morphological analysis of melanocytic lesions. International Journal of Biomedical Imaging 2010, 621357 (2010)
42. Pizzichetta, M.A., Stanganelli, I., Bono, R., Soyer, H.P., Magi, S., Canzonieri, V., Lanzanova, G., Annessi, G., Massone, C., Cerroni, L., Talamini, R.: Dermoscopic features of difficult melanoma. Dermatologic Surgery: Official Publication for American Society for Dermatologic Surgery 33, 91–99 (2007)
43. Ballard, D.H.: Generalizing the hough transform to detect arbitrary shapes. Pattern Recognition 13(2), 111–122 (1981)
44. Ruppertshofen, H., Lorenz, C., Rose, G., Schramm, H.: Discriminative generalized hough transform for object localization in medical images. International Journal of Computer Assisted Radiology and Surgery 8(4), 593–606 (2013)
45. Tsai, A., Yezzi Jr., A., Willsky, A.S.: Curve evolution implementation of the mumford-shah functional for image segmentation, denoising, interpolation, and magnification. IEEE Transactions on Image Processing 10(8), 1169–1186 (2001)
46. de Mauro, C., Diligenti, M., Gori, M., Maggini, M.: Similarity learning for graph-based image representations. Pattern Recognition Letters 24(8), 1115–1122 (2003)
47. Bianchini, M., Gori, M., Mazzoni, P., Sarti, L., Scarselli, F.: Face Localization with Recursive Neural Networks. In: Apolloni, B., Marinaro, M., Tagliaferri, R. (eds.) WIRN 2003. LNCS, vol. 2859, pp. 99–105. Springer, Heidelberg (2003)
48. Chen, C., Freedman, D.: Topology noise removal for curve and surface evolution. In: Menze, B., Langs, G., Tu, Z., Criminisi, A. (eds.) MICCAI 2010. LNCS, vol. 6533, pp. 31–42. Springer, Heidelberg (2011)
49. Vincent, L., Soille, P.: Watersheds in digital spaces: An efficient algorithm based on immersion simulations. IEEE Transactions on Pattern Analysis and Machine Intelligence 13(6), 583–598 (1991)
50. Meyer, F.: The steepest watershed: from graphs to images. arXiv preprint arXiv:1204.2134 (2012)
51. Sonka, M., Hlavac, V., Boyle, R.: Image processing, analysis, and machine vision, 3rd edn. Cengage Learning (2007)

52. Rogowska, J.: Overview and fundamentals of medical image segmentation, pp. 69–85. Academic Press, Inc. (2000)
53. Felzenszwalb, P.F., Huttenlocher, D.P.: Efficient Graph-Based Image Segmentation. International Journal of Computer Vision 59(2), 167–181 (2004)
54. Lee, Y.J., Grauman, K.: Object-graphs for context-aware visual category discovery. IEEE Transactions on Pattern Analysis and Machine Intelligence 34(2), 346–358 (2012)
55. Wiltgen, M., Gerger, A.: Automatic identification of diagnostic significant regions in confocal laser scanning microscopy of melanocytic skin tumors. Methods of Information in Medicine, 14–25 (2008)
56. Oesterling, P., Heine, C., Janicke, H., Scheuermann, G.: Visual analysis of high dimensional point clouds using topological landscapes. In: North, S., Shen, H.W., Vanwijk, J.J. (eds.) IEEE Pacific Visualization Symposium 2010, pp. 113–120. IEEE (2010)
57. Oesterling, P., Heine, C., Janicke, H., Scheuermann, G., Heyer, G.: Visualization of high-dimensional point clouds using their density distribution's topology. IEEE Transactions on Visualization and Computer Graphics 17(11), 1547–1559 (2011)
58. Oesterling, P., Heine, C., Weber, G.H., Scheuermann, G.: Visualizing nd point clouds as topological landscape profiles to guide local data analysis. IEEE Transactions on Visualization and Computer Graphics 19(3), 514–526 (2013)

# Adapted Features and Instance Selection for Improving Co-training

Gilad Katz, Asaf Shabtai, and Lior Rokach

Department of Information Systems Engineering, Ben-Gurion University of the Negev, Israel
{katz,shabtaia,rokach1}@bgu.ac.il

**Abstract.** High quality, labeled data is essential for successfully applying machine learning methods to real-world problems. However, in many cases, the amount of labeled data is insufficient and labeling that data is expensive or time consuming. Co-training algorithms, which use unlabeled data in order to improve classification, have proven to be effective in such cases. Generally, co-training algorithms work by using two classifiers trained on two different views of the data to label large amounts of unlabeled data, and hence they help minimize the human effort required to label new data. In this paper we propose simple and effective strategies for improving the basic co-training framework. The proposed strategies improve two aspects of the co-training algorithm: the manner in which the features set is partitioned and the method of selecting additional instances. An experimental study over 25 datasets, proves that the proposed strategies are especially effective for imbalanced datasets. In addition, in order to better understand the inner workings of the co-training process, we provide an in-depth analysis of the effects of classifier error rates and performance imbalance between the two "views" of the data. We believe this analysis offers insights that could be used for future research.

**Keywords:** Co-training, semi-supervised learning, imbalanced datasets.

## 1 Introduction

High quality and labeled data is essential for successfully applying machine leaning methods to real-world problems. Obtaining a sufficient amount of labeled data is usually difficult, expensive or time consuming. The small number of training items may lead to the creation of inaccurate classifiers, a problem that is usually aggravated in imbalanced datasets.

Co-training [1] is a semi-supervised learning method designed to tackle these types of scenarios. In addition to a small labeled training set, the co-training algorithm assumes that a large "pool" of unlabeled training set is available. The algorithm begins by partitioning the dataset's features into two disjoint sets and creating a classifier from each. Then, iteratively, each classifier selects a few unlabeled instances from the pool for which it has the highest level of certainty in classification. These instances (a few for each class) are added to the labeled training set with the labels the classifier believes they should be assigned (the pool is replenished after each iteration). Thus, the two classifiers "train" each other by feeding to the other classifier samples, which it

A. Holzinger, I. Jurisica (Eds.): Knowledge Discovery and Data Mining, LNCS 8401, pp. 81–100, 2014.
© Springer-Verlag Berlin Heidelberg 2014

may not have chosen on its own. This process continues until some stopping criterion is met, e.g., until a predefined number of iteration is reached or all the unlabeled data are used.

This method has been proven to be effective in the classification of text when additional information is available. For example, in the study by Blum and Mitchel [1] that originally introduced the co-training algorithm, it was used to classify web pages by using the term frequencies of the text as one set and the traits of hyperlinks in the other.

In our view, there are two aspects in which the current co-training framework can be improved:

a) *Flawed feature set partitioning* – in the literature one can find a large variety of techniques used for the purpose of features partitioning – from simple techniques such as Mutual Information and Information Gain [2] to advanced methods such as Hill Climbing [3] and genetic algorithms [4]. However, we believe that whatever method is used, a fundamental problem remains. The small number of the labeled training instances makes it very difficult to optimally partition the features.

b) *Partially random instance selection* – while it is true that the co-training algorithm only selects instances with which has the highest confidence in the current iteration, it is unclear what should be done if a large number of instances have the same confidence level (our experiments show that this number may be as large as hundreds of instances). To the best of our knowledge, only one previous work addressed this problem [5] by using probability calculations in order to increase diversity.

In this paper we propose methods for dealing with these two problems. For the problem of *feature set partitioning* we present two possible strategies – one that utilizes the unlabeled instances in order to improve the feature set partitioning process and another that utilizes the additional instances that are added during the training of the algorithm in order to iteratively repartition the features set.

For the problem of *instance selection*, we propose two strategies: the first strategy ranks the unlabeled instances based on their similarity to the labeled training instances (we present the experimental results of two variations of this strategies). The second strategy attempts to select the instances by integrating input from *both* classifiers (we present two variations of this method as well, one that puts emphasis on error reduction and one that focuses on diversity).

In addition, in an attempt to better understand the effect of our proposed strategies and the co-training process in general, we analyzed the co-training's performance on the iteration level; i.e., in each labeling step. We present some interesting insights regarding the inner workings of the co-training algorithm. In particular, we show that the process of adding new instances has a much higher error rate than expected and we analyze the differences in performance on balanced and imbalanced datasets. To the best of our knowledge, no such analysis has been presented in the past and we believe that it could offer promising directions for future research.

The remainder of this paper is organized as follows. Section 2 introduces related work on co-training and feature set partitioning. In Section 3 we present our proposed methods and in Section 4 we present the evaluation results. In Section 5 we present an in-depth analysis of the co-training algorithm. Lastly, Section 6 presents our conclusions and directions for future research.

## 2     Glossary and Key Terms

In this section we define the main terms used in this paper, in order to avoid a conflict in terminology and to ensure a common understanding.

- *Instance*: A single object of the world from which a model will be learned, or on which a model will be used. An instance is made up of *features* and a *class value*.
- *Feature*: a value (numeric or otherwise) describing one facet of an instance.
- *Class value*: a value (numeric or otherwise) describing the class (i.e. group or affiliation) to which an instance belongs.
- *Classifier*: A structured model that maps unlabeled instances to finite set of classes.
- Feature selection: a process by which the most useful features are chosen from the overall feature set. There exist many criteria for "usefulness", and we elaborate on this subject later on.
- *Feature set partitioning*: the act of splitting the feature set into two (or more) disjoint subsets. This process is an integral part of the co-training process, as we explain in the following section.

## 3     Related Work

The original co-training algorithm consists of the following steps: two independent views of the data are used to train two classifiers. The classifiers are trained on a pool of labeled training instances $L$ and are used to classify a set of unlabeled training instances $U$. Then, iteratively, each classifier selects a few instances of which it is most certain (for each of the target classes) and adds them to the labeled set. Finally, the pool of unlabeled instances is replenished. The process is repeated iteratively until some decision criterion is met. The two classifiers are then used to classify the test set $T$.

The intuition behind this method is that the two classifiers which offer two different views of the data can improve the performance of the other. By feeding the other classifier instances it may not be certain how to classify, the overall performance improves.

Conceptually, the co-training algorithm consists of two parts – feature set partitioning and iterative instance selection. Both of these parts are crucial to the algorithm's success – without a feature set partitioning that generates two different views of the data, the algorithm will produce little (if any) valuable information, and with a poor selection of additional instances the algorithm's performance may deteriorate. We will now review each part in detail.

### 3.1     Feature Partitioning

The co-training algorithm relies on two basic assumptions in order to operate: (a) the dataset's features can be partitioned into (at least) two sets, each containing a sufficient amount of information in order to produce an adequate classifier; (b) the data in the different sets is uncorrelated, so that two different and independent views of the data exist. The fulfillment of these requirements (although it was demonstrated that they could be somewhat relaxed in [6, 7]) needs to be accomplished through the partitioning of the features set.

In some domains the division into two feature sets is clear. For example, in the web page classification problem presented in [1], the features set was divided into two sets: textual and non-textual features. In many other domains, however, finding a satisfying partition is not easy. This difficulty of creating independent feature sets may have a detrimental effect on the performance of the co-training algorithm, as shown in [6].

Previous work in the area of feature set partitioning in co-training can be divided into groups – those that use simple strategies in order to partition the feature set (or just do it randomly), and those that use more advanced methods.

The methods that use a simple strategy usually operate in the following manner: iteratively, for each set, a value function is used in order to rank all the remaining features. There is a large variety of functions that can be used for this purpose: the entropy based methods (Information Gain, Gain Ratio and Mutual Information [8]) are very common, but one can also use Signal-to-Noise (initially used in electrical engineering to determine how degraded a signal has become) [9] and Relief [10]. Advanced methods include Hill climbing [11], Oblivious Trees [12] and genetic algorithms [4].

In this paper we propose two strategies that can be combined with the methods reviewed above in order to improve the partitioning of the feature set. This is possible because our proposed strategies are not focused on finding the best features split but on how to better utilize the available information. One strategy uses the unlabeled data in order to generate a larger set from which more accurate results can be drawn, while the other strategies takes advantage of the information made available with the addition of more instances to the labeled train set.

### 3.2    Instance Selection

The selection of additional instances is an essential part of the co-training algorithm; the additional knowledge that is generated from their addition to the labeled train set is the reason for the co-training algorithm's success (or failure). The selection of instances which are either identical to instances already included in the labeled train set or completely different may actually do more harm than good.

In the area of co-training, a wide variety of methods have been used in order to improve the selection process. Pierce et al. [13], for example, used a statistical estimation of class and diversity in order to choose the instances that will be labeled while [7] used confidence intervals in order to prevent the degradation of the classifiers throughout the co-training process. Another interesting approach includes the use of human experts in order to correct mistaken labels for new instances [13].

In this paper we propose and evaluate a set of simple strategies for better instance selection in co-training. Unlike methods that rely on confidence intervals (which may be sensitive to the distribution of the data or the imbalance of the labeled training set) or other statistical measures, our proposed methods are not data-dependent and can be easily implemented.

Fig. 1 presents the basic (original) co-training algorithm that we use as our baseline. The input to the algorithm is a labeled set or instance ($L$), an unlabeled set of instances ($U$), a test set ($T$), a classification algorithm ($I$), a splitting criterion ($S$) that is used during the partitioning process of the feature set and the number of iterations of the co-training. The output of the algorithm is an extended training set ($ET$) consisted of the initial labeled set ($L$) and a portion of the unlabeled set that was labeled and selected by the co-training procedure.

```
Input:
        L – labeled set
        U – unlabeled set
        T – test set
        I – classification algorithm
        S – feature set partitioning splitting criterion
        n – number of iterations
Output:
        ET – extended training set
        h – classifier


Apply_Co_Training

 1: ET ← L
 2: X ← FeatureSetPartitioning(L , S)
 3: For (i =1; i≤n; i++)
 4:    h₁ ← TrainClassifier(I , πₓ₁(ET))
 5:    h₂ ← TrainClassifier(I , πₓ₂(ET))
          //label all unlabeled instances with classifier h₁
 6:    L₁ ← ApplyClassifier(h₁ , πₓ₁(U))
          //label all unlabeled instances with classifier h₂
 7:    L₂ ← ApplyClassifier(h₂ , πₓ₂(U))
          //add instances with highest confidence in L₁
 8:    ET ← ET ∪ SelectSamplesWithHighestCofidence(L₁)
          //add instances with highest confidence in L₂
 9:    ET ← ET ∪ SelectSamplesWithHighestCofidence(L₂)
          //replenish the "pool" of unlabeled instances
10:    ReplenishUnlabeledSet(U)
11: EvaluateClassifiers(h₁.h₂ , T)
```

**Fig. 1.** The original co-training algorithm

First, the algorithm initializes the extended training set ($ET$) with $L$ (line 1). Then a feature set partitioning procedure is applied on the labeled set $L$ using the splitting criterion $S$ (line 2). The output of the feature set partitioning procedures are $x_1$ and $x_2$, which are two mutually exclusive sets of features that together and constitute the feature set of $L$. Then, the co-training algorithm iteratively adds newly labeled instances to the extended training set (lines 3-9). First, two classifiers $h_1$ and $h_2$ are trained according to the classification algorithm $I$ (lines 3-4). The training sets of $h_1$ and $h_2$ are the result of applying the projection operator ($\pi$) on $ET$ in order to select a subset of features in $ET$ that appear in the feature collection $x_1$ and $x_2$ respectively. Next, $h_1$ and $h_2$ are used in order to label the instances of the unlabeled set $U$ (lines 6-7), where $L_1$ and $L_2$ are the instances of $U$ labeled according to $h_1$ and $h_2$ respectively. Finally, positive instances and negative instances from $L_1$ and $L_2$ having the highest confidence level are added to the extended labeled set $ET$ (lines 8-9). Finally, the pool of unlabeled instances is replenished (line 10). This process is repeated $n$ times. Then, once $ET$ is finalized, the classifiers $h_1$ and $h_2$ are combined and evaluated using test set $T$ (line 11).

# 4     The Proposed Method

In this section we present four strategies for improving the co-training algorithm - unlabeled, iterative, nearest neighbor and certainty-based. The first two strategies - unlabeled and iterative are used in order to improve the feature partitioning process while the nearest neighbor and certainty-based strategies attempt to improve the process by which additional instances are added to the labeled training set. We now review each method in detail.

## 4.1     The Unlabeled Method

Whatever criterion is used to split the feature set (Mutual Information, Information Gain or other), a basic problem exists – the amount of available information (that is, the number of labeled instances) is very limited. This small amount of information may lead to suboptimal splits.

We propose using the unlabeled training set of the co-training algorithm in order to mitigate this problem. Before the initiation of the co-training process we used the labeled set ($L$) to train a classifier and use it (temporarily) in order to label all the unlabeled instances in the unlabeled set ($U$). We then used the new labeled instances in conjunction with the original labeled training set in order to split the feature set. This process is presented in line 1-4 in Fig. 2. We hypothesized that the larger number of instances - even if some were mislabeled – would improve the partitioning of the feature set.

## 4.2     The Iterative Method

Since the number of labeled instances increases with every labeling iteration, we attempt to take advantage of the additional information in order to improve our feature set partitioning. For this reason, we implemented and tested a scenario in which the features set partitioning process is repeated with every iteration (Presented in Fig. 3). We hypothesized that by taking advantage of the newly added information would results in better feature set partitions.

An important benefit of the two feature set partitioning methods presented above (i.e., unlabeled and iterative) is the fact that they can be used in conjunction with other feature partitioning techniques (such as those presented in Section 2). This is the case because the focus of these methods is on obtaining additional information for the set partitioning process rather than the partitioning process itself. It is important to note that the unlabeled method is applied only during the first iteration while the iterative method is used in all other subsequent iterations.

```
Input:
       L – labeled set
       U – unlabeled set
       T – test set
       I – classification algorithm
       S – feature set partitioning splitting criterion
       n – number of iterations
Output:
       ET – extended training set
       h – classifier


Apply_Unlabaeled_ Co_Training

1: h ← TrainClassifier(I , L)
2: L_t ← ApplyClassifier(h , U)
3: ET ← L
4: X ← FeatureSetPartitioning(L∪ L_t , S)
5: For (i=1; i≤n; i++)
6:    h_1 ← TrainClassifier(I , π_{x1}(ET))
7:    h_2 ← TrainClassifier(I , π_{x2}(ET))
8:    L_1 ← ApplyClassifier(h_1 , π_{x1}(U))
9:    L_2 ← ApplyClassifier(h_2 , π_{x2}(U))
10:   ET ← ET ∪ SelectSamplesWithHighestConfidence(L_1)
11:   ET ← ET ∪ SelectSamplesWithHighestConfidence(L_2)
         //replenish the "pool" of unlabeled instances
12:       ReplenishUnlabeledSet(U)
13: EvaluateClassifiers(h_1.h_2 , T)
```

**Fig. 2.** The unlabeled co-training algorithm

## 4.3   The Nearest Neighbors Methods

This strategy (as well as the following one) is designed to improve the selection of the newly labeled instances. Consider the following scenario: when attempting to add two additional instances from the unlabeled instances pool, the co-training algorithm is faced with 10 instances that received the highest certainty. At this point, the algorithm will choose the instances randomly.

We propose using the following strategy in order to improve the instance selection process. Instead of randomly choosing the required number of instances from the "top candidates" (those that received the highest confidence level in the current iteration), we use the distance metric used by the SMOTE algorithm [14], in order to calculate the candidate items' similarities to the labeled items. We tested two variations of this method for ranking the candidate instances:

a)   Selecting the candidates that are most similar to labeled instances from the same class. By doing this, we hope to reduce the classification error.
b)   Selecting the instances that have the highest overall similarity to all labeled instances. By using the overall similarity, we attempt to detect instances that are both similar to those which are already labeled (thus reducing the risk of

a mistaken classification) and are also likely to contribute more to the classification process. By calculating similarity to all labeled items, we aim to select instances whose classification is more likely to assist in the successful partitioning of the two classes. This idea is somewhat similar to that of using active learning [15] with the SVM algorithm, where instances that are closest to the separating line are chosen for labeling by a domain expert.

An overview of the proposed method is presented in Figure 4:

**Input:**
>     $L$ – labeled set
>     $U$ – unlabeled set
>     $T$ – test set
>     $I$ – classification algorithm
>     $S$ – feature set partitioning splitting criterion
>     $n$ – number of iterations
**Output:**
>     $ET$ – extended training set
>     $h$ – classifier

*Apply_Unlabaeled_ Co_Training*

1: $h \leftarrow TrainClassifier(I, L)$
2: $L_t \leftarrow ApplyClassifier(h, U)$
3: $ET \leftarrow L$
4: $X \leftarrow FeatureSetPartitioning(L \cup L_t, S)$
5: For $(i=1; i \leq n; i++)$
6:    $h_1 \leftarrow TrainClassifier(I, \pi_{x1}(ET))$
7:    $h_2 \leftarrow TrainClassifier(I, \pi_{x2}(ET))$
8:    $L_1 \leftarrow ApplyClassifier(h_1, \pi_{x1}(U))$
9:    $L_2 \leftarrow ApplyClassifier(h_2, \pi_{x2}(U))$
10:   $ET \leftarrow ET \cup SelectSamplesWithHighestConfidence(L_1)$
11:   $ET \leftarrow ET \cup SelectSamplesWithHighestConfidence(L_2)$
         //replenish the "pool" of unlabeled instances
12:      $ReplenishUnlabeledSet(U)$
   13: $EvaluateClassifiers(h_1.h_2, T)$

**Fig. 3.** The iterative co-training algorithm

## 4.4     The Certainty Based Method

This method is implemented in the following manner: during every training iteration and for each of the classes of the dataset, each of the two classifiers produces a set of instances for which it has the highest confidence. The final selection of instances from that set, though, will be *done by the other classifier*. The algorithm of the proposed method is presented in Figure 5.

We present two variations of this method – *highest certainty* and *highest uncertainty*:

a) In the *highest certainty* method, the other classifier chooses the instances it is most certain of to have the predicted label (that is, the maximum agreement with the first classifier). The goal of this method is to reduce the error rate of the co-training algorithm by looking for maximum agreement. At the same time, new information is still obtained during the co-training process, because the initial selection of instances is done solely by the first classifier.

In *the highest uncertainty* method, the opposite approach is implemented. In this method, which was inspired by a common idea in active learning [15], the "candidate" instances to be chosen by the other    classifier to be added to the labeled training set are those that the other classifier is least certain of; i.e., the class probability it assigned to the instance is closest to the value that represents no knowledge about the "true label" of the instance (we use the threshold of 0.5 since these are binary classification problem). By doing so, we attempt to maximize the benefit of the second classifier by providing information on the instances it seems least capable of classifying.

---

**Input**:
  $L$ – labeled set
  $U$ – unlabeled set
  $T$ – test set
  $I$ –  classification algorithm
  $S$ – feature set partitioning splitting criterion
  $n$ – number of iterations
**Output**:
  $ET$ – extended training set
  $h$ – classifier

 *Apply_NN_Co_Training*

 1: $ET \leftarrow L$
 2: $X \leftarrow FeatureSetPartitioning(L , S)$
 3: For $(i=1; i \leq n; i++)$
4: $h_1 \leftarrow TrainClassifier(I , \pi_{x1}(ET))$
5: $h_2 \leftarrow TrainClassifier(I , \pi_{x2}(ET))$
   //label all unlabeled instances with classifier $h_1$
6: $L_1 \leftarrow ApplyClassifier(h_1 , \pi_{x1}(U))$
   //from $L_1$ choose instances with highest similarity
7: $L_1\_final \leftarrow SelectInstancesUsingSmote(L_1, ET)$
   //label all unlabeled instances with classifier $h_2$
8: $L_2 \leftarrow ApplyClassifier(h_2 , \pi_{x2}(U))$
   // from $L_2$ choose instances with highest similarity
9: $L_2\_final \leftarrow SelectInstancesUsingSmote(L_2, ET)$
   //add instances with highest confidence in $L_1$
8: $ET \leftarrow ET \cup SelectSamplesWithHighestCofidence(L_1\_final)$
   //add instances with highest confidence in $L_2$
9: $ET \leftarrow ET \cup SelectSamplesWithHighestCofidence(L_2\_final)$
   //replenish the "pool" of unlabeled instances
10: $ReplenishUnlabeledSet(U)$
 11: $EvaluateClassifiers(h_1.h_2 , T)$

**Fig. 4.** The nearest neighbors co-training algorithm

**Input**:
  $L$ – labeled set
  $U$ – classification algorithm
  $T$ – test set
  $I$ – classification algorithm
  $S$ – feature set partitioning splitting criterion
  $n$ – number of iterations
**Output**:
  $ET$ – extended training set
  $h$ – classifier

*Apply_Certainty_Based_Co_Training*
1: $ET \leftarrow L$
2: $X \leftarrow FeatureSetPartitioning(L , S)$
3: For $(i=1; i{\leq}n; i{+}{+})$
4: $h_1 \leftarrow TrainClassifier(I , \pi_{x1}(ET))$
5: $h_2 \leftarrow TrainClassifier(I , \pi_{x2}(ET))$
6: $L_1 \leftarrow ApplyClassifier(h_1 , \pi_{x1}(U))$
7: $L_2 \leftarrow ApplyClassifier(h_2 , \pi_{x2}(U))$
  // select instances for $L_1$ based on their certainty in $L_2$
8: $L_1\_final \leftarrow SelectInstancesUsingOtherSetCertainty(L_1, L_2)$
  // select instances for $L_2$ based on their certainty in $L_1$
9: $L_2\_final \leftarrow SelectInstancesUsingOtherSetCertainty(L_2, L_1)$
  //add the chosen instances
10: $ET \leftarrow ET \cup SelectSamplesWithHighestCofidence(L_1\_final)$
11: $ET \leftarrow ET \cup SelectSamplesWithHighestCofidence(L_2\_final)$
  //replenish the "pool" of unlabeled instances
12: $ReplenishUnlabeledSet(U)$
 13: $EvaluateClassifiers(h_1.h_2 , T)$

**Fig. 5.** The certainty-based co-training algorithm

# 5 Evaluation

## 5.1 Experiment Setup

The proposed strategies were tested on 17 two-class datasets (binary problems) and 8 multi-class datasets, which were converted to a two-class problem (with the majority class being in one group and all other classes in another) – 25 datasets overall. All datasets are well known and available online (from the UCI repository1). We chose datasets which bore a large variety in size, number of attributes, number of numeric attributes and imbalance (the properties of the various datasets are presented in Table 1) in order to evaluate the proposed methods on a variety of cases. The original co-training algorithm [1] (hereinafter called "standard" co-training algorithm) is used as the baseline algorithm.

  This evaluation is organized as follows. We begin by comparing the performance of our proposed strategies on all the datasets presented in Table 1, analyzing their strengths and weaknesses and proposing a strategy for their application. Then, in Section 5, we analyze the results and test hypotheses regarding the "inner workings" of the co-training algorithm.

---

[1] http://archive.ics.uci.edu/ml/

**Table 1.** Datasets Used in the Evaluation Process

| | Number of item | Number of attributes | Number of numeric | Percentage of numeric | Imbalance |
|---|---|---|---|---|---|
| adult | 32561 | 14 | 6 | 0.43 | 3.15 |
| bank | 45211 | 16 | 7 | 0.44 | 7.54 |
| cancer | 569 | 30 | 30 | 1.00 | 1.68 |
| cardiography | 2126 | 22 | 22 | 1.00 | 3.51 |
| contraceptive | 1473 | 9 | 6 | 0.67 | 3.42 |
| credit | 690 | 15 | 6 | 0.40 | 1.25 |
| diabetes | 768 | 8 | 8 | 1.00 | 1.87 |
| german credit | 1000 | 20 | 7 | 0.35 | 2.33 |
| heart | 270 | 13 | 6 | 0.46 | 1.25 |
| horse | 368 | 22 | 7 | 0.32 | 1.70 |
| house votes | 435 | 16 | 0 | 0.00 | 1.59 |
| ionosphere | 351 | 34 | 34 | 1.00 | 1.79 |
| letter | 20000 | 16 | 16 | 1.00 | 23.60 |
| magic | 19020 | 10 | 10 | 1.00 | 1.84 |
| nursery | 12960 | 8 | 0 | 0.00 | 2.00 |
| page_block | 5473 | 10 | 10 | 1.00 | 8.70 |
| pima | 768 | 8 | 8 | 1.00 | 1.87 |
| segment | 2310 | 19 | 19 | 1.00 | 6.00 |
| sonar | 208 | 60 | 60 | 1.00 | 1.14 |
| soy_bean | 683 | 35 | 0 | 0.00 | 6.42 |
| spam | 4601 | 57 | 57 | 1.00 | 1.54 |
| tic_tac_toe | 958 | 9 | 0 | 0.00 | 1.89 |
| vehicle | 846 | 18 | 18 | 1.00 | 2.88 |
| waveform | 5000 | 40 | 40 | 1.00 | 1.95 |
| yeast | 1004 | 8 | 8 | 1.00 | 9.14 |

For the purpose of assessing the performance of the proposed strategies, we chose to use the AUC (area under the ROC curve) measure. The proposed methods were implemented using the open source machine learning platform Weka [17] and all experiments were run on it[2]. The experiments were conducted using the following settings:

1. Two algorithms were used to evaluate the proposed method: a) Naïve Bayes, which was used in the original co-training paper [1] (and is the most commonly used classifier in papers in this field); b) the C4.5 algorithm, which is one of the most commonly used decision trees algorithms.
2. For each dataset 20 experiments were conducted.
3. Each dataset was split into three disjoint sets – labeled (training set), unlabeled (training set) and test.
   a. We used two labeled training set sizes in order to evaluate the performance of the model – both 2% and 5% of the overall number of instances (in order to assess the proposed methods' performance with different levels of available information). The instances were chosen randomly.
   b. We required that at least one instance from each class be present in the labeled set.
   c. All remaining instances were split between the unlabeled and test sets – 75% to the former, 25% to the latter.

---

[2] We plan to make the source code of our prototype co-training implementation available on the website of the authors.

4. Each co-training experiment consisted of 30 iterations. During each iteration each classifier adds two instances of each class to the labeled instances "pool". This means that for each experiment, a total of 120 instances were added.
5. For each experiment, the initial labeled training set was used by both the proposed method and by the standard co-training algorithms (the benchmark).

## 5.2     Comparing the Performance of the Proposed Methods

Evaluation results of the proposed methods are presented in Table 2. We chose to show not only the average performance of the proposed methods over all the datasets, but to also divide them into two groups based on their level of imbalance, as we found this division to be informative. Datasets whose class ratio was 2:1 or lower were defined as "balanced" while datasets with a higher ratio were defined as "imbalanced". As can be seen in Table 2, the proposed methods produce very different results for each group.

From the results we were able to conclude the following:

a) *The feature partitioning methods – unlabeled and iterative – are the ones that show the most significant improvement for imbalanced datasets.* These results support our hypothesis that high imbalance in the dataset makes feature selection and partitioning more difficult.

b) *Both the highest-certainty and highest-uncertainty methods show statistically significant improvement in many cases.* This is interesting, since the sample selection strategy of the two methods is completely opposite (certainty vs. diversity). This leads us to conclude that in many cases of co-training, a consistent selection strategy – even if it is not optimal - is better than no strategy at all.

c) *The nearest neighbors methods (especially the overall similarity version) show improvement in the largest number of scenarios.* In addition, this type of algorithms is the only one that achieved improvement in the majority of the scenarios involving the balanced datasets.

d) *The proposed methods seem to show larger improvement for imbalanced datasets.* This fact is very interesting, since imbalanced datasets are considered to be a more difficult problem, especially when the number of labeled training instances is small. We believe this issue warrants additional research which will be addressed in future work.

Based on the analysis presented above, we were able to propose a strategy for the implementation of the proposed methods: for datasets whose imbalance is equal to or smaller than 2, we recommend using the *nearest neighbors overall similarity* method and for datasets with higher imbalance we recommend that the *iterative* method be used. For other datasets, we recommend using the iterative method. If applied on the datasets presented here, this strategy would yield an overall improvement of 7% on the 25 datasets used in our experiments (proven to be statistically significant using a paired $t$-test with $p<0.05$).

**Table 2.** The Relative Performance of the Proposed Methods to the "Original" Cotraining Algorithm. for Each Algorithm We Show the Results for the Balanced Datasets (Ratio of 2:1 or Lower), Imbalanced Datasets and Overall Average Performance. Results are Shown for Experiments Where the Size of the Labeled Training Set is 2% and 5%. Fields Marked with an Asteriks are Fields Where the improvement has been Proven to be Statistically Significant with P<0.05.

| Algorithm & Training Set Size | Imbalance Level | Unlabeled | Iterative | Highest Certainty | Highest Uncertainty | NN Overall Similarity | NN Same Class Similarity |
|---|---|---|---|---|---|---|---|
| Naïve Bayes - 2% Labeled Learning Set Size | low imbalance | -2.9% | -2.1% | -1.8% | -0.1% | -0.1% | 2.1%* |
| | high imbalance | 5.2%* | 7.8%* | -1.2% | 1.2% | 5.1%* | -0.1% |
| | average | 0.6% | 2.3%* | -1.5% | 0.1% | 1.8% | 1.1% |
| Naïve Bayes - 5% Labeled Learning Set Size | low imbalance | 1.3% | 0.9% | 1.9% | 3.5%* | 4.2%* | 2.7%* |
| | high imbalance | 1.1% | 5.8%* | -1.1% | 2.7%* | 6.9%* | 1.7% |
| | average | 1.2% | 3% | 0.5% | 3.1% | 5.4%* | 2.3%* |
| C4.5 - 2 % Labeled Learning Set Size | low imbalance | -5.6% | -7.1% | 2.1%* | -1.2% | 3.1%* | -6.8% |
| | high imbalance | 5.2%* | 6%* | 2.8%* | 7.1%* | 0.6% | -5% |
| | average | -0.1% | -1.4% | 2.5%* | 2.5%* | 2% | -6.3% |
| C4.5 - 5%Labeled Learning Set Size | low imbalance | -4.5% | -5% | 0.8% | -2.3%* | -4.9% | -2.2% |
| | high imbalance | 10.5%* | 7.4%* | 6.9%* | 1.5% | 3.3%* | 5.3%* |
| | average | 2.1%* | 0.4% | 3.6%* | -0.7% | -1.2% | 1.1% |

# 6    Analysis of Labeling Accuracy

The performance of the iterative strategy (as shown in the previous section) as well as an interest in a better understanding of the inner workings of the co-training algorithm led us to the conduct additional analysis. We defined a set of questions that we believed could help us better understand the co-training process and tried to answer them by analyzing our experiment logs. The purpose of this analysis is two-fold: a) to identify factors and patterns that affect the performance of the co-training algorithm (for better or for worse); b) to propose future research directions.

Since analyzing all the proposed strategies would be difficult to follow, we decided to analyze three algorithms: the standard co-training algorithm, the iterative method (which performed best on imbalanced sets) and the most-similar similarity method (which fared best on balanced datasets). The analysis was conducted for the Naïve Bayes method which is both the most commonly used algorithm for co-training and the algorithm whose overall performance (in terms of absolute AUC) was better than that of the C4.5 algorithm. Following are five questions that we attempt to address.

1) What percentage of the instances added during the co-training learning phase are assigned with the wrong label?

Table 3 presents the percentage of instances that were added during the learning phase to the co-training algorithms with wrong labels. It is clear that the co-training algorithm, which supposedly labels only "safe" instances, has a high error rate (41% on average). It is also clear that despite its superior performance in imbalanced datasets, the iterative method does not display a lower error rate – an interesting fact in itself, which warrants future research. The nearest neighbors method, on the other hand, shows a significantly lower error rate (but still around 30% of all added instances).

The vastly superior performance of the nearest neighbors method led us to hypothesize that most of the misclassifications were reported in outliers, namely instances that have one or more abnormal values that may "derail" a classifier. Because of the small training set, co-training algorithms are not well suited to deal with this kind of challenge.

This analysis, however, suggests an interesting possible direction for future research: it has been shown that identifying the abnormal attribute values and addressing them can lead to substantial improvement in performance, especially when small training sets are used [18]. It may pay off to pursue a similar approach in the context of co-training.

**Table 3.** Percentage of Mistakenly Labeled Instances Added During the Learning Phase to the Co-Training Algorithms

|  | Original | | Iterative | | NN Overall Similarity | |
|---|---|---|---|---|---|---|
|  | 2% | 5% | 2% | 5% | 2% | 5% |
| Balanced datasets average | 41.06% | 37.42% | 42.08% | 39.53% | 27.76% | 31.28% |
| Imbalanced datasets average | 42.08% | 38.26% | 41.85% | 39.17% | 30.77% | 36.03% |
| Overall average | 41.51% | 37.79% | 41.98% | 39.37% | 29.09% | 33.37% |

2) How would the co-training algorithm perform if no wrong instances were added?

After reviewing these results, we decided to assess what would the performance of the co-training algorithm be had no mistakes been made during the instance selections. The purpose of this analysis was not to prove that a smaller number of errors lead to better results, but to determine the algorithm's "upper bound" for improvement. By doing so, we were attempting to assess the possible benefits of investing time and effort in error reduction in the co-training process.

We ran a set of experiments in which an "oracle" prevented the algorithm from wrongly labeling instances such that instead of the rejected instance, the next instance with the highest degree of certainty was chosen. The results are presented in Table 4 and contain a comparison both to the "standard" co-training algorithm and to the baseline method (obtained by using two classifiers on the original labeled training set).

The results show (not surprisingly) that avoiding mistakes in the selection of instances can significantly improve the co-training algorithm's performance. The conclusion we draw from this analysis is that future work should focus not only on better instance selection but also on error reduction, which appears to have gotten lesser attention in comparison.

3)  Is there a correlation between the percentages of these misclassified added instances and the performance of various co-training algorithms?

**Table 4.** Comparing the Performance of the Original Co-Training Algorithm and the Co-Training Algorithm with an "Oracle" (no Mistakenly Labeled Instances Added)

|  | AUC (original) | AUC (oracle) | Oracle / Original |
|---|---|---|---|
| sonar | 0.312 | 0.785 | 2.514 |
| credit | 0.729 | 0.873 | 1.197 |
| heart | 0.810 | 0.915 | 1.129 |
| spam | 0.726 | 0.900 | 1.240 |
| house votes | 0.945 | 0.958 | 1.013 |
| cancer | 0.937 | 0.953 | 1.017 |
| horse | 0.666 | 0.849 | 1.275 |
| ionosphere | 0.603 | 0.726 | 1.204 |
| magic | 0.495 | 0.529 | 1.068 |
| diabetes | 0.662 | 0.750 | 1.133 |
| pima | 0.627 | 0.757 | 1.207 |
| tic tac toe | 0.587 | 0.668 | 1.138 |
| waveform | 0.517 | 0.615 | 1.190 |
| nursery | 0.682 | 0.964 | 1.412 |
| german credit | 0.582 | 0.693 | 1.191 |
| vehicle | 0.436 | 0.560 | 1.283 |
| adult | 0.779 | 0.868 | 1.115 |
| contraceptive | 0.640 | 0.707 | 1.105 |
| cardiography | 0.630 | 0.759 | 1.205 |
| segment | 0.897 | 0.941 | 1.048 |
| soy_bean | 0.645 | 0.707 | 1.095 |
| bank | 0.589 | 0.633 | 1.076 |
| page_block | 0.824 | 0.858 | 1.041 |
| yeast | 0.864 | 0.926 | 1.072 |
| letter | 0.489 | 0.482 | 0.984 |
|  |  |  | **1.198** |

In Table 5 we compare the performance (in AUC) of the two analyzed methods to the "standard" co-training. The comparison is based on the relative error rate in the labeling of new instances – datasets in which the proposed methods (iterative and NN overall similarity) had a lower error rate are in one group and datasets in which the error rate was higher are in another. It is clear that there is a strong correlation between a lower error rate during the co-training process and the performance of the algorithm.

4)  Are mistakes that are made during the early iterations of the co-training algorithm more detrimental to the co-training algorithm's performance?

In order to answer this question, for each dataset (and for each method) we calculated the following value $\frac{\%\ of\ errors\ in\ the\ first\ 5\ trainin\ iteration}{\%\ of\ errors\ in\ all\ training\ iterations}$ , which indicates whether more errors were made in the first 5 iterations than in later ones. Then, for each dataset we divided the values obtained for the two novel methods (iterative

**Table 5.** The Relative Performance of the Iterative and "NN Overall Similarity" Methods Compared to the "Standard" Cotraining Algorithm, Grouped by the Relative Percentage of Mistaken Instances Labeling During the Training Process

| | Iterative | | NN Overall Similarity | |
|---|---|---|---|---|
| | 2% Labeled Learning Set | 5% Labeled Learning Set | 2% Labeled Learning Set | 5% Labeled Learning Set |
| **Smaller error compared to standard" co-training** | 7.85% | 5.8% | 5.1% | 6.9% |
| **Larger error compared to "standard" co-training** | -2.1% | 0.9% | -0.7% | 4.2% |

and NN overall similarity) by the value obtained for the "standard" co-training. Our goal in so doing was to check whether there is a correlation between reduced error rates in the first co-training iterations and improved classification performance.

The results of the evaluation are presented in Table 6. We show the average relative improvement for datasets on which the relative error rate for the first iterations was below and above 1. The results of the analysis clearly show that a low error rate in these iterations is critical for the performance of the co-training algorithm.

We believe this conclusion regarding the importance of the initial iterations could be used to develop new methods for the prediction and improvement of co-training results. By paying closer attention to the early iterations it might be possible to reduce the required number of training iterations, improve classification accuracy and even evaluate early on the benefits of using co-training for a certain dataset.

5) Does a significant difference between the performances of the two classifiers correlate with the performance of the co-training algorithm?

In order to answer this question, we divided (for each dataset) the error rates of the two classifiers that make up the co-training algorithm. The lower error rate was divided by the higher one. Then, as we did before, we divided the values obtained for the two novel methods by the value obtained for the "original" co-training method. Those values were then paired with the relative improvement of the novel methods (over the standard co-training algorithm) in search of correlation.

The results are presented in Table 7. It is clear from the results (3 out of 4 cases) that "balanced" co-training method – those whose classifiers have a similar error rate – outperforms "imbalanced" ones.

We believe that this conclusion regarding the performance of the classifier could be used to develop additional methods for the improvement of the co-training process. One option that comes to mind is the use of sampling (with or without the involvement of human experts) in order to evaluate the relative performance of the classifiers.

**Table 6.** The Relative Performance of the Proposed Methods Compared to the "Standard" Co-Training Algorithm, Grouped by the Relative Error Rate of Labeled Instances Added in the First Five Iterations Compared to the Overall Error Rate

|  | Iterative | | NN Overall Similarity | |
|---|---|---|---|---|
|  | 2% Labeled Learning Set | 5% Labeled Learning Set | 2% Labeled Learning Set | 5% Labeled Learning Set |
| **Relative error rate in first 5 iterations < 1** | 1.8% | 7.4% | 1.25% | 12% |
| **relative error rate in first 5 iterations >= 1** | -1.1% | 0.6% | -1.2% | -3% |

**Table 7.** The Relative Performance of the Proposed Methods Compared to the "Standard" Co-Training Algorithm, Based the Relative Error Ratio of the Two Classifiers to the Original, Iterative and Most Similar Methods

|  | Iterative | | NN Overall Similarity | |
|---|---|---|---|---|
|  | 2% Labeled Learning Set | 5% Labeled Learning Set | 2% Labeled Learning Set | 5% Labeled Learning Set |
| **ratio <1** | 3.4% | 2.6% | 3.6% | 14% |
| **ratio >=1** | 0.9% | 3.3% | -4.9% | -2.3% |

# 7    Open Problems

The purpose of this section is to define the problems and challenges whose solutions – we believe – will enable us to advance the field of co-training in a significant manner. The analysis presented in the previous section has led us to define the following problems as the ones that are – in our view – most pressing:

a)    **Reducing the error rate in the labeling process** – as shown in our analysis, this is possibly the greatest problem currently inflicting the field of co-training. Despite its importance, the large majority of papers seem to ignore it by simply assuming that all the labeled instances are correct. As shown by our analysis, this assumption is not only false but possibly detrimental, especially if a high error rate is incurred in the initial iterations.

b)    **Intelligently selecting the instances to be labeled** – another issue that we believe that has been underrepresented in existing works is the matter of selecting the best instances to be labeled. We believe that other than choosing the instances that are "safest" or "most informative"  [15] there are also other issues to be considered: the imbalance of the data, maintaining a training set that is characteristic of the overall dataset, etc. These issues are currently not addressed by any existing work, to the best of our knowledge.

c)   **Preventing "concept drift"** – it is quite possible for the co-training algo-
     rithm to become adept at classifying a subset of the data while becoming in-
     ept at classifying other subsets. This may be due to pure chance (because of
     the partially random selection of new instances) or because some subsets are
     easier to classify than others. To the best of our knowledge, no solution is
     proposed to this problem.

## 8    Future Outlook

Because of its semi-supervised nature, co-training may be very suitable for scenarios
in which the cost of obtaining additional labeled instances is high or time consuming
– medicine and biology, for example. The capabilities presented by Big Data and its
already proven applications to the abovementioned fields open the way for some very
interesting   research directions, which may also be able to address at least some of
the problems raised in the previous section:

a)   **Co-training and ensemble** – instead of using the two classifiers presented
     by the "original" co-training method, it is possible to generate a much larger
     number of classifiers and use them in an ensemble  [16]. The proposed en-
     semble could be applied both "horizontally" - multiple pairs tagging different
     instances - and "vertically" - using only a single pair of classifiers while reus-
     ing the classification models from previous iterations.

b)   **Adaptation to multi-class problems** – co-training is almost always applied
     to binary classification problems. Even when faced with multi-class problems,
     they are often represented as a set of binary problems by iteratively grouping
     together all classes but one. The computational power presented by Big Data
     platforms can enable more advanced models. Two options come to mind:

     • Represent all possible problem combination simultaneously – generate
       all "leave one out" combinations and train them simultaneously. When
       choosing the new items to label, the different classifiers can "consult"
       with each other.

     • Train each representation separately, and combine the results once the
       training has been completed – the combination can be done by voting,
       averaging or more advanced methods such as regression or principal
       component analysis (PCA).

c)   **Advances feature partitioning methods** – as shown in this paper, existing
     feature partitioning methods still leave much to be desired. By taking advan-
     tage of the computational power of new platforms, multiple feature partitions
     can be simulated and test simultaneously, making finding the optimal fea-
     tures split easier.

## 9    Conclusions

In this paper we propose strategies for improving the co-training algorithm, which
were evaluated and showed an overall improvement of 7% in the AUC measure when
compared to the original/standard co-training algorithm.

The contribution of this paper is three-fold. First, we propose novel strategies for both "parts" of the co-training algorithm - feature set partitioning and instance selection. Second, we analyze the performance of the proposed methods and show how they can be optimally combined. Finally, we analyze the co-training process itself and present findings that may form the base for future research – particularly the importance of the early iterations for the success of the co-training process, and the advantages of both classifiers having a similar error rate.

# References

1. Blum, A., Mitchell, T.: Combining labeled and unlabeled data with co-training. In: Proceedings of the Eleventh Annual Conference on Computational Learning Theory, pp. 92–100. ACM (1998)
2. Duda, R.O., Hart, P.E., Stork, D.G.: Pattern Classification and Scene Analysis, 2nd edn. Wiley (1995)
3. Hoffmann, J.: A heuristic for domain independent planning and its use in an enforced hill-climbing algorithm. In: Ohsuga, S., Raś, Z.W. (eds.) ISMIS 2000. LNCS (LNAI), vol. 1932, pp. 216–227. Springer, Heidelberg (2010)
4. Rokach, L.: Mining manufacturing data using genetic algorithm-based feature set decomposition. International Journal of Intelligent Systems Technologies and Applications 4(1), 57–78 (2008)
5. Xu, J., He, H., Man, H.: DCPE co-training: Co-training based on diversity of class probability estimation. In: The 2010 International Joint Conference on Neural Networks (IJCNN), pp. 1–7. IEEE (2010)
6. Nigam, K., Ghani, R.: Analyzing the effectiveness and applicability of co-training. In: Proceedings of the Ninth International Conference on Information and Knowledge Management, pp. 86–93. ACM (2000)
7. Goldman, S., Zhou, Y.: Enhancing supervised learning with unlabeled data. In: Proceeding of the International Conference on Machine Learning (ICML), pp. 327–334 (2000)
8. Witten, I.H., Frank, E.: Data Mining: Practical machine learning tools and techniques. Morgan Kaufmann (2005)
9. Yang, C.-H., Huang, C.-C., Wu, K.-C., Chang, H.-Y.: A novel ga-taguchi-based feature selection method. In: Fyfe, C., Kim, D., Lee, S.-Y., Yin, H. (eds.) IDEAL 2008. LNCS, vol. 5326, pp. 112–119. Springer, Heidelberg (2008)
10. Kira, K., Rendell, L.A.: A practical approach to feature selection. In: Proceedings of the Ninth International Workshop on Machine Learning, pp. 249–256. Morgan Kaufmann Publishers Inc. (1992)
11. Ling, C.X., Du, J., Zhou, Z.-H.: When does co-training work in real data? In: Theeramunkong, T., Kijsirikul, B., Cercone, N., Ho, T.-B. (eds.) PAKDD 2009. LNCS, vol. 5476, pp. 596–603. Springer, Heidelberg (2009)
12. Rokach, L., Maimon, O.: Theory and applications of attribute decomposition. In: Proceedings IEEE International Conference on Data Mining, ICDM 2001, pp. 473–480 (2001)
13. Pierce, D., Cardie, C.: Limitations of co-training for natural language learning from large datasets. In: Proceedings of the 2001 Conference on Empirical Methods in Natural Language Processing, pp. 1–9 (2001)
14. Bowyer, K.W., Chawla, N.V., Hall, L.O., Kegelmeyer, W.P.: SMOTE: Synthetic Minority Over-sampling Technique. Journal of Artificial Intelligence Research 16, 321–357 (2002)

15. Cohn, D., Atlas, L., Ladner, R.: Improving generalization with active learning. Machine Learning 15(2), 201–221 (1994)
16. Menahem, E., Rokach, L., Elovici, Y.: Troika–An improved stacking schema for classification tasks. Information Sciences 179(24), 4097–4122 (2009)
17. Hall, M., Frank, E., Holmes, G., Pfahringer, B., Reutemann, P., Witten, I.H.: The WEKA Data Mining Software: An Update. SIGKDD Explorations 11(1), 10–18 (2009)
18. Katz, G., Shabtai, A., Rokach, L., Ofek, N.: ConfDTree: Improving Decision Trees Using Confidence Intervals. In: IEEE 12th International Conference on Data Mining, ICDM 2012, pp. 339–348. IEEE (2012)

# Knowledge Discovery and Visualization of Clusters for Erythromycin Related Adverse Events in the FDA Drug Adverse Event Reporting System

Pinar Yildirim[1], Marcus Bloice[2], and Andreas Holzinger[2]

[1] Department of Computer Engineering, Faculty of Engineering & Architecture,
Okan University, Istanbul, Turkey
pinar.yildirim@okan.edu.tr
[2] Medical University Graz, Institute for Medical Informatics, Statistics and Documentation
Research Unit HCI, Auenbruggerplatz 2/V, A-8036 Graz, Austria
marcus.bloice@medunigraz.at, a.holzinger@hci4all.at

**Abstract.** In this paper, a research study to discover hidden knowledge in the reports of the public release of the Food and Drug Administration (FDA)'s Adverse Event Reporting System (FAERS) for erythromycin is presented. Erythromycin is an antibiotic used to treat certain infections caused by bacteria. Bacterial infections can cause significant morbidity, mortality, and the costs of treatment are known to be detrimental to health institutions around the world. Since erythromycin is of great interest in medical research, the relationships between patient demographics, adverse event outcomes, and the adverse events of this drug were analyzed. The FDA's FAERS database was used to create a dataset for cluster analysis in order to gain some statistical insights. The reports contained within the dataset consist of 3792 (44.1%) female and 4798 (55.8%) male patients. The mean age of each patient is 41.759. The most frequent adverse event reported is oligohtdramnios and the most frequent adverse event outcome is OT(Other). Cluster analysis was used for the analysis of the dataset using the DBSCAN algorithm, and according to the results, a number of clusters and associations were obtained, which are reported here. It is believed medical researchers and pharmaceutical companies can utilize these results and test these relationships within their clinical studies.

**Keywords:** Open medical data, knowledge discovery, biomedical data mining, bacteria, drug adverse event, erythromycin, cluster analysis, clustering algorithms.

## 1 Introduction

Modern technology has increased the power of data by facilitating linking and sharing. Politics has embraced transparency and the citizens' rights to data access; the top down culture is being challenged. Many governments around the world now release large quantities of data into the public domain, often free of charge and without administrative overhead.

A. Holzinger, I. Jurisica (Eds.): Knowledge Discovery and Data Mining, LNCS 8401, pp. 101–116, 2014.
© Springer-Verlag Berlin Heidelberg 2014

This allows citizen-centered service delivery and design and improves accountability of public services, leading to better public service outcomes [1]. Therefore, open data has been of increasingly great interest to several scientific communities and is a big opportunity for biomedical research [2], [3], [4].

The US Food and Drug Administration (FDA) Adverse Event Reporting System (FAERS) is such a public database and contains information on adverse events and medication error reports submitted to the FDA [5]. The database is designed to support the FDA's post marketing safety surveillance program for drug and therapeutic biologic products [6], [7], [8]. Adverse events and medication errors are coded using terms from the Medical Dictionary for Regulatory Activities (MedDRA) terminology [9]. Reports can be submitted by health care professionals and the public through the "MedWatch" program. Since the original system was started in 1969, reporting has been markedly increasing. To date, the FAERS is the largest repository of spontaneously reported adverse events in the world with more than 4 million reports [10], [11].

The FDA releases the data to the public, and public access offers the possibility to external researchers and/or pharmacovigilance experts to explore this data source for conducting pharmacoepidemiological studies and/or pharmacovigilance analyses [5].

This study was carried out to describe the safety profile of erythromycin. This is of great importance as erythromycin is one of the main medications for bacterial diseases. Bacterial diseases are of particular interest due to the high morbidity, mortality, and costs of disease management [12]. Previous work has investigated the adverse events of erythromycin. Manchia et al. presented a case of a young man who had symptoms of psychotic mania after the administration of erythromycin and acetaminophen with codeine on 2 separate occasions [13]. Varughese et al. reported antibiotic-associated diarrhea (AAD) associated with the use of an antibiotic such as erythromycin [14].

Bearing the importance of any new insights into erythromycin in mind, the data from the FDA's FAERS was used to discover associations between patient information such as demographics (e.g., age and gender), the route of the drug, indication for use, the adverse event outcomes (death, hospitalization, disability, etc.), and the adverse events of erythromycin were explored. A number of statistically significant relations in the event reports were detected. The automated acquisition, integration, and management of disease-specific knowledge from disparate and heterogeneous sources are of high interest in the data mining community [15].

In the project which this paper describes, data mining experts and clinicians worked closely together to achieve these results.

## 2     Glossary and Key Terms

*Bacteria:* are living organisms that have only one cell. Under a microscope, they look like spheres, rods, or spirals. They are so small that a line of 1,000 could fit across a pencil eraser. Most bacteria do no harm - less than 1 percent of bacteria species cause any illnesses in humans. Many are helpful. Some bacteria help to digest food, destroy disease-causing cells, and give the body needed vitamins [42].

*Cluster analysis*: is the process of grouping data into classes or clusters so that objects within a cluster have high similarity in comparison to other objects in that cluster, but are very dissimilar to objects in other clusters [36].

*DBSCAN:* a density-based clustering algorithm. A density-based cluster is a set of density-connected objects that is maximal with respect to density-reachability. Every object not contained in any cluster is considered to be noise [36].

*Drug adverse event:* An appreciably harmful or unpleasant reaction, resulting from an intervention related to the use of a medicinal product, which predicts hazard from future administration and warrants prevention or specific treatment, or alteration of the dosage regimen, or withdrawal of the product [43].

*FDA FAERS (Food and Drug Administration Adverse Event Reporting System):* is a public database that contains information on adverse event and medication error reports submitted to the FDA [5].

*Open data:* Data that can be freely used, reused and redistributed by anyone – subject only, at most, to the requirement to attribute and share alike [44].

*Pharmacovigilance:* is the science relating to prevention of adverse effects with drugs.

## 3    Related Work

Several studies have been carried out regarding data mining on drug adverse event relations in the biomedical domain. Kadoyama et al. mined the FDA's FAERS for side-effect profiles of tigecycline. They used standardized, official pharmacovigilance tools using of a number of measures such as proportional ratio, the reporting odds ratio, the information component given by a Bayesian confidence propagation neural network, and the empirical Bayes geometric mean. They found some adverse events with relatively high frequency including nausea, vomiting, and hepatic failure [16].

Malla et al. investigated trabectedin related muscular and other adverse effects in the FDA FAERS database. Adverse event reports submitted to the database from 2007 to September 2011 were retrospectively reviewed and the entire safety profile of trabectedin was explored. They detected that rhabdomyolysis is a life-threatening adverse toxicity of trabectedin [17].

Raschi et al. searched macrolides and torsadogenic risk and analyzed cases of drug induced Torsade de Pointes (TdP) submitted to the publicly available FDA FAERS database. They collected patient demographic, drug, and reaction and outcome information for the 2004-2011 period and performed statistical analyses by using the statistical package SPSS. They concluded that in clinical practice azithromycin carries a level of risk similar to other macrolides; the notable proportion of fatal cases and the occurrence of TdP-related events in middle-aged patients strengthen the view that caution is needed before considering azithromycin as a safer therapeutic option among macrolides. Appropriate prescription of all macrolides is therefore vital and should be based on the underlying disease, patient's risk factors, concomitant drugs, and local pattern of drug resistance [18].

Harpaz et al. have performed a number of studies on data mining for adverse drug events (ADEs). They provide an overview of recent methodological innovations and data sources used to support ADE discovery and analysis [19]. Multi-item ADE associations are associations relating multiple drugs to possibly multiple adverse events. The current standard in pharmacovigilance is bivariate association analysis, where each single ADE combination is studied separately. The importance and difficulty in the detection of multi-item ADE associations was noted in several prominent pharmacovigilance studies. The application of a well-established data mining method known as association rule mining was applied to the FDA's spontaneous adverse event reporting system (FAERS). Several potentially novel ADEs were identified [20]. Harpaz et al. also present a new pharmacovigilance data mining technique based on the biclustering paradigm, which is designed to identify drug groups that share a common set of adverse events in the FDA's spontaneous reporting system. A taxonomy of biclusters was developed, revealing that a significant number of verified adverse drug event (ADE) biclusters were identified. Statistical tests indicate that it is extremely unlikely that the discovered bicluster structures as well as their content arose by chance. Some of the biclusters classified as indeterminate provide support for previously unrecognized and potentially novel ADEs [21].

Vilar et al. developed a new methodology that combines existing data mining algorithms with chemical information through the analysis of molecular fingerprints. This was done to enhance initial ADE signals generated from FAERS to provide a decision support mechanism to facilitate the identification of novel adverse events. Their method achieved a significant improvement in precision for identifying known ADEs, and a more than twofold signal enhancement when applied to the rhabdomyolysis ADE. The simplicity of the method assists in highlighting the etiology of the ADE by identifying structurally similar drugs [22].

The creation and updating of medical knowledge is challenging. Therefore, it is important to automatically create and update executable drug-related knowledge bases so that they can be used for automated applications. Wang et al. suggest that the drug indication knowledge generated by integrating complementary databases was comparable to the manually curated gold standard. Knowledge automatically acquired from these disparate sources could be applied to many clinical applications, such as pharmacovigilance and document summarization [23].

# 4     Methods

## 4.1     Data Sources

Input data for our study was taken from the public release of the FDA's FAERS database, which covers the period from the third quarter of 2005 through to the second quarter of 2012. The data structure of FAERS consists of 7 datasets: patient demographic and administrative information (DEMO), drug/biologic information (DRUG), adverse events (REAC), patient outcomes (OUTC), report sources (RPSR), drug therapy start and end dates (THER), and indications for use/diagnosis (INDI). The adverse events in REAC are coded using preferred terms (PTs) from the Medical Dictionary for Regulatory Activities (MedDRA) terminology. All ASCII data files are linked using an ISR, a unique number for identifying an AER. Three of seven files are linked using DRUG_SEQ, a unique number for identifying a drug for an ISR [24], [25].

**Table 1.** Characteristics of dataset

| Attribute | Type |
|---|---|
| Age | **Numeric** <br> Minimum: 6 <br> Maximum: 91 <br> Mean: 41.759 <br> StdDev: 23.409 |
| Gender | **Nominal** <br> Male, <br> Female, <br> NS |
| Route | **Nominal** <br> Oral, <br> Transplacental, <br> Ophthalmic, <br> Intravenous, <br> Topical, <br> Parenteral, <br> Disc, Nos |
| Indication for use | **Nominal** <br> 48 distinct values (MedDRA terms) |
| Adverse event outcome | **Nominal** <br> HO-Hospitalization, <br> OT-Other, <br> DE-Death, <br> DS-Disability, <br> LT-Life threatening, <br> RI- Required Intervention to Prevent Permanent Impairment/Damage, <br> CA- Congenital Anomaly |
| Adverse event | **Nominal** <br> 220 distinct values (MedDRA terms) |

The data in this study was created from the public release of the FDA's FAERS database by collecting data from the DEMO, DRUG, REAC, OUTC and INDI datasets [17]. The data, in ASCII format, were combined and stored in a database using Microsoft SQL Server 2012. Erythromycin related records were then selected to create a dataset for cluster analysis. In total, 8592 patients involved in adverse event reports for erythromycin were collected from the FDA database [25].

The dataset contains patient demographics such as age, gender, route, indication for use, adverse event outcome, and adverse event (Table 1). The attributes of the dataset were directly collected from the database. The dataset consists of 8592 instances.

## 4.2    Cluster Analysis by DBSCAN Algorithm

Cluster analysis is one area of unsupervised machine learning of particular interest for data mining and knowledge discovery. Clustering techniques have been applied to medical problems for some time and there are many different algorithms available, all with very different performances and use cases [26], [27], [28], [29].

Cluster analysis provides the means for the organization of a collection of patterns into clusters based on the similarity between these patterns, where each pattern is represented as a vector in multidimensional space [30], [31].

In clustering schemes, data entities are usually represented as vectors of feature-value pairs. Features represent certain attributes of the entities that are known to be useful for the clustering task. In numeric clustering methods, a distance measure is used to find the dissimilarity between the instances [32]. The Euclidean distance is one of the common similarity measures and is defined as the square root of the squared discrepancies between two entities summed over all variables (i.e., features) measured. For any two entities A and B and k=2 features, say, $X_1$ and $X_2$, $d_{ab}$ is the length of the hypotenuse of a right triangle. The square of the distance between the points representing A and B is obtained as follows:

$$d^2_{ab} = (X_{a1}\text{-}X_{b1})^2 + (X_{a2} \text{-} X_{b2})^2 \quad [1]$$

The square root of this expression is the distance between the two entities [33], [34].

In this study, we used the DBSCAN algorithm to analyze adverse events reports. DBSCAN (Density-Based Spatial Clustering of Applications with Noise) is a density-based clustering algorithm. A density-based cluster is a set of density-connected objects that is maximal with respect to density-reachability. Any object not contained in a cluster is considered to be noise. The DBSCAN algorithm grows regions with sufficiently high density into clusters and discovers clusters of arbitrary shape in spatial databases, even those that contain noise. It defines a cluster as a maximal set of density-connected points. The basic principles of density-based clustering involve a number of definitions, as shown in the following:

- The neighborhood within a radius ε-neighborhood of the object.
- If the ε-neighborhood of an object contains at least a minimum number, *MinPts*, of objects, then the object is called a core object.

- Given a set of objects, $D$, we say that an object $p$ is the directly density-reachable from object $q$ if $p$ is within the $\varepsilon$-neighborhood of $q$, and $q$ is a core object.
- An object $p$ is density-reachable from object $q$ with respect to $\varepsilon$ and *MinPts* in a set of objects, if there is a chain of objects $p_1,...,p_n$, $p_1=q$ and $p_n=p$ such as $p_{i+1}$ is directly density-reachable from $p_i$ with respect to $\varepsilon$ and *MinPts*, for $1 \leq i \leq n, p_i \in D$.

Density reachability is the transitive closure of direct density reachability, and this relationship is asymmetric. Only core objects are mutually density reachable. Density connectivity, however, is a symmetric relation.

DBSCAN searches for clusters by checking the $\varepsilon$-neighborhood of each point in the database. If the $\varepsilon$-neighborhood of a point $p$ contains more than *MinPts*, a new cluster with $p$ as a core object is created. DBSCAN then iteratively collects directly density-reachable objects from these core objects, which may involve the merger of some density-reachable clusters. The process terminates when no new point can be added to any cluster [37]. If a spatial index is used, the computational complexity of DBSCAN is $O(nlogn)$, where $n$ is the number of database objects. Otherwise, it is $O(n^2)$. The algorithm is therefore sensitive to the user-defined parameters [38].

The DBSCAN algorithm was used to perform cluster analysis on the dataset. Table 1 show the attributes used in the dataset. Weka 3.6.8 was used for the analysis. Weka is a collection of machine learning algorithms for data mining tasks and is open source software. The software contains tools for data pre-processing, classification, regression, clustering, association rules, and visualization [38]. The application of the DBSCAN algorithm on the dataset generated 336 clusters (Fig. 3). Some of these are shown in Table 6. The results of the application of the DBSCAN algorithm when run in Weka is as follows:

```
Clustered data objects: 8592
Number of attributes: 6
Epsilon(ε): 0.9;   minPoints(MinPts) : 6
Number of generated  clusters: 336
Elapsed time: 34.97
```

## 5    Experimental Results and Discussion

We investigated the DrugBank database to get detailed information regarding erythromycin, which is shown in Table 2. The DrugBank database is a bioinformatics and cheminformatics resource that combines detailed drug data (i.e. chemical, pharmacological, and pharmaceutical data) with comprehensive drug target information (i.e. sequence, structure, and pathway data) [39]. In the database, each drug has a DrugCard that provides extensive information on the drug's properties.

The majority of the adverse event reports in the dataset are for males (55.8%) (Table 3) with an average age of 41.759 years (Table 1) [14]. The most frequent indication for erythromycin use was for ill-defined disorders, followed by rosacea, rhinitis allergic, and diabetes mellitus (Table 4). Oral use occurs with the highest frequency (Table 5).

The ten most frequent adverse events associated with erythromycin are shown in Fig 1. Oligohtdramnios is at the top of the list, followed by intra-uterine death, gestational diabetes, and C-reactive protein increase. Fig. 2 shows the graphical representation of the top ten co-occurrences of adverse event outcomes with erythromycin. According to Fig. 2, the most observed outcome is OT(Other) (47%), followed by HO(Hospitalization) (25.4%), DE(Death) (16%), LT(Life-Threatening) (5%), DS(Disability) (3%), RI(Required Intervention to Prevent Permanent Impairment/Damage) (1%), CA(Congenital Anomaly) (0.8%), and Unknown(0.01%) in this order.

Table 2. Erythromycin in the DrugBank database

| Drugbank ID | DB00199 |
|---|---|
| Drug name | Erythromycin |
| Some synonyms | Erythromycin oxime, EM, Erythrocin Stearate |
| Some brand names | Ak-mycin, Akne-Mycin, Benzamycin, Dotycin |
| Categories | Anti-Bacterial Agents, Macrolides |
| ATC Codes | D10AF02, J01FA01, S01AA17 |

Table 3. The number of reports by gender

| Gender | The number of reports |
|---|---|
| Female | 3792 (44.1%) |
| Male | 4798(55.8%) |
| NS(Not Specified) | 2(0.2%) |

Table 4. Top ten indications for use

| No | Indication for use | The number of co-occurrences (N) |
|---|---|---|
| 1 | Ill-defined disorder | 2948(39%) |
| 2 | Rosacea | 1887(25%) |
| 3 | Rhinitis allergic | 579(7.7%) |
| 4 | Diabetes mellitus | 528(7%) |
| 5 | Drug use for unknown indication | 500(6%) |
| 6 | Lower respiratory tract infection | 420(5%) |
| 7 | Infection | 205(2%) |
| 8 | Prophylaxis | 144(1.9%) |
| 9 | Enterobacter infection | 126(1.6%) |
| 10 | Acne | 101(1.3%) |

**Table 5.** Route of drug administration

| Route | The number of reports |
|---|---|
| Oral | 7875(91%) |
| Transplacental | 279(3%) |
| Ophthalmic | 270(3%) |
| Intravenous | 96(1%) |
| Topical | 42(0.4%) |
| Parenteral | 18(0.2%) |
| Disc, Nos | 12(0.1%) |

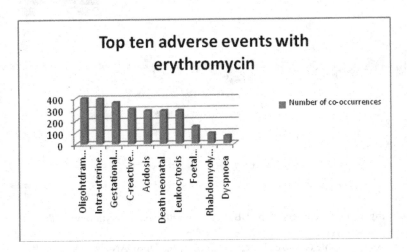

**Fig. 1.** The number of co-occurrences of adverse events (MedDRA terms) with erythromycin

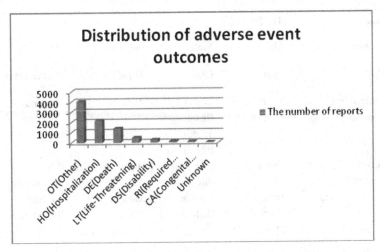

**Fig. 2.** The number of co-occurrences of adverse event outcomes with erythromycin

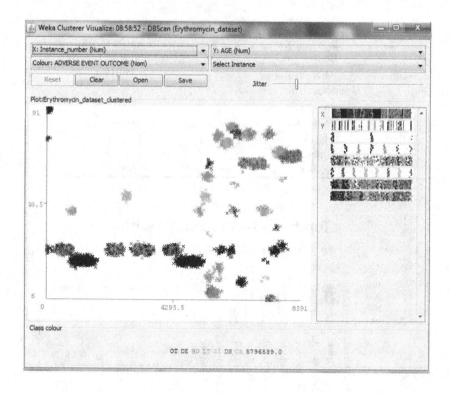

**Fig. 3.** Visual clusters of the DBSCAN algorithm on the erythromycin dataset

**Table 6.** Some clusters obtained by the DBSCAN algorithm

| Attributes | Cluster1 | Cluster2 | Cluster3 | Cluster4 |
|---|---|---|---|---|
| Age | 41.758 | 52 | 20 | 83 |
| Gender | Male | Male | Female | Male |
| Route | Oral | Oral | Topical | Intravenous |
| Indication for use | Rosacea | Lower Respiratory Tract Infection | Acne | Pneumonia Primary Atypical |
| Adverse event outcome | Other | Life threatening | Hospitalization | Life threatening |
| Adverse event | Intra-Uterine Death | Cardiac Failure | Rash Pruritic | Weight Decreased |

Erythromycin has some well-known adverse events such as vomiting, diarrhea, and mild skin rash [40]. According to our results, some events such as intra-uterine death, cardiac failure, rash pruritic, and weight decrease, are also seen in the clusters obtained by the DBSCAN algorithm. For example, intra-uterine death has a relationship with middle aged and male patients who are diagnosed with rosacea disease (cluster 1). In addition, young female patients form a cluster and the rash pruritic adverse event is seen with acne disease in the same cluster (cluster 3). Clinicians and researchers can search our results and perform clinical studies to find new hypotheses for the evaluation of drug safety of erythromycin.

The FDA's FAERS database is an important resource, but it has some limitations. For example, the database has many missing attribute values such as age and adverse events. We therefore omitted some records containing missing values. In addition, we faced some data quality and compatibility problems with the datasets created during different time periods. We therefore merged the datasets that covered the third quarter of 2005 through to the second quarter of 2012. Apart from the FDA's FAERS database, medical records that are created in hospital information systems are also an important resource for determining drug adverse events and their outcomes. Wang X et al analyzed narrative discharge summaries collected from the Clinical Information System at New York Presbyterian Hospital (NYPH). They applied MedLEE, a natural language processing system, to the collection in order to identify medication events and entities which could be potential adverse drug events. Co-occurrence statistics with adjusted volume tests were used to detect associations between the two types of entities, to calculate the strengths of the associations, and to determine their cutoff thresholds. Seven drugs/drug classes (ibuprofen, morphine, warfarin, bupropion, paroxetine, rosiglitazone, and angiotensin-converting-enzyme inhibitors) with known ADEs were selected to evaluate the system [41]. Medical records can therefore be used to reveal any serious risks involving a drug in the future [25].

# 6    Conclusion

Pharmacovigilance aims to search for previously unknown patterns and automatically detect important signals, such as drug-associated adverse events, from large databases [17]. The FDA's FAERS is a large resource for pharmacovigilance and can be used to detect hidden relationships between drugs and adverse events. In this study, the adverse event profile for erythromycin was analyzed and a research study based on patient demographics, route for drug administration, indication for use, adverse events, and adverse event outcome relationships in the FAERS reports was carried out. Erythromycin is commonly used for the treatment of bacterial diseases and bacterial diseases are one of the most serious causes for health problems in the world. Therefore, the prevention and treatment of these diseases is an important research issue in the medical domain.

We analyzed FAERS reports through the use of computational methods, and subsequently applied the DBSCAN algorithm to the dataset in order to discover clusters. The clusters highlighted that patient demographics can have some relationships with certain adverse events and event outcomes of erythromycin use. Medical researchers must be made aware of these results and the information obtained in this study could lead to new research studies for the evaluation of erythromycin drug safety.

## 7    Open Problems

The FDA FAERS database offers a rich opportunity to discover novel post-market drug adverse events. However, the exploration of the FDA Adverse Event Reporting System's data by a wider scientific community is limited due to several factors.

**Problem 1.** FAERS data must be intensively preprocessed to be converted into analyzable and unified format [45]. While preprocessing is common for the effective machine learning analysis of any data, for complex medical datasets this can often require domain-specific medical expertise. This is especially true during, for example, the feature selection phase of data preprocessing. Open datasets, without proper preprocessing, can also be extremely large. Running times for quadratic machine learning algorithms can grow quickly, and when working with medical data that have been made available with no particular research question in mind, proper data preprocessing is especially important to reduce their size.

**Problem 2.** The data has some data quality issues. For example, the data has many missing attribute values such as age and adverse events. Missing data and noise are two hindrances to using machine learning methods on open data. Open data sets, while free and publicly available, mean no possibility of retroactive refinement by the authors. They must be taken as is, and cannot normally be expanded, refined, or corrected. In the case of medical data, open data is almost always de-identified, which—depending on the research question—can result in too much missing data to make it useful or usable. However, missing values and noise are a reality of any data analysis or collection process. Machine learning techniques and algorithms that are especially designed for data that contain missing values is an active area of research, and specific solutions have been developed in the past.

**Problem 3.** There are few existing methods and tools to access the data and improve hypothesis generation with respect to potential drug adverse event associations. Those that exist are usually based on limited techniques such as proportional reporting ratios and reporting adds ratios. A generalized method or piece of software for the analysis of adverse event data is not yet available. Whether such a generalized approach would even be feasible, considering for example the level of dataset fragmentation, is fertile ground for future research. With the numbers of datasets that are being made available constantly increasing, novel approaches to properly and more easily analyze this data are sure to increase alongside it.

## 8    Future Outlook

The FDA FAERS database is used to analyze the safety profiles of several drugs. A number of commercial tools, such as query engines, are now available to analyze the FDA FAERS. These tools provide free-text search query abilities that allow for the primary safety profile of drugs to be viewed. Other tools calculate the probability of an adverse event being associated with a drug. They also allows searching the FDA FAERS database by providing interpretable graphics for the adverse events reported over time, stratified by relevant category, ages, and gender, thus allowing for clinicians to quickly check drug safety information. This would be of benefit for the entire drug safety assessment [46]. However, these tools offer limited statistical techniques and data mining algorithms. Therefore, the automatic preprocessing of data, temporal analysis, and interactive data mining [47], [48] of drug adverse events through the use of state of the art data mining techniques is sorely needed. By increasing access to, and through the analysis of such drug-safety data new insights into ADEs will be discovered, but only when novel approaches in searching, mining, and analysis are discovered and implemented.

**Acknowledgements.** We would like to thank Ozgur Ilyas Ekmekci for help and Dr. Cinar Ceken for medical expert advice.

## References

1. Shadbolt, N., O'Hara, K., Berners-Lee, T., Gibbins, N., Glaser, H.: Linked Open Government Data: Lessons from Data.gov.uk. IEEE Intelligent Systems, 1541–1672 (2012)
2. Boulton, G., Rawlins, M., Vallance, P., Walport, M.: Science as a public enterprise: The case for open data. The Lancet 377, 1633–1635 (2011)
3. Rowen, L., Wong, G.K.S., Lane, R.P., Hood, L.: Intellectual property - Publication rights in the era of open data release policies. Science 289, 1881 (2000)
4. Thompson, M., Heneghan, C.: BMJ OPEN DATA CAMPAIGN We need to move the debate on open clinical trial data forward. British Medical Journal, 345 (2012)
5. Sakaeda, T., Tamon, A., Kadoyama, K., Okuno, Y.: Data mining of the Public Version of the FDA Adverse Event Reporting System. International Journal of Medical Sciences 10(7), 796–803 (2013)
6. Rodriguez, E.M., Staffa, J.A., Graham, D.J.: The role of databases in drug postmarketing surveillance. Pharmacoepidemiol Drug Saf. 10, 407–410 (2001)
7. Wysowski, D.K., Swartz, L.: Adverse drug event surveillance and drug withdrawals in the United States, 1969-2002: The importance of reporting suspected reactions. Arch Intern Med. 165, 1363–1369 (2005)
8. [Internet] (Internet) U.S. Food and Drug Administration (FDA),
   http://www.fda.gov/Drugs/
   GuidanceComplianceRegulatoryInformation/Surveillance/
   AdverseDrugEffects/default.htm
9. [Internet] (Internet) MedDRA MSSO, http://www.meddramsso.com/index.asp

10. Moore, T.J., Cohen, M.R., Furberg, C.D.: Serious adverse drug events reported to the Food and Drug Administration, 1998-2005. Arch. Intern. Med. 167, 1752–1759 (2007)
11. Weiss-Smith, S., Deshpande, G., Chung, S., et al.: The FDA drug safety surveillance program: Adverse event reporting trends. Arch. Intern. Med. 171, 591–593 (2011)
12. (Internet) Bacterial Infections,
    http://www.who.int/vaccine_research/diseases/soa_bacterial/en/index4.html
13. Manchia, M., Alda, M., Calkin, C.V.: Repeated erythromycin/codeine-induced psychotic mania. Clin. Neuropharmacol. 36(5), 177–178 (2013)
14. Varughese, C.A., Vakil, N.H., Phillips, K.M.: Antibiotic-associated diarrhea: A refresher on causes and possible prevention with probiotics–continuing education article. J. Pharm. Pract. 26(5), 476–482 (2013)
15. Chen, E.S., Hripcsak, G., Xu, H., Markatou, M., Friedman, C.: Automated Acquisition of Disease–Drug Knowledge from Biomedical and Clinical Documents: An Initial Study. J. Am. Med. Inf. Assoc. 15, 87–98 (2008)
16. Kadoyama, K., Sakaeda, T., Tamon, A., Okuno, Y.: Adverse event profile of Tigecycline:Data mining of the public version of the U.S. Food and Drug Administration Adverse Event Reporting System. Biological & Pharmaceutical Bulletin 35(6), 967–970 (2012)
17. Malla, S., Banda, S., Bansal, D., Gudala, K.: Trabectedin related muscular and other adverse effects; data from public version of the FDA Adverse Event Reporting System. Internatial Journal of Medical and Pharmaceutical Sciences 03(07), 11–17 (2013)
18. Raschi, E., Poluzzi, E., Koci, A., Moretti, U., Sturkenboom, M., De Ponti, F.: Macrolides and Torsadogenic Risk: Emerging Issues from the FDA Pharmacovigilance Database. Journal of Pharmacovigilance 1(104), 1–4 (2013)
19. Harpaz, R., DuMouchel, W., Shah, N.H., Madigan, D., Ryan, P., Friedman, C.: Novel data-mining methodologies for adverse drug event discovery and analysis. Clin. Pharmacol. Ther. 91(6), 1010–1021 (2012)
20. Harpaz, R., Chase, H.S., Friedman, C.: Mining multi-item drug adverse effect associations in spontaneous reporting systems. BMC Bioinformatics 11(suppl. 9), S7 (2010)
21. Harpaz, R., Perez, H., Chase, H.S., Rabadan, R., Hripcsak, G., Friedman, C.: Biclustering of adverse drug events in the FDA's spontaneous reporting system. Clin. Pharmacol. Ther. 89(2), 243–250 (2011)
22. Vilar, S., Harpaz, R., Chase, H.S., Costanzi, S., Rabadan, R., Friedman, C.: Facilitating adverse drug event detection in pharmacovigilance databases using molecular structure similarity: Application to rhabdomyolysis. J. Am. Med. Inform. Assoc. 18(suppl. 1) (December 2011)
23. Wang, X., Chase, H.S., Li, J., Hripcsak, G., Friedman, C.: Integrating heterogeneous knowledge sources to acquire executable drug-related knowledge. In: AMIA Annu. Symp. Proc. 2010, pp. 852–856 (2010)
24. Kadoyama, K., Miki, I., Tamura, T., Brown, J.B., Sakaeda, T., Okuno, Y.: Adverse Event Profiles of 5-Fluorouracil and Capecitabine: Data Mining of the Public Version of the FDA Adverse Event Reporting System, AERS, and Reproducibility of Clinical Observations. Int. J. Med. Sci. 9(1), 33–39 (2012)
25. Yildirim, P., Ekmekci, I.O., Holzinger, A.: On Knowledge Discovery in Open Medical Data on the Example of the FDA Drug Adverse Event Reporting System for Alendronate (Fosamax). In: Holzinger, A., Pasi, G. (eds.) HCI-KDD 2013. LNCS, vol. 7947, pp. 195–206. Springer, Heidelberg (2013)

26. Belciug, S., Gorunescu, F., Salem, A.B., Gorunescu, M.: Clustering-based approach for detecting breast cancer recurrence. Intelligent Systems Design and Applications (ISDA), 533–538 (2010)

27. Belciug, S., Gorunescu, F., Gorunescu, M., Salem, A.: Assessing performances of unsupervised and supervised neural networks in breast cancer detection. In: 7th International Conference on Informatics and Systems (INFOS), pp. 1–8 (2010)

28. Emmert-Streib, F., de Matos Simoes, R., Glazko, G., McDade, S., Haibe-Kains, B., Holzinger, A., Dehmer, M., Campbell, F.: Functional and genetic analysis of the colon cancer network. BMC Bioinformatics 15(suppl. 6), S6 (2014)

29. Yildirim, P., Majnaric, L., Ekmekci, O., Holzinger, A.: Knowledge discovery of drug data on the example of adverse reaction prediction. BMC Bioinformatics 15(suppl. 6), S7 (2014)

30. Reynolds, A.P., Richards, G., de la Iglesia, B., Rayward-Smith, V.J.: Clustering rules: a comparison of partitioning and hierarchical clustering algorithms. Journal of Mathematical Modelling and Algorithms 5, 475–504 (2006)

31. Yıldırım, P., Ceken, K., Saka, O.: Discovering similarities fort he treatments of liver specific parasites. In: Proceedings of the Federated Conference on Computer Science and Information Systems, FedCSIS 2011, Szczecin, Poland, September 18-21, pp. 165–168. IEEE Xplore (2011) ISBN 978-83-60810-22-4

32. Holland, S.M.: Cluster Analysis, Department of Geology, University of Georgia, Athens, GA 30602-2501 (2006)

33. Hammouda, K., Kamel, M.: Data Mining using Conceptual Clustering, SYDE 622: Machine Intelligence, Course Project (2000)

34. Beckstead, J.W.: Using Hierarchical Cluster Analysis in Nursing Research. Western Journal of Nursing Research 24, 307–319 (2002)

35. Yıldırım, P., Ceken, C., Hassanpour, R., Tolun, M.R.: Prediction of Similarities among Rheumatic Diseases. Journal of Medical Systems 36(3), 1485–1490 (2012)

36. Han, J., Micheline, K.: Data mining: concepts and techniques. Morgan Kaufmann (2001)

37. Yang, C., Wang, F., Huang, B.: Internet Traffic Classification Using DBSCAN. In: 2009 WASE International Conference on Information Engineering, pp. 163–166 (2009)

38. Hall, M., Frank, E., Holmes, G., Pfahringe, B., Reutemann, P., Witten, I.E.: The WEKA data mining software: an update. ACM SIGKDD Explorations Newsletter 11, 1 (2009)

39. [Internet] (internet) Drugbank, http://www.drugbank.ca

40. [Internet] (internet) Erythromycin, http://www.drugs.com

41. Wang, X., Hripcsak, G., Markatou, M., Friedman, C.: Active Computerized Pharmacovigilance Using Natural Language Processing, Statistics, and Electronic Health Records: A Feasibility Study. Journal of the American Medical Informatics Association 16(3), 328–337 (2009)

42. [Internet] (internet) Bacterial infections, http://www.nlm.nih.gov/medlineplus/bacterialinfections.html

43. Edwards, I.R., Aronson, J.K.: Adverse drug reactions: Definitions, diagnosis, and management. Lancet 356(9237), 1255–1259 (2000)

44. [Internet] (internet) Open Knowledge Foundation,Open data introduction, http://okfn.org/opendata/

45. [Internet] (internet) http://www.chemoprofiling.org/AERS/t1.html

46. Poluzzi, E., Raschi, E., Piccinni, C., De Ponti, F.: Data mining techniques in Pharmacovigilance: Intech, Open Science (2012)

47. Holzinger, A., Dehmer, M., Jurisica, I.: Knowledge Discovery and interactive Data Mining in Bioinformatics - State-of-the-Art, future challenges and research directions. BMC Bioinformatics 15(suppl. 6), I1 (2014)
48. Otasek, D., Pastrello, C., Holzinger, A., Jurisica, I.: Visual Data Mining: Effective Exploration ofthe Biological Universe. In: Holzinger, A., Jurisica, I. (eds.) Interactive Knowledge Discovery and Data Mining in Biomedical Informatics: State-of-the-Art and Future Challenges. LNCS, vol. 8401, pp. 19–33. Springer, Heidelberg (2014)

# On Computationally-Enhanced Visual Analysis of Heterogeneous Data and Its Application in Biomedical Informatics

Cagatay Turkay[1], Fleur Jeanquartier[2]
Andreas Holzinger[2], and Helwig Hauser[3]

[1] giCentre, Department of Computer Science, City University, London, UK
Cagatay.Turkay.1@city.ac.uk
[2] Research Unit HCI, Institute for Medical Informatics, Statistics and
Documentation Medical University Graz, Austria
{f.jeanquartier,a.holzinger}@hci4all.at
[3] Visualization Group, Department of Informatics, University of Bergen, Norway
Helwig.Hauser@uib.no

**Abstract.** With the advance of new data acquisition and generation technologies, the biomedical domain is becoming increasingly data-driven. Thus, understanding the information in large and complex data sets has been in the focus of several research fields such as statistics, data mining, machine learning, and visualization. While the first three fields predominantly rely on computational power, visualization relies mainly on human perceptual and cognitive capabilities for extracting information. Data visualization, similar to Human–Computer Interaction, attempts an appropriate interaction between human and data to interactively exploit data sets. Specifically within the analysis of complex data sets, visualization researchers have integrated computational methods to enhance the interactive processes. In this state-of-the-art report, we investigate how such an integration is carried out. We study the related literature with respect to the underlying analytical tasks and methods of integration. In addition, we focus on how such methods are applied to the biomedical domain and present a concise overview within our taxonomy. Finally, we discuss some open problems and future challenges.

**Keywords:** Visualization, Visual Analytics, Heterogenous Data, Complex Data, Future Challenges, Open Problems.

## 1 Introduction and Motivation

Our society is becoming increasingly information-driven due to new technologies that provide data at an immense speed and scale. Even scientific practices are going under significant changes to adapt to this tremendous availability of data and data analysis is an important part in answering scientific questions. One of the fields where data analysis is especially important is biomedicine. In this domain, data sets are often structured in terms of both the scales they relate to,

A. Holzinger, I. Jurisica (Eds.): Knowledge Discovery and Data Mining, LNCS 8401, pp. 117–140, 2014.

e.g., from molecular interactions to how biological systems in the human body, and the inherent characteristics they carry, e.g., images from different medical devices. Such structures are both a challenge and a opportunity for scientists and significant efforts are put in several domains to understand these data. In this paper, we focus on how visualization, in particular those that incorporate computational analysis, approaches and enhances the analysis of structured information sources. We start with a section that discusses our goals and move on to more specific discussions on understanding information in data.

## 1.1   Goals

The best way of beginning such a paper, would be to start with the definition of Visualization and discuss the **goal of visualization**: A classical goal of visualization is, in an interactive, visual representation of abstract data, to amplify the acquisition or use of knowledge [1] and to enable humans to gain *insight* into complex data sets, either for the purpose of data exploration and analysis, or for data presentation [2], [3] (see section Glossary and Key Terms for more discussions). Visualization is a form of computing that provides new scientific insight through visual methods and therefore of enormous importance within the entire knowledge discovery process [4].

The **goal of this paper** is to provide a concise introduction into the visualization of large and heterogeneous data sets, in particular from the biomedical domain. For this purpose we provide a glossary to foster a common understanding, give a short nutshell-like overview about the current state-of-the-art and finally focus on open problems and future challenges. We base our taxonomy on a 2D structure on the different analytical tasks and on how computational methods can be integrated in visualizations. All the relevant works are then grouped under these categories. In addition to studies that do not have a specific application domain, we categorize visualization methods that specifically aimed at solving biomedical problems. Such subsets of work are presented under each category.

The **goal of this dual focus strategy** is to identify areas where visualization methods have shown to be successful but have not yet been applied to problems in the biomedical domain.

## 1.2   Understanding Information in Data

Understanding the relevant information in large and complex data sets has been in the focus of several research fields for quite a time; studies in statistics [5], data mining [6], machine learning [7], and in visualization have devised methods to help analysts in extracting valuable information from a large variety of challenging data sets. While the first three fields predominantly rely on computational power, visualization relies mainly on the perceptual and cognitive capabilities of the human for extracting information. Although these research activities have followed separate paths, there have been significant studies to bring together the strengths from these fields [8–10]. Tukey [11] led the way in integrating visualization and statistics with his work on **exploratory data analysis**. Earlier research on integrating statistics [12] and data mining [8] with information visualization have taken Tukey's ideas further.

This vision of integrating the best of both worlds has been a highly praised goal in visualization research [13–15] and parallels the emergence of *visual analytics* as a field on its own, which brings together research from visualization, data mining, data management, and human computer interaction [14]. In visual analytics research, the integration of automated and interactive methods is considered to be the main mechanism to foster the construction of knowledge in data analysis. In that respect, Keim [16] describes the details of a visual analysis process, where the data, the visualization, hypotheses, and interactive methods are integrated to extract relevant information. In their sense-making loop, based on the model introduced by van Wijk [17], the analytical process is carried out iteratively where the computational results are investigated through interactive visualizations. Such a loop aims to provide a better understanding of the data that will ultimately help the analyst to build new hypotheses. However, previously presented approaches still lack considering certain research issues to support a truly cross-disciplinary, seamless and holistic approach for the process chain of *data > information > knowledge*. Research needs to deal with data integration, fusion, preprocessing and data mapping as well as issues of privacy and data protection. These issues are being addressed in the HCI-KDD approach by Holzinger [18], [19] and is supported by the international expert network HCI-KDD (see hci4all.at).

## 1.3   Understanding Information in Biomedical Data

Interactive visual methods have been utilized within a wide spectrum of domains. In biomedicine, visualization is specifically required to support data analysts in tackling with problems inherent in this domain [19–21]. These can be summarized in three specific and general challenges:

*Challenge 1:* Due to the trend towards a data-centric medicine, data analysts have to deal with increasingly growing volumes and a diversity of highly complex, multi-dimensional and often weakly-structured and noisy data sets and increasing amounts of unstructured information.

*Challenge 2:* Due to the increasing trend towards precision medicine (P4 medicine: Predictive, Preventive, Participatory, Personalized (Hood and Friend, 2011)), biomedical data analysts have to deal with results from various sources in different structural dimensions, ranging from the microscopic world (systems biology, see below), and in particular from the "Omics-world" (data from genomics, proteomics, metabolomics, lipidomics, transcriptomics, epigenetics, microbiomics, fluxomics, phenomics, etc.) to the macroscopic world (e.g., disease spreading data of populations in public health informatics).

*Challenge 3:* The growing need for *integrative* solutions for interactive visualization of the data mentioned in challenge 1 and 2. Note that, although there are many sophisticated results and paradigms from the visualization community, integrated solutions, e.g. within business hospital information systems, are rare today.

An example from the biological domain can emphasize the aforementioned challenges: Biologists deal with data of different scale and resolution, ranging from tissues at the molecular and cellular scale ("the microscopic") up to organ scale ("the macroscopic"), as well as data from a diversity of databases of genomes and expression profiles, protein-protein interaction and pathways [22]. As understood by *systems biology*, the biological parts do not act alone, but in a strongly interwoven fashion, therefore biologists need to bridge and map different data types and analyze interactions [23]. Biomedicine has reached a point where the task of analyzing data is replacing the task of generating data [24]. At this point, visual analysis methods that support knowledge discovery in complex data become extremely important.

## 2   Glossary and Key Terms

In this section, we try to capture visualization and data analysis related terms that are only referenced explicitly within this paper. We do not cover the whole spectrum of visualization and analysis terms.

*Visualization:* is a visual representation of data sets intended to help people carry out some task more effectively according to Tamara Munzner [25]. Ward describes visualization as the graphical presentation of information, with the goal of providing the viewer with a qualitative understanding of the information contents [3].

*Space:* A set of points a $\in \mathbb{S}$ which satisfy some geometric postulate.

*Topological Visualization:* a prominent trend in current visualization research, driven by the data deluge. A topological abstraction provides a common mathematical language to identify structures and contexts [26], [27].

*Visual Analytics:* is an integrated approach combining visualization, human factors and data analysis to achieve a deep understanding of the data [13, 14].

*Interactive Visual Analysis (IVA):* is a set of methods that have overlaps with visual analytics. It combines the computational power of computers with the perceptive and cognitive capabilities of humans to extract knowledge from large and complex data sets. These techniques involve looking at data sets through different, linked views and iteratively selecting and examining features the user finds interesting.

*Heterogeneous Data:* composed of data objects carrying different characteristics and coming from different sources. The heterogeneity can manifest itself in several forms such as different *scales of measure*, i.e., being categorical, discrete or continuous, or challenging to relate representations, e.g., genomic activity through gene expression vs. molecular pathways; a recent example of such data sets is described by Emmert-Streib et al. [28].

*Classification:* Methods that identify which subpopulation a new observation belongs on the basis of a training set of observations with known categories.

*Factor Analysis and Dimension Reduction:* is a statistical method that aims to describe the information in the data by preserving most of the variety. This process often leads to derived, unobserved variables called the factors [5]. Similarly, there exist dimension reduction methods, such as Principal Component Analysis (PCA) and Multi-Dimensional Scaling (MDS) that project higher dimensional data onto lower dimensional spaces by preserving the variance in the data [5].

*Decision Tree:* is a predictive statical model that enhances classification tasks [29]. It is often represented visually as a tree to support decision making tasks (see Figure 4).

*Regression Analysis:* is a statistical method that aims to estimate the relations between data variables. In other words, it tries to model how dependent certain factors are on others in the data [30].

# 3    State of the Art

There are a number of surveys that characterize how the integration of automated methods and interactive visualizations are accomplished. Crouser and Chang [31] characterize the human computer collaboration by identifying what contributions are made to the process by the two sides. In their survey, several papers are grouped according to these types of contributions. According to the authors, humans contribute to the analytical processes mainly by *visual perception, visuospatial thinking, creativity* and *domain knowledge*. On the other side, the computer contributes by *data manipulation, collection and storing*, and *bias-free analysis routines*. Bertini and Lalanne [15] categorize methods involving data mining and visualization into three: *computationally enhanced visualization, visually enhanced mining*, and *integrated visualization and mining*. Their categorization depends on whether it is the visualization or the automated method that plays the major role in the analysis.

In this state of the art analysis, we categorize the related literature in two perspectives. Our first perspective relates to the analytical task that is being carried out. After an investigation of literature from the computational data analysis domain [5, 32, 33], we identify a general categorization of the most common data analysis tasks as follows: *summarizing information, finding groups &*

*classification*, and *investigating relations & prediction*. We discuss these tasks briefly under each subsection in the following. Our second perspective relates to how the integration of computational tools in visual analysis is achieved. We identify three different categories to characterize the level of integration of computational tools in visualization, namely, *visualization as a presentation medium*, *semi-interactive use of computational methods* and the *tight integration of interactive visual and computational tools*. These levels are discussed in detail in Section 3.1.

In the following, we firstly organize the literature under the three analytical task categories and then group the related works further in sub-categories relating to the levels of integration. Before we move on to the literature review, we describe the three levels of integration introduced above. Even though we describe each analysis task separately, the categorization into the three common analysis tasks can be seen as a series of steps within a single analysis flow. Starting with summarizing information, proceeding with finding groups and last but not least finding relations and trends. One aspect that we do not cover explicitly is the consideration of outliers. Outlier analysis focuses on finding elements that do not follow the common properties of the data and needs to be part of a comprehensive data analysis process [34]. In this paper, we consider outlier analysis as an inherent part of summarizing information although there are works that are targeted at treating outliers explicitly [35].

Table 1 groups the investigated literature under the categories listed here. One important point to make with respect to the allocations to sub-groups in this table is that the borders within the categories are not always clear and there is rather a smooth transition between the categories. There are methods that try to address more than one analytical question. For such works, we try to identify the core questions tackled to place them in the right locations in this table. Similar smooth transitions also existent for the levels of integration, and our decision criteria is discussed in the following section.

## 3.1   Levels of Integration

On the first level of integration of computational tools within visual data analysis, visualization is used as a presentation medium to communicate the results of computational tools. These visualizations are either static representations, or only allow limited interaction possibilities such as zooming, panning, or making selections to highlight interesting parts of the data. A typical example for this category is the use of graphical plotting capabilities of statistical analysis software such as R [36]. In this system, users often refer to static visualizations to observe the results from computational procedures, such as clustering or fitting a regression line.

The second level of integration involves the use of the computational tool as a separate entity within the analysis where the tool's inner working is not transparent to the user. In this setting, the user interacts with the computational mechanism either through *modifying parameters* or *altering the data domain* being analyzed. The results are then presented to the user through different

**Table 1.** Analytical Tasks vs. Levels of Integration. This 2D structure is used to categorize the reviewed literature in this paper.

| | Visualization as presentation | Semi-interactive Methods | Tight Integration |
|---|---|---|---|
| Summarizing Information | [37], [24] | [38], [39], [40], [41], [42], [43], [44], [45], [46], [47], [48], [49] [50] | [51], [52], [53], [54], [55], [56] |
| Groups & Classification | [57] [58], [59] | [60], [61], [62], [63], [64], [65], [66], [67], [68], [69], [70], [71], [72], [73], [74] | [75], [76], [77], [78], [79], [80] |
| Dependence & Prediction | [81], [82], [46] | [83], [84], [85], [86], [87], [88], [89] | [90], [91], [92] |

visual encodings that are often accompanied by interaction. One potential benefit here is that if problems are just too large so that a comprehensive computational approach is totally unfeasible, for ex., exhaustively searching a high-dimensional parameter space, then some directed steering by the intelligent expert user can help.

The third level constitutes mechanisms where a tight integration of interactive methods and computational tools is achieved. In these approaches, the automated methods are used seamlessly within interactive visual analysis. Sophisticated interaction mechanisms make the automated tools an integral part of the visualization. Methods in this category also interfere with the inner working of the algorithms and the results of automated tools are communicated immediately to the user.

When the second and the third levels are considered, we observe that categorizing a paper is not straightforward since the boundaries between these levels are smooth rather than discrete. In that respect, our classification criteria for level three is whether the integration allows for flexibility and done in a seamless way. If the integration is done at a manner where the automated method exists explicitly as a black-box that allows interaction to a certain level, we categorize the method under level two.

## 3.2  Summarizing Information

Data sets are becoming large and complex both in terms of the number of items and the number of modalities, i.e., data measured/collected from several sources, they contain. In order to tackle with the related visualization challenges, methods that are based on the summarization of underlying information are widely used in both automated and interactive visual data analysis [93]. Methods in this category involve the integration of descriptive statistics, dimension reduction, and factor analysis methods in general.

## Visualization as Presentation

For this category, we focus only on visualization tools in the biomedical context where there are many examples for visualization as presentation. As databases have become an integral part of dissemination and mining in biomedicine, the consolidation of such experiments data already brought up comprehensive tools for managing and sharing data. To name one, the Cell Centered Database [37] is a public image repository for managing and sharing (3D) imaging data. Next to image databases there is also a wide variety of different visualization tools, including interaction networks, pathway visualizations, multivariate omics data visualizations and multiple sequence alignments that have been reviewed recently by others [23, 24, 94]. In this context, visualization is most commonly used for exploration (hypothesis generation). Common visualization methods in addition to network visualization include scatter plots, profile plots/parallel coordinates and heatmaps with dendograms, while many tools provide combinations of those as linked views. Comprehensive summaries of visualization tools exist for certain areas. Nielsen et al. [24] present a review on tools for visualizing genomes, in particular tools for visualizing sequencing data, genome browsers and comparative genomics. Gehlenborg et al. [23] present a table of visualization tools in the area of systems biology, categorized by the different focusses of omics data. While most tools still lack in usability and integration, some of the listed tools already provide sophisticated interactive possibilities like annotating, comparing and showing confidence measures and prediction results next to view manipulations such as navigating, zooming and filtering. There is also a trend towards implementing web-based solutions to facilitate collaboration.

## Semi-interactive Methods

Perer and Shneiderman [45] discuss the importance of combining computational analysis methods, in particular statistics, with visualization to improve exploratory data analysis. Jänicke et al. [38] utilize a two-dimensional projection method (see Figure 1) where the analysis is performed on a projected 2D space called the attribute cloud. The resulting point cloud is then used as the medium for interaction where the user is able to brush and link the selections to other views of the data. Johansson and Johansson [39] enable the user to interactively reduce the dimensionality of a data set with the help of quality metrics. The visually guided variable ordering and filtering reduces the complexity of the data in a transparent manner where the user has a control over the whole process. The authors later use this methodology in the analysis of high-dimensional data sets involving microbial populations [40]. Fuchs et al. [41] integrate methods from machine learning with interactive visual analysis to assist the user in knowledge discovery. Performing the high-dimensional data analysis on derived attributes is a strategy utilized in a number of studies. Kehrer et al. [49] integrate statistical moments and aggregates to interactively analyze collections of multivariate data sets. In the VAR display by Yang et al. [48], the authors

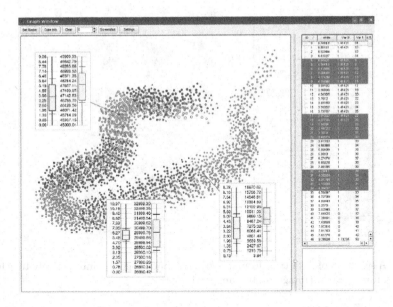

**Fig. 1.** Data can be visually analyzed on interactively created 2D spaces. (Image by Jänicke et al. [38]).

represent the dimensions as glyphs on a 2D projection of the dimensions. A multidimensional scaling operation is performed on the glyphs where the distances between the dimensions are optimally preserved in the projection.

In Biomedicine there are only a few visualization tools that are being used to construct integrated web applications for interactive data analysis. Next to the UCSC Genome Browser [46], the IGV [47] is another common genome browser that integrates many different and large data sets and supports a wide variety of data types to be explored interactively. A few similar tools that are tightly integrated with public databases for systems biology are listed by Gehlenborg et al. [23].

In MulteeSum, Meyer et al. [50] used visual summaries to investigate the relations between linked multiple data sets relating to gene expression data. Artemis [43] supports the annotation and visual inspection, comparison and analysis of high-throughput sequencing experimental data sets. The String-DB [44] is a commonly used public comprehensive database for protein-protein interaction that supports visual data analysis by providing interactive network visualizations.

Otasek et al. [95] present a work on Visual Data Mining (VDM), which is supported by interactive and scalable network visualization and analysis. Otasek et al. emphasize that knowledge discovery within complex data sets involves many workflows, including accurately representing many formats of source data, merging heterogeneous and distributed data sources, complex database searching,

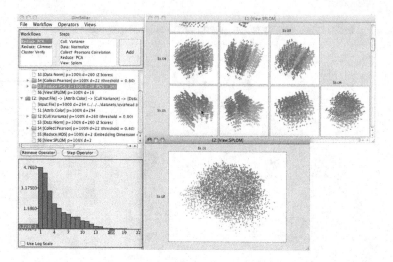

**Fig. 2.** A selection of data transformations are chained together interactively to achieve dimension reduction. (Image by Ingram et al. [54]).

integrating results from multiple computational and mathematical analyses, and effectively visualizing properties and results.

Mueller et al. report in a recent work [96] on the successful application of data Glyphs in a disease analyser for the analysis of big medical data sets with automatic validation of the data mapping, selection of subgroups within histograms and a visual comparison of the value distributions.

**Tight Integration**

Nam and Mueller [51] provides the user with an interface where a high-dimensional projection method can be steered according to user input. In MDSteer [52], an embedding is guided with user interaction leading to an adapted multidimensional scaling of multivariate data sets. Such a mechanism enables the analyst to steer the computational resources accordingly to areas where more precision is needed. Ingram et al. [54] present a system called DimStiller, where a selection of data transformations are chained together interactively to achieve dimension reduction (see Figure 2). Endert et al. [53] introduce observation level interactions to assist computational analysis tools to deliver more reliable results. The authors describe such operations as enabling the *direct manipulation* for visual analytics [55]. Turkay et al. introduce the dual-analysis approach [56] to support analysis processes where computational methods such as dimension reduction [92] are used.

## 3.3    Finding Groups and Classification

One of the most common analytical tasks in data analysis is to determine the different groups and classifications [5]. Analysts often employ cluster analysis methods that divide data into clusters where data items are assigned to groups that are similar with respect to certain criteria [97]. One aspect of cluster analysis is that it is an unsupervised method, i.e., the number of groups or their labels are not known a priori. However, when the analyst has information on class labels beforehand, often referred to as *the training set*, classification algorithms can be utilized instead. Below, we list interactive visualization methods where cluster analysis tools and/or classification algorithms are utilized.

### Visualization as Presentation

Parallel Sets by Kosara et al. [58] is a successful example where the overlaps between groups is presented with a limited amount of interaction. In the software visualization domain, Telea and Auber [59] represent the changes in code structures using a flow layout where they identify steady code blocks and when splits occur in the code of a software. Demvsar et al. [57] present a visualization approach for exploratory data analysis of multidimensional data sets and show it's utility for classification on several biomedical data sets.

### Semi-interactive Methods

May and Kohlhammer [64] present a conceptual framework that improves the classification of data using decision trees in an interactive manner. The authors later proposed a technique called SmartStripes [65] where they investigate the relations between different subsets of features and entities. Interactive systems have also been used to help create decision trees [98] (see Figure 4). Guo et al. [70] enable the interactive exploration of multivariate model parameters. They visualize the model space together with the data to reveal the trends in the data. Kandogan [71] discusses how clusters can be found and annotated through an image-based technique. Rinzivillo et al. [72] use a visual technique called progressive clustering where the clustering is done using different distance functions in consecutive steps. Schreck et al. [73] propose a framework to interactively monitor and control Kohonen maps to cluster trajectory data. The authors state the importance of integrating the expert within the clustering process in achieving good results. gCluto [74] is an interactive clustering and visualization system where the authors incorporate a wide range of clustering algorithms.

In *Hierarchical Clustering Explorer* [69], Seo and Shneiderman describe the use of an interactive dendogram coupled with a colored heatmap to represent clustering information within a coordinated multiple view system. Other examples include works accomplished within the Caleydo software for pathway analysis and associated experimental data by Lex et al. [60–62]. In a recent work (see Figure 3), the integrated use of statistical computations is shown to

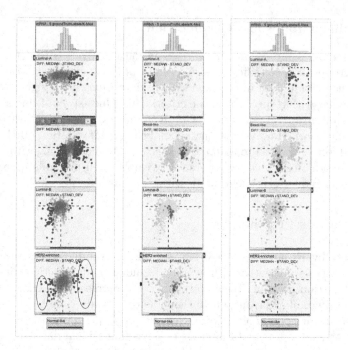

**Fig. 3.** Results of statistical test computations are communicated through visual encodings to support the identification of discriminative elements in subgroups. (Image by Turkay et al. [63]).

be useful to characterize the groupings in the data [63]. Gehlenborg et al. [23] identified that scatter plots, profile plots and heat maps are the most common visualization techniques used in interactive visualization tools for tasks like gene expression analysis. Younesy et al. [66] presents a framework where users have the ability to steer clustering algorithms and visually compare the results. Dynamically evolving clusters, in the domain of molecular dynamics, are analyzed through interactive visual tools by Grottel et al. [67]. The authors describe flow groups and a schematic view that display cluster evolution over time. Mayday is one framework example where a visual analytics framework supports clustering of gene expression data sets [68].

## Tight Integration

Turkay et al. presents an interactive system that addresses both the generation and evaluation stages in a clustering process [79]. Another example is the iVisClassifier by Choo et al. [80] where the authors improve classifitcation performance through interactive visualizations. Ahmed and Weaver [75] discuss how the clustering process can be embedded within an highly interactive system. Examples in biomedical domain are rare in this category. One example is by Rubel

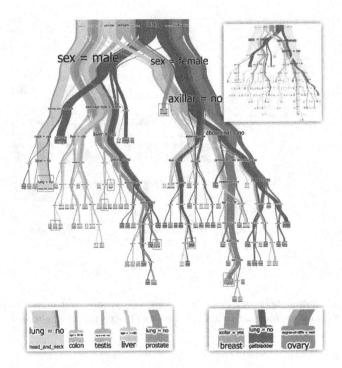

**Fig. 4.** Interactive systems have been used to help create and evaluate decision trees (Image by van den Elzen and van Wijk [98])

et al. [76], who present a framework for clustering and visually exploring (3D) expression data. In the domain of molecular dynamics simulation, there are some examples of tight integrations of interactive visualizations, clustering algorithms, and statistics to support the validity of the resulting structures [77], [78].

### 3.4  Investigating Dependence

An often performed task in data analysis is the investigation of relations within different features in a data set [99]. This task is important to build cause and effect relations, understanding the level of dependence between features, and predicting the possible outcomes based on available information. In this category, we list interactive methods that incorporate computational tools to facilitate such tasks. Often employed mechanisms are: regression, correlation, and predictive analysis approaches. In the biomedical domain, Secrier et al. [100] present a list of tools that deal with the issue of time, however, they note that it is yet an open challenge in comparative genomics to find tools for analyzing time series data that can handle both the visualization of changes as well as showing trends and predictions for insightful inferences and correlations.

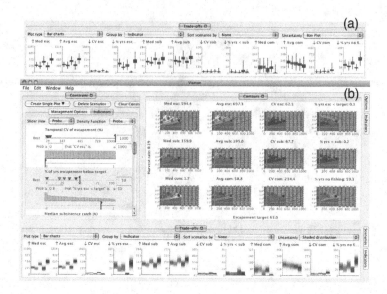

**Fig. 5.** Visualization helps analysts in making predictions and investigating uncertainties in relations within simulation parameters (Image by Booshehrian et al. [86])

## 3.5   Visualization as Presentation

In this category, we focus mainly on works from biomedical domain. Krzywinski et al. [81] presents a tool for comparative genomics by visualizing variation in genome structure. Karr et al. [82] present a promising topic, namely computing comprehensive whole-cell model and presenting model predictions for cellular and molecular properties.

Nielsen et al. [24] reviews tools for the visual comparison of genomes. The list of referenced tools includes Circos [81], a visualization presentation method for visualizing synteny (genetic linkage) in a circular layout. One example referenced is the already mentioned UCSC genome browser [46] that also provides simple phylogenetic tree graphs. The list also includes tools that integrate computational methods and support the visual analysis of comparative genomics more interactively, which are discussed in the next level of integration.

## 3.6   Semi Interactive Visualization

Visualization has shown to be effective in validating predictive models through interactive means [84]. Mühlbacher and Piringer [85] (see Figure 6) discuss how the process of building regression models can benefit from integrating domain knowledge. In the framework called Vismon, visualization has helped analysts to make predictions and investigate the uncertainties that are existent in relations within simulation parameters [86] (see Figure 5). Interaction methods facilitate the investigation of multivariate relations in multi-variate data sets [88]. Yang

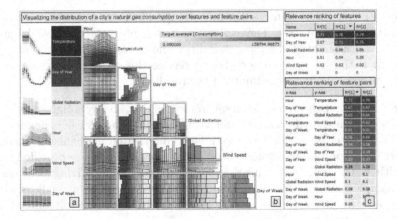

**Fig. 6.** The process of building regression models can benefit from integrating domain knowledge through interactive visualizations. (Image by Mühlbacher and Piringer [85]).

et al. [89] analyze the relations between the dimensions of a data set to create a hierarchy that they later use to create lower-dimensional spaces.

Within biomedical applications, Meyer et al. [83] present a synteny browser called MizBee, that provides circular views for the interactive exploration and analysis of conserved synteny relationships at multiple scales. In a later paper, they investigate the dependencies within signals coming from related data sets and present a comparative framework [87].

### 3.7 Tight Integration

Berger et al. [90] introduce an interactive approach that enables the investigation of the parameter space with respect to multiple target values. Malik et al. [91] describe a framework for interactive auto-correlation. This is an example where the correlation analysis is tightly coupled with the interactive elements in the visualization solution. Correlation analysis have been integrated as an internal mechanism to investigate how well lower-dimensioal projections relate to the data that they represent [92].

## 4  Open Problems

Nearly 10 years ago, Chaomei Chen (2005) [101] raised a list of top 10 unsolved information visualization problems, interestingly on top are usability issues, which are particularly relevant for the biomedical domain, and still unsolved today, as a recent study has shown [102]. This is mostly due to the fact that usability engineering methods are still considered as nice add-on and not yet an integrated part in the software development process [103]. Here we list a number of open problems in relation to the literature we cover in this report.

*Problem 1.* A topic that needs further attention is to address the uncertainty within the analysis process. The explorative nature of interactive visual analysis creates a vast amount of analysis possibilities and often leads to several plausible results. It is thus of great importance to reduce this space of possibilities and inform the user about the certainty of the results.

*Problem 2.* Although we have seen several works that involve a tight integration between computational methods and visualization, examples of *seamless integrations* are rare. With this term, we refer to interaction mechanisms where the support from appropriate sophisticated computational tools are provided to the user without the analyst noticing the complexities of the underlying mechanisms. One example to clarify this term could be: applying regression analysis locally on a selection within a 2D scatterplot and presenting the result immediately with a regression line.

*Problem 3.* One aspect that needs to be investigated further in the integration of interactive and automated methods is the *issue of usability*. Most of the solutions introduced here require significant literacy in statistics and skills in using different computational methods – which can lead to a demanding learning curve.

*Problem 4.* We have seen that most of the visual analysis methods are focussed at particular data types. However, given the current state of data collection and data recording facilities, there are often several data sets related to a phenomenon. There is the need for advanced mechanisms that can harness these various sources of information and help experts to run analysis that stretches over several data sets. This issue relates to the goal of developing an integrated visualization environment spanning several biological dimensions, from micro to macro towards an integrated approach. The recent survey by Kehrer and Hauser [104], which illustrates the many different axes along which data complexity evolves and how visualization can address these complexities, is a starting point to identify suitable approaches.

*Problem 5.* One observation we make is that the visualization methods often use the support from a single, specific computational mechanism. However, in order to achieve a comprehensive data analysis session, one needs to address all of the analysis tasks we present in our discussions above from summarizing information up to finding cause and effect [22, 100]. Especially, when works relating to biomedical applications are considered, we notice that studies that involve the tight integration of computational tools are rare. Given the successful application of such methods in other domains, it is expected that biomedical applications can also benefit significantly from these approaches.

## 5   Future Outlook

As stated within the open problems above, there is a certain need for mechanisms to improve the interpretability and usability of interactive visual analysis techniques. Possible methods could be to employ *smart labeling and annotation,* creating *templates that analysts can follow* for easier progress, and *computationally guided interaction* mechanisms where automated methods are *integrated seamlessly.* Such methods need to utilize computational tools as underlying support mechanism for users, one aspect that needs attention in this respect is to maintain the interactivity of the systems. Appropriate computation and sampling mechanisms needs to be developed to achieve such systems.

In order to address the uncertainties in visual data analysis, mechanisms that communicate the reliability of the observations made through interactive visualizations need to be developed, e.g., what happens to the observation if the selection is moved slightly along the x-axis of a scatter plot? If such questions are addressed, interactive and visual methods could easily place themselves in the everyday routine of analysts that require precise results.

The ability to define features interactively and refine feature definitions based on insights gained during visual exploration and analysis provides an extremely powerful and versatile tool for knowledge discovery. Future challenges lie in the integration of alternate feature detection methods and their utilization in intelligent brushes. Furthermore, integrating IVA and simulations, thus supporting computational steering, offers a wide range of new possibilities for knowledge discovery [105].

An interesting direction for future research relates to improving the usability of analysis processes. Current usability studies often focus on specific parts of a technique. However in order to evaluate the effectiveness of the whole analysis process, there is the need to perform comprehensive investigations on the interpretability of each step of the analysis and study the effects of using computational tools interactively. Such studies can be carried out in forms of controlled experiments where the analysts are given well-determined tasks and are asked to employ particular types of analysis routes. These routes can then be evaluated and compared against non-interactive processes where possible.

A challenging future research avenue for effective HCI is to find answers to the question "What is interesting?" as *Interest* is an essentially human construct [106], a perspective on relationships between data that is influenced by context, tasks, personal preferences, previous knowledge (=expectations) and past experience [107]. For a correct semantic interpretation, a computer would need to understand the *context* in which a visualization is presented; however, comprehension of a complex context is still beyond computation. In order for a data mining system to be generically useful, it must therefore have some way in which one can indicate what is interesting, and for that to be dynamic and changeable [108].

A recent research route in HCI is *Attention Routing*, which is a novel idea introduced by Polo Chau [109] and goes back to models of attentional mechanisms for forming position-invariant and scale-invariant representations of objects in the visual world [110]. Attention routing is a promising approach to overcome one very critical problem in visual analytics, particularly of large and heterogeneous data sets: to help users locate good starting points for their analysis. Based on *anomaly detection* [111], attention routing methods channel the end-users to interesting data subsets which do not conform to standard behaviour. This is a very promising and important research direction for Knowledge Discovery and Data Mining [18].

Top end research routes encompassing uncountable research challenges are in the application of computational topology [26], [112], [113] approaches for data visualization. Topology-based methods for visualization and visual analysis of data are becoming increasingly popular, having their major advantages in the capability to provide a concise description of the overall *structure* of a scientific data set, because subtle features can easily be missed when using traditional visualization methods (e.g. volume rendering or isocontouring), unless correct transfer functions and isovalues are chosen. By visualizing a topology directly, one can guarantee that no feature is missed and most of all solid mathematical principles can be applied to simplify a topological structure. The topology of functions is also often used for feature detection and segmentation (e.g., in surface segmentation based on curvature) [114].

In this state-of-the-art report, we investigated the literature on how visualization and computation support each other to help analysts in understanding complex, heterogeneous data sets. We also focused on to what degree these methods have been applied to biomedical domain. When the three different levels of integration are considered, we have observed that there are not yet many works falling under the third integration level. We have seen that existing applications in this category have significant potential to address the challenges discussed earlier in the paper. However, there exist several open problems, which can motivate the visualization and knowledge discovery community to carry out research on achieving a tight integration of computational power and capabilities of human experts.

# References

1. Card, S.K., Mackinlay, J.D., Shneiderman, B.: Information Visualization: Using Vision to Think. Morgan Kaufmann, San Francisco (1999)
2. Moeller, T., Hamann, B., Russell, R.D.: Mathematical foundations of scientific visualization, computer graphics, and massive data exploration. Springer (2009)
3. Ward, M., Grinstein, G., Keim, D.: Interactive data visualization: Foundations, techniques, and applications. AK Peters, Ltd. (2010)
4. Holzinger, A., Dehmer, M., Jurisica, I.: Knowledge discovery and interactive data mining in bioinformatics - state-of-the-art, future challenges and research directions. BMC Bioinformatics 15(suppl. 6), I1 (2014)
5. Johnson, R., Wichern, D.: Applied multivariate statistical analysis, vol. 6. Prentice Hall, Upper Saddle River (2007)
6. Tan, P.N., Steinbach, M., Kumar, V.: Introduction to Data Mining. Addison-Wesley Longman Publishing Co., Inc. (2005)
7. Alpaydin, E.: Introduction to machine learning. MIT press (2004)
8. Keim, D.: Information visualization and visual data mining. IEEE Transactions on Visualization and Computer Graphics 8(1), 1–8 (2002)

9.  Shneiderman, B.: Inventing discovery tools: Combining information visualization with data mining. Information Visualization 1(1), 5–12 (2002)
10. Ma, K.L.: Machine learning to boost the next generation of visualization technology. IEEE Computer Graphics and Applications 27(5), 6–9 (2007)
11. Tukey, J.W.: Exploratory Data Analysis. Addison-Wesley (1977)
12. Cleveland, W.S., Mac Gill, M.E.: Dynamic graphics for statistics. CRC Press (1988)
13. Thomas, J.J., Cook, K.A.: Illuminating the Path: The Research and Development Agenda for Visual Analytics. National Visualization and Analytics Ctr (2005)
14. Keim, D.A., Kohlhammer, J., Ellis, G., Mansmann, F.: Mastering The Information Age-Solving Problems with Visual Analytics. Florian Mansmann (2010)
15. Bertini, E., Lalanne, D.: Investigating and reflecting on the integration of automatic data analysis and visualization in knowledge discovery. SIGKDD Explor. Newsl. 11(2), 9–18 (2010)
16. Keim, D.A., Andrienko, G., Fekete, J.-D., Görg, C., Kohlhammer, J., Melançon, G.: Visual analytics: Definition, process, and challenges. In: Kerren, A., Stasko, J.T., Fekete, J.-D., North, C. (eds.) Information Visualization. LNCS, vol. 4950, pp. 154–175. Springer, Heidelberg (2008)
17. van Wijk, J.J.: The value of visualization. In: IEEE Visualization, VIS 2005, pp. 79–86. IEEE (2005)
18. Holzinger, A.: Human-computer interaction and knowledge discovery (hci-kdd): What is the benefit of bringing those two fields to work together? In: Cuzzocrea, A., Kittl, C., Simos, D.E., Weippl, E., Xu, L. (eds.) CD-ARES 2013. LNCS, vol. 8127, pp. 319–328. Springer, Heidelberg (2013)
19. Holzinger, A., Jurisica, I.: Knowledge discovery and data mining in biomedical informatics: The future is in integrative, interactive machine learning solutions. In: Holzinger, A., Jurisica, I. (eds.) Interactive Knowledge Discovery and Data Mining in Biomedical Informatics: State-of-the-Art and Future Challenges. LNCS, vol. 8401, pp. 1–17. Springer, Heidelberg (2014)
20. Holzinger, A.: On knowledge discovery and interactive intelligent visualization of biomedical data - challenges in humancomputer interaction and biomedical informatics. In: DATA 2012, pp. 9–20. INSTICC (2012)
21. Fernald, G.H., Capriotti, E., Daneshjou, R., Karczewski, K.J., Altman, R.B.: Bioinformatics challenges for personalized medicine. Bioinformatics 27(13), 1741–1748 (2011)
22. O'Donoghue, S.I., Gavin, A.C., Gehlenborg, N., Goodsell, D.S., Hériché, J.K., Nielsen, C.B., North, C., Olson, A.J., Procter, J.B., Shattuck, D.W., et al.: Visualizing biological datanow and in the future. Nature Methods 7, S2–S4 (2010)
23. Gehlenborg, N., O'Donoghue, S., Baliga, N., Goesmann, A., Hibbs, M., Kitano, H., Kohlbacher, O., Neuweger, H., Schneider, R., Tenenbaum, D., et al.: Visualization of omics data for systems biology. Nature Methods 7, S56–S68 (2010)
24. Nielsen, C.B., Cantor, M., Dubchak, I., Gordon, D., Wang, T.: Visualizing genomes: techniques and challenges. Nature Methods 7, S5–S15 (2010)
25. Munzner, T.: Visualization principles. Presented at VIZBI 2011: Workshop on Visualizing Biological Data (2011)
26. Hauser, H., Hagen, H., Theisel, H.: Topology-based methods in visualization (Mathematics+Visualization). Springer, Heidelberg (2007)
27. Pascucci, V., Tricoche, X., Hagen, H., Tierny, J.: Topological Methods in Data Analysis and Visualization: Theory, Algorithms, and Applications (Mathematics+Visualization). Springer, Heidelberg (2011)

28. Emmert-Streib, F., de Matos Simoes, R., Glazko, G., McDade, S., Haibe-Kains, B., Holzinger, A., Dehmer, M., Campbell, F.: Functional and genetic analysis of the colon cancer network. BMC Bioinformatics 15(suppl. 6), S6 (2014)

29. Olshen, L.B.J.F.R., Stone, C.J.: Classification and regression trees. Wadsworth International Group (1984)

30. Cohen, J., Cohen, P., West, S.G., Aiken, L.S.: Applied multiple regression/correlation analysis for the behavioral sciences. Lawrence Erlbaum (2003)

31. Crouser, R.J., Chang, R.: An affordance-based framework for human computation and human-computer collaboration. IEEE Transactions on Visualization and Computer Graphics 18(12), 2859–2868 (2012)

32. Brehmer, M., Munzner, T.: A multi-level typology of abstract visualization tasks. IEEE Transactions on Visualization and Computer Graphics 19(12), 2376–2385 (2013)

33. Kerren, A., Ebert, A., Meyer, J. (eds.): GI-Dagstuhl Research Seminar 2007. LNCS, vol. 4417. Springer, Heidelberg (2007)

34. Filzmoser, P., Hron, K., Reimann, C.: Principal component analysis for compositional data with outliers. Environmetrics 20(6), 621–632 (2009)

35. Novotný, M., Hauser, H.: Outlier-preserving focus+context visualization in parallel coordinates. IEEE Transactions on Visualization and Computer Graphics 12(5), 893–900 (2006)

36. R Core Team: R: A Language and Environment for Statistical Computing. R Foundation for Statistical Computing, Vienna, Austria (2013)

37. Martone, M.E., Tran, J., Wong, W.W., Sargis, J., Fong, L., Larson, S., Lamont, S.P., Gupta, A., Ellisman, M.H.: The cell centered database project: An update on building community resources for managing and sharing 3d imaging data. Journal of Structural Biology 161(3), 220–231 (2008)

38. Jänicke, H., Böttinger, M., Scheuermann, G.: Brushing of attribute clouds for the visualization of multivariate data. IEEE Transactions on Visualization and Computer Graphics, 1459–1466 (2008)

39. Johansson, S., Johansson, J.: Interactive dimensionality reduction through user-defined combinations of quality metrics. IEEE Transactions on Visualization and Computer Graphics 15(6), 993–1000 (2009)

40. Fernstad, S., Johansson, J., Adams, S., Shaw, J., Taylor, D.: Visual exploration of microbial populations. In: 2011 IEEE Symposium on Biological Data Visualization (BioVis), pp. 127–134 (2011)

41. Fuchs, R., Waser, J., Gröller, M.E.: Visual human+machine learning. IEEE TVCG 15(6), 1327–1334 (2009)

42. Oeltze, S., Doleisch, H., Hauser, H., Muigg, P., Preim, B.: Interactive visual analysis of perfusion data. IEEE Transactions on Visualization and Computer Graphics 13(6), 1392–1399 (2007)

43. Carver, T., Harris, S.R., Berriman, M., Parkhill, J., McQuillan, J.A.: Artemis: An integrated platform for visualization and analysis of high-throughput sequence-based experimental data. Bioinformatics 28(4), 464–469 (2012)

44. Franceschini, A., Szklarczyk, D., Frankild, S., Kuhn, M., Simonovic, M., Roth, A., Lin, J., Minguez, P., Bork, P., von Mering, C., et al.: String v9. 1: Protein-protein interaction networks, with increased coverage and integration. Nucleic Acids Research 41(D1), D808–D815 (2013)

45. Perer, A., Shneiderman, B.: Integrating statistics and visualization for exploratory power: From long-term case studies to design guidelines. IEEE Computer Graphics and Applications 29(3), 39–51 (2009)

46. Kuhn, R.M., Haussler, D., Kent, W.J.: The ucsc genome browser and associated tools. Briefings in Bioinformatics 14(2), 144–161 (2013)
47. Thorvaldsdóttir, H., Robinson, J.T., Mesirov, J.P.: Integrative genomics viewer (igv): High-performance genomics data visualization and exploration. Briefings in Bioinformatics 14(2), 178–192 (2013)
48. Yang, J., Hubball, D., Ward, M., Rundensteiner, E., Ribarsky, W.: Value and relation display: Interactive visual exploration of large data sets with hundreds of dimensions. IEEE Transactions on Visualization and Computer Graphics 13(3), 494–507 (2007)
49. Kehrer, J., Filzmoser, P., Hauser, H.: Brushing moments in interactive visual analysis. Computer Graphics Forum 29(3), 813–822 (2010)
50. Meyer, M., Munzner, T., DePace, A., Pfister, H.: Multeesum: A tool for comparative spatial and temporal gene expression data. IEEE Transactions on Visualization and Computer Graphics 16(6), 908–917 (2010)
51. Nam, J., Mueller, K.: Tripadvisorn-d: A tourism-inspired high-dimensional space exploration framework with overview and detail. IEEE Transactions on Visualization and Computer Graphics 19(2), 291–305 (2013)
52. Williams, M., Munzner, T.: Steerable, progressive multidimensional scaling. In: Proceedings of the IEEE Symposium on Information Visualization, pp. 57–64. IEEE Computer Society, Washington, DC (2004)
53. Endert, A., Han, C., Maiti, D., House, L., North, C.: Observation-level interaction with statistical models for visual analytics. In: 2011 IEEE Conference on Visual Analytics Science and Technology (VAST), pp. 121–130. IEEE (2011)
54. Ingram, S., Munzner, T., Irvine, V., Tory, M., Bergner, S., Möller, T.: Dimstiller: Workflows for dimensional analysis and reduction. In: 2010 IEEE Symposium on Visual Analytics Science and Technology (VAST), pp. 3–10 (2010)
55. Endert, A., Bradel, L., North, C.: Beyond control panels: Direct manipulation for visual analytics. IEEE Computer Graphics and Applications 33(4), 6–13 (2013)
56. Turkay, C., Filzmoser, P., Hauser, H.: Brushing dimensions – a dual visual analysis model for high-dimensional data. IEEE Transactions on Visualization and Computer Graphics 17(12), 2591–2599 (2011)
57. Demšar, J., Leban, G., Zupan, B.: Freeviz - an intelligent multivariate visualization approach to explorative analysis of biomedical data. Journal of Biomedical Informatics 40(6), 661–671 (2007)
58. Kosara, R., Bendix, F., Hauser, H.: Parallel sets: Interactive exploration and visual analysis of categorical data. IEEE Transactions on Visualization and Computer Graphics 12(4), 558–568 (2006)
59. Telea, A., Auber, D.: Code flows: Visualizing structural evolution of source code. Computer Graphics Forum 27(3), 831–838 (2008)
60. Lex, A., Streit, M., Schulz, H.J., Partl, C., Schmalstieg, D., Park, P.J., Gehlenborg, N.: StratomeX: Visual analysis of large-scale heterogeneous genomics data for cancer subtype characterization. Computer Graphics Forum (EuroVis 2012) 31(3), 1175–1184 (2012)
61. Lex, A., Streit, M., Partl, C., Kashofer, K., Schmalstieg, D.: Comparative analysis of multidimensional, quantitative data. IEEE Transactions on Visualization and Computer Graphics (Proceedings Visualization / Information Visualization 2010) 16(6), 1027–1035 (2010)
62. Partl, C., Kalkofen, D., Lex, A., Kashofer, K., Streit, M., Schmalstieg, D.: Enroute: Dynamic path extraction from biological pathway maps for in-depth experimental data analysis. In: 2012 IEEE Symposium on Biological Data Visualization (BioVis), pp. 107–114. IEEE (2012)

63. Turkay, C., Lex, A., Streit, M., Pfister, H., Hauser, H.: Characterizing cancer subtypes using dual analysis in caleydo stratomex. IEEE Computer Graphics and Applications 34(2), 38–47 (2014)

64. May, T., Kohlhammer, J.: Towards closing the analysis gap: Visual generation of decision supporting schemes from raw data. In: Computer Graphics Forum, vol. 27, pp. 911–918. Wiley Online Library (2008)

65. May, T., Bannach, A., Davey, J., Ruppert, T., Kohlhammer, J.: Guiding feature subset selection with an interactive visualization. In: 2011 IEEE Conference on Visual Analytics Science and Technology (VAST), pp. 111–120. IEEE (2011)

66. Younesy, H., Nielsen, C.B., Möller, T., Alder, O., Cullum, R., Lorincz, M.C., Karimi, M.M., Jones, S.J.: An interactive analysis and exploration tool for epigenomic data. In: Computer Graphics Forum, vol. 32, pp. 91–100. Wiley Online Library (2013)

67. Grottel, S., Reina, G., Vrabec, J., Ertl, T.: Visual verification and analysis of cluster detection for molecular dynamics. IEEE Transactions on Visualization and Computer Graphics 13(6), 1624–1631 (2007)

68. Dietzsch, J., Gehlenborg, N., Nieselt, K.: Mayday-a microarray data analysis workbench. Bioinformatics 22(8), 1010–1012 (2006)

69. Seo, J., Shneiderman, B.: Interactively exploring hierarchical clustering results. IEEE Computer 35(7), 80–86 (2002)

70. Guo, Z., Ward, M.O., Rundensteiner, E.A.: Model space visualization for multivariate linear trend discovery. In: Proc. IEEE Symp. Visual Analytics Science and Technology VAST 2009, pp. 75–82 (2009)

71. Kandogan, E.: Just-in-time annotation of clusters, outliers, and trends in point-based data visualizations. In: 2012 IEEE Conference on Visual Analytics Science and Technology (VAST), pp. 73–82. IEEE (2012)

72. Rinzivillo, S., Pedreschi, D., Nanni, M., Giannotti, F., Andrienko, N., Andrienko, G.: Visually driven analysis of movement data by progressive clustering. Information Visualization 7(3), 225–239 (2008)

73. Schreck, T., Bernard, J., Tekusova, T., Kohlhammer, J.: Visual cluster analysis of trajectory data with interactive Kohonen Maps. In: IEEE Symposium on Visual Analytics Science and Technology, VAST 2008, pp. 3–10 (2008)

74. Rasmussen, M., Karypis, G.: gCLUTO–An Interactive Clustering, Visualization, and Analysis System., University of Minnesota, Department of Computer Science and Engineering, CSE. Technical report, UMN Technical Report: TR (2004)

75. Ahmed, Z., Weaver, C.: An Adaptive Parameter Space-Filling Algorithm for Highly Interactive Cluster Exploration. In: Procedings of IEEE Symposium on Visual Analytics Science and Technology, VAST (2012)

76. Rubel, O., Weber, G., Huang, M.Y., Bethel, E., Biggin, M., Fowlkes, C., Luengo Hendriks, C., Keranen, S., Eisen, M., Knowles, D., Malik, J., Hagen, H., Hamann, B.: Integrating data clustering and visualization for the analysis of 3D gene expression data. IEEE/ACM Transactions on Computational Biology and Bioinformatics 7(1), 64–79 (2010)

77. Turkay, C., Parulek, J., Reuter, N., Hauser, H.: Interactive visual analysis of temporal cluster structures. Computer Graphics Forum 30(3), 711–720 (2011)

78. Parulek, J., Turkay, C., Reuter, N., Viola, I.: Visual cavity analysis in molecular simulations. BMC Bioinformatics 14(19), 1–15 (2013)

79. Turkay, C., Parulek, J., Reuter, N., Hauser, H.: Integrating cluster formation and cluster evaluation in interactive visual analysis. In: Proceedings of the 27th Spring Conference on Computer Graphics, pp. 77–86. ACM (2011)

80. Choo, J., Lee, H., Kihm, J., Park, H.: ivisclassifier: An interactive visual analytics system for classification based on supervised dimension reduction. In: 2010 IEEE Symposium on Visual Analytics Science and Technology (VAST), pp. 27–34. IEEE (2010)
81. Krzywinski, M., Schein, J., Birol, İ., Connors, J., Gascoyne, R., Horsman, D., Jones, S.J., Marra, M.A.: Circos: An information aesthetic for comparative genomics. Genome Research 19(9), 1639–1645 (2009)
82. Karr, J.R., Sanghvi, J.C., Macklin, D.N., Gutschow, M.V., Jacobs, J.M., Bolival Jr., B., Assad-Garcia, N., Glass, J.I., Covert, M.W.: A whole-cell computational model predicts phenotype from genotype. Cell 150(2), 389–401 (2012)
83. Meyer, M., Munzner, T., Pfister, H.: Mizbee: A multiscale synteny browser. IEEE Transactions on Visualization and Computer Graphics 15(6), 897–904 (2009)
84. Piringer, H., Berger, W., Krasser, J.: Hypermoval: Interactive visual validation of regression models for real-time simulation. In: Proceedings of the 12th Eurographics / IEEE - VGTC Conference on Visualization. EuroVis 2010, pp. 983–992. Eurographics Association, Aire-la-Ville (2010)
85. Muhlbacher, T., Piringer, H.: A partition-based framework for building and validating regression models. IEEE Transactions on Visualization and Computer Graphics 19(12), 1962–1971 (2013)
86. Booshehrian, M., Möller, T., Peterman, R.M., Munzner, T.: Vismon: Facilitating analysis of trade-offs, uncertainty, and sensitivity in fisheries management decision making. In: Computer Graphics Forum, vol. 31, pp. 1235–1244. Wiley Online Library (2012)
87. Meyer, M., Wong, B., Styczynski, M., Munzner, T., Pfister, H.: Pathline: A tool for comparative functional genomics. In: Computer Graphics Forum, vol. 29, pp. 1043–1052. Wiley Online Library (2010)
88. Elmqvist, N., Dragicevic, P., Fekete, J.: Rolling the dice: Multidimensional visual exploration using scatterplot matrix navigation. IEEE Transactions on Visualization and Computer Graphics 14(6), 1539–1148 (2008)
89. Yang, J., Ward, M.O., Rundensteiner, E.A., Huang, S.: Visual hierarchical dimension reduction for exploration of high dimensional datasets. In: VISSYM 2003: Proceedings of the Symposium on Data Visualisation 2003, pp. 19–28 (2003)
90. Berger, W., Piringer, H., Filzmoser, P., Gröller, E.: Uncertainty-aware exploration of continuous parameter spaces using multivariate prediction. Computer Graphics Forum 30(3), 911–920 (2011)
91. Malik, A., Maciejewski, R., Elmqvist, N., Jang, Y., Ebert, D.S., Huang, W.: A correlative analysis process in a visual analytics environment. In: 2012 IEEE Conference on Visual Analytics Science and Technology (VAST), pp. 33–42. IEEE (2012)
92. Turkay, C., Lundervold, A., Lundervold, A., Hauser, H.: Representative factor generation for the interactive visual analysis of high-dimensional data. IEEE Transactions on Visualization and Computer Graphics 18(12), 2621–2630 (2012)
93. Mirkin, B.: Core Concepts in Data Analysis: Summarization, Correlation and Visualization. Springer (2011)
94. Procter, J.B., Thompson, J., Letunic, I., Creevey, C., Jossinet, F., Barton, G.J.: Visualization of multiple alignments, phylogenies and gene family evolution. Nature Methods 7, S16–S25 (2010)
95. Otasek, D., Pastrello, C., Holzinger, A., Jurisica, I.: Visual Data Mining: Effective Exploration of the Biological Universe. In: Holzinger, A., Jurisica, I. (eds.) Knowledge Discovery and Data Mining. LNCS, vol. 8401, pp. 19–34. Springer, Heidelberg (2014)

96. Mueller, H., Reihs, R., Zatloukal, K., Holzinger, A.: Analysis of biomedical data with multilevel glyphs. BMC Bioinformatics 15(suppl. 6), S5 (2014)

97. Tan, P., Steinbach, M., Kumar, V.: Introduction to data mining. Pearson Addison Wesley, Boston (2006)

98. van den Elzen, S., van Wijk, J.J.: Baobabview: Interactive construction and analysis of decision trees. In: 2011 IEEE Conference on Visual Analytics Science and Technology (VAST), pp. 151–160. IEEE (2011)

99. Hair, J., Anderson, R.: Multivariate data analysis. Prentice Hall (2010)

100. Secrier, M., Schneider, R.: Visualizing time-related data in biology, a review. Briefings in Bioinformatics, bbt021 (2013)

101. Chen, C.: Top 10 unsolved information visualization problems. IEEE Computer Graphics and Applications 25(4), 12–16 (2005)

102. Jeanquartier, F., Holzinger, A.: On Visual Analytics And Evaluation In Cell Physiology: A Case Study. In: Cuzzocrea, A., Kittl, C., Simos, D.E., Weippl, E., Xu, L. (eds.) CD-ARES 2013. LNCS, vol. 8127, pp. 495–502. Springer, Heidelberg (2013)

103. Holzinger, A.: Usability engineering methods for software developers. Communications of the ACM 48(1), 71–74 (2005)

104. Kehrer, J., Hauser, H.: Visualization and visual analysis of multifaceted scientific data: A survey. IEEE Transactions on Visualization and Computer Graphics 19(3), 495–513 (2013)

105. Matkovic, K., Gracanin, D., Jelovic, M., Hauser, H.: Interactive visual steering-rapid visual prototyping of a common rail injection system. IEEE Transactions on Visualization and Computer Graphics 14(6), 1699–1706 (2008)

106. Beale, R.: Supporting serendipity: Using ambient intelligence to augment user exploration for data mining and web browsing. International Journal of Human-Computer Studies 65(5), 421–433 (2007)

107. Holzinger, A., Kickmeier-Rust, M., Albert, D.: Dynamic media in computer science education; content complexity and learning performance: Is less more? Educational Technology & Society 11(1), 279–290 (2008)

108. Ceglar, A., Roddick, J.F., Calder, P.: Guiding knowledge discovery through interactive data mining. Managing Data Mining Technologies in Organizations: Techniques and Applications, 45–87 (2003)

109. Chau, D.H., Myers, B., Faulring, A.: What to do when search fails: finding information by association. In: Proceeding of the Twenty-Sixth Annual SIGCHI Conference on Human Factors in Computing Systems, pp. 999–1008. ACM (2008)

110. Olshausen, B.A., Anderson, C.H., Vanessen, D.C.: A neurobiological model of visual-attention and invariant pattern-recognition based on dynamic routing of information. Journal of Neuroscience 13(11), 4700–4719 (1993)

111. Chandola, V., Banerjee, A., Kumar, V.: Anomaly detection: A survey. ACM Computing Surveys (CSUR) 41(3), 15 (2009)

112. Edelsbrunner, H., Harer, J.L.: Computational Topology: An Introduction. American Mathematical Society, Providence (2010)

113. Holzinger, A.: On topological data mining. In: Holzinger, A., Jurisica, I. (eds.) Knowledge Discovery and Data Mining. LNCS, vol. 8401, pp. 331–356. Springer, Heidelberg (2014)

114. Bremer, P.T., Pascucci, V., Hamann, B.: Maximizing Adaptivity in Hierarchical Topological Models Using Cancellation Trees, pp. 1–18. Springer (2009)

# A Policy-Based Cleansing and Integration Framework for Labour and Healthcare Data

Roberto Boselli[1,2], Mirko Cesarini[1,2], Fabio Mercorio[2], and Mario Mezzanzanica[1,2]

[1] Department of Statistics and Quantitative Methods - University of Milano Bicocca, Milan, Italy
[2] CRISP Research Centre - University of Milano Bicocca, Milan, Italy
{firstname.lastname}@unimib.it

**Abstract.** Large amounts of data are collected by public administrations and healthcare organizations, the integration of the data scattered in several information systems can facilitate the comprehension of complex scenarios and support the activities of decision makers.

Unfortunately, the quality of information system archives is very poor, as widely stated by the existing literature. Data cleansing is one of the most frequently used data improvement technique. Data can be cleansed in several ways, the optimal choice however is strictly dependent on the integration and analysis processes to be performed. Therefore, the design of a data analysis process should consider in a holistic way the data integration, cleansing, and analysis activities. However, in the existing literature, the data integration and cleansing issues have been mostly addressed in isolation.

In this paper we describe how a model based cleansing framework is extended to address also integration activities. The combined approach facilitates the rapid prototyping, development, and evaluation of data pre-processing activities. Furthermore, the combined use of formal methods and visualization techniques strongly empower the data analyst which can effectively evaluate how cleansing and integration activities can affect the data analysis. An example focusing on labour and healthcare data integration is showed.

**Keywords:** Data Quality, Data Integration, Model-based Reasoning, Data Visualisation.

## 1 Introduction and Motivation

Organizations and public administrations have been collecting huge amount of data in the last years. Several public services and business processes make use of ICT (Information and Communication Technologies) e.g., the back-office activities are supported by Information Systems, coordination information are exchanged using networked systems, several services and goods are purchased using the Web. The ICT have opened the frontiers for collecting and managing data in an unforeseeable manner. Methodologies, infrastructures, and tools for handling and analysing huge amount of data are now available. Such data can be used to deeply describe and understand social, economic, and business phenomena.

A. Holzinger, I. Jurisica (Eds.): Knowledge Discovery and Data Mining, LNCS 8401, pp. 141–168, 2014.

Unfortunately, turning those data into information useful for decision making still represents a challenging task. Focusing on information systems, their data quality is frequently very poor [1] and, due to the "garbage in, garbage out" principle, dirty data strongly affect the information derived from them e.g., see [2]. The causes of such poor data quality are not further investigated in this paper, they are well described in the literature, the interested reader can see [3–5]. Data cleansing is frequently performed in analytical contexts to address the data quality issues, since accessing the real data or alternative and trusted data sources is rarely feasible. Indeed, as remarked in [6] while introducing the KDD process, "the value of storing volumes of data depends on our ability to extract useful reports, spot events and trends, support decisions and policy based on statistical analysis and inference." In the last years, the data quality improvement and analysis techniques have become an essential part of the KDD process as they contribute to guarantee the believability of the overall knowledge process, making the reasoning over data a very significant concern [7–11]. In this paper we aim to draw the attention to data quality and integration in the context of KDD.

Furthermore, several data sources should be considered to obtain a holistic vision of a phenomenon. However the data quality issues of the involved archives may negatively affect each other, complicating even more the scenario. An example is provided to clarify such mutual interaction.

*A Motivating Example.* The relationships between the working conditions and some illnesses (especially mental illness) can be investigated using two archives: a medical registry and a labour administrative archive. The latter records job start and cessation dates while the former stores data about drug prescriptions used to treat mental illnesses. The data are collected for administrative purposes by different public administrations who agree to share their data.

An example of the labour archive content is reported in Table 1. A data quality examination on the labour data is shortly introduced. A rule can be inferred by the country law and common practice: an employer can't have more than one full time contract active at the same time.

The reader would notice that the working history reported in Table 1 is inconsistent with respect to the semantic just introduced: a Full Time Cessation is missing for the contract started by *event 03*. A typical cleansing approach would add a Full Time Cessation event in a date between *event 03* and *event 04*.

**Table 1.** An example of data describing the working career of a person

| Event # | Event Type | Employer-ID | Date |
|---------|------------|-------------|------|
| 01 | Part Time Start | Firm 1 | $12^{th}$/01/2010 |
| 02 | Part Time Cessation | Firm 1 | $31^{st}$/03/2011 |
| 03 | Full Time Start | Firm 2 | $1^{st}$/04/2011 |
| 04 | Full Time Start | Firm 3 | $1^{st}$/10/2012 |
| 05 | Full Time Cessation | Firm 3 | $1^{st}$/06/2013 |
| ... | ... | ... | ... |

**Table 2.** Data describing the drug prescription about a mental illness

| Event # | Drug Description | Quantity | Date |
|---------|------------------|----------|------|
| 01 | Drug X | ... | $9^{th}$/01/2012 |
| 02 | Drug X | ... | $13^{th}$/02/2012 |
| 03 | Drug X | ... | $12^{th}$/03/2012 |
| 04 | Drug X | ... | $9^{th}$/04/2012 |
| ... | ... | ... | ... |

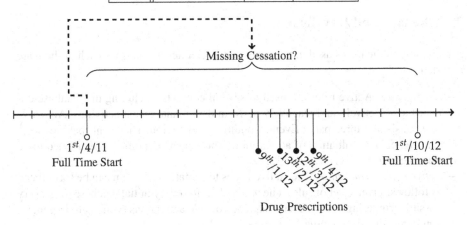

**Fig. 1.** A timeline showing the possible range of dates for a missing Full Time Cessation Event

Unfortunately the *corrections* performed on a single data source can affect the other archives. Let us suppose that the labour archive content just introduced should be integrated with data describing drug prescriptions for mental illness. Table 2 reports the drug prescriptions of the same person whose career has been described in Table 1. The reader can see that the person started receiving precriptions from $9^{th}$/01/2012. Let us suppose a researcher is investigating the relationships (if any) between unemployment and mental illness. In such a case, the Full Time Cessation event to be added by the cleansing procedure is paramount. Depending on the date chosen, the person may be considered receiving the treatment as a worker or as an unemployed, as showed in Figure 1. Considering the time slot where the cessation can be placed, the unemployment can start long before or far after the treatment. The reader may argue that a single inconsistency may be fixed by accessing the real data (e.g., by interviewing the person). Unfortunately, these data are frequently provided in anonymised version, and even when contact details were available, similar problems can occur a lot of times making the interview option unfeasible.

*Research Perspective and Goal.* This paper draws on a previous work [12] where a model based framework for data cleansing can be customized specifying a cleansing policy. The (already) existing framework recognises the actual data inconsistencies and for each of them identifies the set of possible corrections, then a policy is used to select the correction to perform. This paper outlines how the framework can be extended to perform also data integration, taking into account the mutual influences between data cleansing and data integration tasks. The extended framework empowers the data analysts with a swiss army knife that can be used to evaluate different cleansing policies and how they impact on the analysis performed on data coming from several sources. The extended framework is discussed in the context of a real world case where data coming from heterogeneous sources (labour and healthcare archives) have to be cleansed, integrated, and analysed.

## 2  Glossary and Key Terms

A taxonomy of the terms used in the paper and a brief descriptions for each of them are reported.

- *Active rules*. Active rules are used in several contexts (including the database domain) to selectively and reactively perform data management activities. An active rule consists of three parts: Event, Condition and Action. The event specifies what can trigger the evaluation of a condition. Then, if the condition is evaluated to be true, the action is performed [13, 14].
- *Active rules termination*. The Active Rules termination problem can be formulated as follows: given a set of rules, check whether, for every initial database (and every possible triggering event), every sequence of rule activations (which are in general non-deterministic) eventually terminates [15].
- *AI Complete Problem* (Artificial Intelligence Complete Problem). Solving an AI-complete problem is equivalent to solving the entire AI problem i.e., producing a generally intelligent computer program that can pass the Turing Test [16]. The latter test is successful if a human interrogator cannot tell whether the responses are returned from a person or not [17].
- *Business Rules*. Business rules are constraints that define conditions which must hold true in specified situations [18]. They are used in the data quality domain to identify data inconsistencies. E.g., in a country where the minimal age for getting a driving license is 18 years old, a business rule can be derived and used to identify the inconsistent records of a driving license owners database. An inconsistent record example is the following: name="Laura" and age="4".
- *Data Cleansing* (or data cleaning, or data scrubbing). According to [19] Real-word data tend to be incomplete, noisy, and inconsistent. Data cleansing routines attempt to fill in missing values, smooth out noise, identify outliers, correct inconsistencies, and improve data to address quality issues.
- *Data Consistency* is a quality dimension which refer to the violation of semantic rules defined over (a set of) data items [5] e.g., items can be tuples of relational tables or records in a file.
- *Data Fusion* is the last step of a data integration proces [20] where the data coming from heterogeneous sources are combined and fused into a single representation, while duplicate and inconsistencies in the data are resolved. This is also called *data extensional integration* in the database domain [21].
- *Data Integration* is the problem of combining data residing at different sources, and providing the user with a unified view of these data [22–25].

- *Dataspace* systems seek to provide a unified view of several data sources that aim to overcome some of the problems encountered in traditional data integration systems. The aim is to reduce the integration effort by providing base functionality over all data sources e.g., key-word search (similar to that provided by existing desktop search systems) [26]. In contrast with other information-integration systems, dataspaces systems offer best-effort answers before complete semantic mappings are provided to the system [27]. When more sophisticated operations are required, such as relational-style queries or data mining then additional effort can be applied, postponing the labor-intensive aspects of data integration until they are absolutely needed [26].
- *Data Quality Dimensions*. Data quality can be intuitively characterized as fitness for use [28]. Some specific quality dimensions have been identified to fully understand the concept, the more common are accuracy, completeness, currency and consistency as discussed by [29], Accuracy is a measure of the distance between the data value and the value which is considered correct. Completeness measures "the extent to which data are of sufficient breadth, depth and scope for the task at hand" [29, 30]. The percentage of null values in a column table is an example of (in)completeness. Currency measures how promptly data are updated [29]. Consistency was introduced in the item *data consistency* of this glossary.
- *Extraction-Transformation-Loading* (ETL) is the process responsible for the extraction of data from several sources, their cleansing, customization and insertion into a destination repository [31] which very frequently is a data warehouse. In the data warehouse field the term ETL is used to refer both to the process, tools, and software used.
- *Functional Dependency* (FD), *Conditional Functional dependency* (CFD). A Functional Dependency is a constraint between two sets of attributes in a database relation [32]. Traditional FDs are to hold on all the tuples in a relation while CFDs [33] are supposed to hold only for the subset of tuples matching a given data pattern. CFDs can be used for data cleansing over relational data [34].
- *Global-as-View* (GaV) is an approach for data integration, it requires the global schema to be expressed in terms of the data sources [22] i.e., the global schema is a view of the local schemata.
- *Linked Data*. The term linked data refers to a set of best practices for publishing and connecting structured data on the web, specifically to create typed links between data from different sources. [27].
- *Local-as-View* (LaV) is an approach for data integration where the global schema is specified independently from the sources and every source is defined as a view over the global schema [22].
- *Mediator/Wrapper*. Most of the works focusing on data integration conceptually refer to a mediator/wrapper based architecture as described in [35, 36]. A mediator can be described as a software module that performs the tasks of query submission, planning, decomposition and results integration. Wrappers (also called translators) allow for the description of source contents and allow user queries to be converted into source-specific queries [36].
- *Ontology*. While there are many definitions of what an ontology is [37], the common thread in these definitions is that an ontology is some formal description of

a domain of discourse, intended for sharing among different applications, and expressed in a language that can be used for reasoning [38].

- *Schema integration* in a database is the activity of integrating the schemas of existing databases into a global, unified schema [39].
- *Schema mapping problem* is a problem where a source (legacy) database is mapped into a different, but fixed, target schema. Schema mapping involves the discovery of a query or set of queries that transform the source data into the new structure [40].

## 3   State-of-the-Art

The proliferation of information sources and the increasing volumes of data available from information systems provides challenges and opportunities to several research communities. The task of extracting, cleaning, and reconciling data coming from multiple sources requires large amounts of effort and is often underestimated by the scientific and the research community as discussed by [41].

Most researchers agree that quality of data archives is frequently poor, and because of the "garbage in, garbage out" principle, dirty data can have unpredictable effects on the information derived from them, as noted by [42–47]. A few real-life causes of poor data quality are described in the following (the examples are not exhaustive and focus on the medicine and biomedical field).

- The medical data is generally collected for patient-care purposes and research is only a secondary consideration. As a result, medical databases contain many features that create problems for the data mining tools and techniques [48].
- Patient records collected for diagnosis and prognosis are characterised by their incompleteness (missing parameter values), incorrectness (systematic or random noise in the data), sparseness (few or non-representable patient records), and inexactness (inappropriate selection of parameters for the given task) [49].
- Considering microarray gene expression data, microarrays often miss to produce data for a considerable amount of genes, therefore missing values imputation is required [50] before performing the following step of data analysis.

The need for data integration and data quality improvement activities, the intrinsic difficulties os such tasks, and the call for tools and methodologies has been extensively acknowledged in the literature e.g., [50–56]. Furthermore, the data quality and integration techniques have become an essential part of the KDD process, making the reasoning over data very significant concern [7–11].

Although several works call for a holistic approach dealing with data integration and data quality issues, the two problems have been mostly addressed in isolation in the scientific literature. E.g., data mining algorithms implicitly assume data to originate from a single source although very frequently several ones are considered [50]. Different formats and different semantics in disparate data sources require semantic integration effort, which form long-standing challenges for the database community [57]. Researchers and practitioners in the fields of databases and information integration have produced a large body of research to facilitate interoperability between different systems [38], an overview of the state of the art is proved in subsection 3.1.

Data quality problems have been addressed in several sectors, including the database community too, a survey is presented in Subsection 3.2. The combined data cleansing and integration approach described in this paper aims to build a bridge between the data integration and data quality research fields.

## 3.1  Data Integration

*Data integration* is the problem of combining data residing at different sources, and providing the user with a unified view of these data [22–25]. The relevant theoretical issues in data integration are outlined in [22]. The goal of information integration is to enable rapid development of new applications requiring information from multiple sources. This simple goal hides many challenges: identifying the best data sources to use; creating an appropriate interface to (or schema for) the integrated data; how to query diverse sources with differing capabilities; how to deal with uncertainty; how to identify the same object in different data sources [58].

In the classical data integration scenario, the main elements are: a source database schema (or schemas), a target schema, a collection of schema mappings relating source and target schemas, and a source database instance (or instances) [59].

A three-steps data integration process is described in [20], the identified steps are: *Schema Mapping*, *Duplicate Detection*, and *Data Fusion*.

- *Schema Mapping* is the detection of equivalent schema elements in different sources to turn the data into a common representation.
  Schema mapping is a very complex task, it is an Artificial Intelligence Complete (AI-Complete) problem [60] i.e., human intelligence is strongly required. In such a context there is a call to reduce the amount of human effort and to speed up the creation of integrated solutions e.g., [40,61]. Furthermore, there is little support for iteration between schema-level and data-level tasks in the integration process [61]. According to [22] two basic approaches for specifying the mapping in a data integration system have been proposed in the literature, called local-as-view (LaV), and global-as-view (GaV), respectively [25] and [23]. According to [62], the GaV integration model expresses a global schema as views of local schemata, whereas LaV expresses local schemata as views on the global schema. In both cases, the effort required to create the mappings between the sources and the unified schema is a bottleneck in setting up a data integration application.
- *Duplicate Detection* focuses on identifying the multiple representations of the same real-world objects. Duplicate detection will be detailed in Section 3.2.
- In *Data Fusion*, the duplicate representations are combined and fused into a single representation while inconsistencies in the data are resolved.
  In [62] the strategies for handling the data fusion conflicts are outlined and the existing tools and frameworks are classified according to the strategy they can adopt [1]. A survey on how existing tools and frameworks manage the previously re-

---

[1] The possible options are: 1) *Conflict ignoring* strategies do not make a decision and sometimes the data management processes are not even aware of data conflicts; 2) *Conflict avoiding* strategies handle conflicting data by applying a general decision equally to all data, such as preferring data from a special source; 3) *Conflict resolution* strategies do regard all the data and each conflict is managed appropriately.

ported strategies is presented in [62], as the authors state, user defined aggregation functions are supported by database management systems only in a very limited way, if at all. E.g., the aggregation functions (max, min, sum, count, etc.) of the SQL standard allow only for limited possibilities in resolving conflicts, the FraQL project [63–65] addresses the problem by defining four additional 2-parameter aggregation functions, each aggregating one column depending on the values of another column.

Most of the works focusing on data integration either assume the integrated data to be materialized in a target repository or refer to a *mediator*/*wrapper* based architecture as described in [35, 36]. A *mediator* can be described as a software module that performs the tasks of query submission, planning, decomposition and results integration, *wrappers* (also called translators) describe source contents and allow user queries to be converted into source-specific queries [36].

Several other approaches can be used to manage data originating from several sources. The approaches listed next are discussed in [58], the considerations previously outlined on schema mapping, duplicate detection, and data fusion can also be extended to the next approaches (when applicable).

- *Materialization*. The result of data integration is created and stored. Materialization can be achieved through:
  - *ETL* (Extract/Transform/Load) jobs which extract data from one or more data sources, transform them and then store the result in a destination repository.
  - *Replication* which makes and maintains a copy of data, often differentially by reading database log files.
  - *Caching* which captures query results for future reuse.
- *Federation* creates a virtual representation of the integrated datasets.
- *Indexing*/*Search* creates a single index over the data being integrated, which will be used to dynamically identify and fetch relevant documents at the user's request.

In a *Materialization* or *Federation* approach, the data system has to know the precise relationships between the terms used in each data schema (both local and global) before any services can be provided. As a result, a significant up-front effort is required in order to set up an integrated system [26]. However, users often need only base functionalities over all the involved data sources [66] and not full integration. Therefore, researchers have been investigating on lightweight approaches in the past years.

The works on *Indexing*/*Search* [41, 67] started as a way to find unstructured information, but they rapidly shifted to information integration [68]. *Search* poses an imprecise query to one or more sources, and returns a ranked list of results. Nevertheless, *search* can be "good enough" for integration scenarios, while requiring much less work than traditional integration [58].

In the streamline of lightweight systems, the DataSpace Systems and DataSpace Support Platforms (DSSPs) [26] have been proposed. The goal of dataspace support is to provide base functionality over all data sources e.g., a DSSP can provide key-word search over all of its data sources (similar to that provided by existing desktop search systems). When more sophisticated operations are required, such as relational style queries or data mining, then additional effort can be applied, postponing the labor-intensive aspects of data integration until they are absolutely needed [26]. In contrast with other information-integration systems, dataspaces systems offer best-effort answers before complete semantic mappings are provided to the system [27].

The *linked data* and the *web of data* research fields seek to pursue on a global scale the same goals of the dataspace works previously outlined, relying on a specific set of web standards [27] e.g., ontologies. Ontologies have been investigated to address semantic heterogeneity in structured data [38], unfortunately most researchers agree that automatic mapping between ontologies is far from being achieved [38]. In [69] a detailed discussion is reported on the uses of ontologies, their differences from database schemas, and the semantic integration challenges to be faced.

In [70] the authors propose to use description logic to deal with data integration in a context where the global view is expressed using an ontology. Since the use of a full-fledged expressive description logic is infeasible due to the high computational complexity, the authors of [70] work on identifying a restricted language balancing expressive power and computational complexity.

## 3.2 Data Quality

The data quality analysis and improvement tasks have been the focus of a large body of research in different domains, that involve statisticians, mathematicians and computer scientists, working in close cooperation with application domain experts, each one focusing on its own perspective [8, 71].

To give a few examples, statisticians always fought for better data quality by applying: data mining and machine learning techniques for data edits (also known as data imputation) [72–74], probabilistic record linkage [75–77], and error detection [78, 79]. On the other side, computer scientists developed algorithms and tools to ensure data correctness by paying attention to the whole Knowledge Discovery process, from the collection or entry stage to data visualisation [42, 80–82], exploiting both hard and soft computing techniques, see e.g. [45, 83–85].

The quality improving task in the literature has been frequently associated with the data *cleansing* (or *cleaning*) problem, which basically consists in the identification of a set of activities to cleanse a dirty dataset. In this regard, common technique are:

- *record linkage* (also known as *object identification, record matching, merge-purge problem, duplicate detection*) which aims to bring together corresponding records from two or more data sources (the purpose is to link the data to a corresponding higher quality version and to compare them [78]) or to find duplicates within the same source.
- dealing with *missing data*, four conventional approaches are described in [86] however, both of them fail to take into account the patterns of missing data and the impact on the data mining results.
- an alternative approach uses *Business Rules* identified by domain experts to cleanse the dirty data. The cleansing procedures can be implemented in SQL or in other tool specific languages.

A lot of works have been focusing on *constraint-based data repair* for identifying errors by exploiting FDs (Functional Dependencies). Two approaches based on FDs are *database repair* [87, 88] and *consistent query answering* [83, 89]. The former aims to find a *repair* (namely a database instance that satisfies integrity constraints) that minimally differs from the original (inconsistent) one. The latter approach tries to compute *consistent query answers* in response to a query, namely answers that are true in every repair of the given database, but the source data is not fixed. Unfortunately, finding consistent answers to aggregate queries is a NP-complete problem already using two (or more) FDs [83, 84]. To mitigate this problem, recently a number of works have exploited heuristics to find a database repair, as [90–92]. They seem to be very promising approaches, even though their effectiveness have not been evaluated on real-world domains.

It is worth noting that the FDs expressiveness may be not able to specify constraints on longitudinal or historical data [93–95]. To give a few examples, in [93] Vardi motivates the usefulness of formal systems in databases by observing that FDs are only a fragment of the first-order logic used in formal methods. Furthermore, as observed in [96], even though FDs allow one to detect the presence of errors, they have a limited usefulness since they fall short of guiding one in correcting the errors.

Recently the NADEEF [97] and LLUNATIC [98] tools have been developed for unifying the most used cleansing and analysis solutions by both academy and industry through variants of FDs. As [97] argue, the consistency requirements are usually defined on either a single tuple, two tuples or a set of tuples. While the first two classes can be modelled through FDs and their variants, the latter class of quality constraints requires reasoning with a (finite but not bounded) set of data items over time as the case of longitudinal data, and this makes the exploration-based technique (as Model Checking and Planning) a good candidate for that task [99].

This paper deals with data quality issues modelled in terms of *consistency* by mapping both the data dynamics and the consistency constraints over a Finite State System, then using model checking to verify them. Finite State Systems in the context of data (and Formal Methods in general) have been investigated in the areas of *Databases* and *Artificial Intelligence*. The work in [94] basically encodes bounded database history over Büchi automata to check temporal constraints. The purpose of [94] is to build an efficient framework for performing temporal queries on databases, but no attention is paid to the data quality issues. Indeed, the author declares that the work focuses on transaction time databases and it is assumed that the stored data *exactly* correspond to the real world ones.

Formal verification techniques were applied to databases with the aim to prove the termination of triggers by exploiting both *explicit* model checking [100] and *symbolic* techniques [101]. The use of CTL model checking has been investigated for semistructured data retrieval, whether XML based [102] or web based [103] as well as to solve queries on semistructured data [103–105].

A method for addressing the genomic nomenclature problem by using phylogenetic tools along with the BIO-AJAX data cleaning framework [106] is proposed in [107]. A framework for the application of data mining tools to data cleaning in the biological domain has been presented [108]. They focused on tuple constraints and functional dependencies detection in representative biological databases by means of association rule mining. By analysing association rules they can deduce not only constraints and dependencies (which provide structural knowledge on a dataset) but also the anomalies in the system, which could be errors or interesting information to highlight to domain experts [109].

An XML-based active rule language named BioRL for declarative specification of biological semantics was presented in [14]. In [110], heterogeneous biological data in several files and relational databases were converted into XML under a unified XML Schema using XML-based active rules. Unfortunately, active rules termination decidability can be guaranteed only in special cases or restrictions of the language [15].

It is widely recognized that data visual exploration play a key role in the knowledge discovery process, since it provides an effective understanding of the data and of the information managed [81]. To this aim, a number of data visualisation techniques are currently explored in several contexts, from healthcare to management information systems e.g., [82, 111–113]. Data visualization can be very helpful for data quality and integration tasks.

Finally it is worth of mentioning the Knodwat tool [114] i.e., a very promising framework for testing KDD methods in the context of Biomedical data.

# 4 Preliminaries

Huge amounts of data describing people behaviours are collected by the Information Systems of enterprises and organizations. Such data often have an unexpressed informative power, indeed the study of relations and correlations among them allows domain experts to understand the evolution of subtended behaviours or phenomena over time, as recently outlined by [115–118]. Among the time-related data, the *longitudinal data* (i.e., repeated observations of a given subject, object or phenomena at distinct time points) have received much attention from several academic research communities as they are well-suited to model many real-world instances, including labour and healthcare domains, see, e.g. [114, 115, 118–121].

In such a context graphs or tree formalisms, which are exploited to model *weakly-structured* data, are deemed also appropriate to model the expected data behaviour, that formalise how the data should evolve over time. In this regard, [115] has recently clarified that a relationship exists between weakly-structured data and time-related data. Namely, let $Y(t)$ be an ordered sequence of observed data, e.g., subject data sampled at different time $t \in T$, the observed data $Y(t)$ are weakly structured if and only if the trajectory of $Y(t)$ resembles a random walk (on a graph).

## 4.1 Model-Based Universal Cleansing

The longitudinal data evolution can be described, formalised, and checked using the framework presented in [122]. Intuitively, let us consider an events sequence $\epsilon = e_1, e_2, \ldots, e_n$. Each event $e_i$ will contain a number of observation variables whose evaluation can be used to determine a snapshot of the subject's *state* at time point $i$, namely $s_i$. Then, each further event $e_{i+1}$ may change the value of one or more state variables of $s_i$, generating a new state[2] $s_{i+1}$. More generally, a sequence of $n$ <state,event> pairs $\pi = s_1 e_1 \ldots s_n e_n$ determines a *trajectory* describing the subject behaviour during the time. In [12, 122] a well-known graph-based formalism, namely Finite State Systems (FSS), has been used to model the data behaviour, then the model-checking algorithms have been used to verify and cleanse the dirty data. Specifically, the UP-Murphi tool [123] has been used. More precisely, once a trajectory has been modelled through an FSS, the authors evaluate if it follows an *allowed* behaviour (with respect to the model) or not. Although UPMurphi is a model-checking-based planner, it has proved its effectiveness in dealing with several AI planning problems in both deterministic and non-deterministic domains (see. e.g., [124–130]) as well as in the KDD context [12, 99, 131, 132].

*Universal Cleanser (UC).* More recently, this approach has been enhanced to identify the corrective events able to cleanse an inconsistent dataset formalised in both AI Planning and Model Checking paradigms respectively [131, 132]. The authors focus on the inconsistency data quality dimension, to clarify the matter, let us consider an inconsistent event sequence having an event $e_i$ that leads to an inconsistent state $s_j$ when applied on a state $s_i$. Intuitively, a *cleansing event sequence* represents an alternative trajectory leading the subject's state from $s_i$ to a state where the event $e_i$ can be applied (without violating the consistency rules).

Informally speaking, the *Universal Cleanser* is a table which summarises, for each *pair* <state, event> leading to an inconsistent state, the set $E'$ of *all* the feasible cleansing event sequences. Note that the UC represents a repository of *all* the cleansing interventions. As a consequence, when several interventions are available, a *policy* is required to identify the one to perform, taking into account the data analysis purposes.

The UC has been considered in this work since it presents some relevant characteristics: (1) it is computed off-line only once. (2) It is *data-independent* since, once the UC has been synthesised, it can be used to cleanse *any* dataset conforming to the model. Finally, (3) it is *policy-dependent* since the cleansed results may vary as the policy varies.

## 5    The Labour and Healthcare Datasets

In the following we introduce the main elements of two administrative datasets, namely the *Labour* and the *Healthcare* datasets, which are actually supported within a Research Project granted by the CRISP institute [3].

The methodology proposed in this paper is being used in a project performed in collaboration with a European country (regional) public administration.The aim is to jointly use the data collected for administrative purposes about employment contracts and drug prescriptions. The two archives can describe in detail both the working and the health history of the reference area population.

---

[2] The term "state" here is considered in terms of a value assignment to a set of finite-domain state variables.

[3] http://www.crisp-org.it/english/

## 5.1   The Labour Market Database

The scenario we are presenting focuses on a European country labour market domain. According to the country law, every time an employer hires or dismisses an employee, or an employment contract is modified (e.g. from part-time to full-time, or from fixed-term to unlimited-term), a *communication* (i.e., an event) is sent to a job registry. The country public administration has developed an ICT infrastructure for recording the *communications*, generating an administrative archive useful for studying the labour market dynamics. Each mandatory communication is stored into a record which can be broken down into the following attributes:

**e_id:** it represents an id identifying the communication;
**w_id:** it represents an id identifying the person involved;
**e_date:** it is the event occurrence date;
**e_type:** it describes the event type occurring to the worker career. Events types are the *start* or the *cessation* of a working contract, the *extension* of a fixed-term contract, or the *conversion* from a contract type to a different one;
**c_flag:** it states whether the event is related to a full-time or a part-time contract;
**c_type:** describes the contract type with respect to the country law. In this context, the *limited* (i.e. fixed-term), and *unlimited* (i.e. unlimited-term) contracts are considered.
**empr_id:** it uniquely identifies the employer involved.

In our context a *communication* represents an *event*, whilst a career can be modelled as an *event sequence*. Finally, the *consistency* of a career has been derived from the country labour law and from the domain knowledge, as reported in the following.

**c1:** an employee can have no more than one full-time contract at the same time;
**c2:** an employee cannot have more than $K$ part-time contracts (signed by different employers), in our context we assume $K = 2$;
**c3:** an *unlimited term* contract cannot be extended;
**c4:** a contract extension can change neither the existing contract type ($c\_type$) nor the part-time/full-time status ($c\_flag$) e.g., a part-time and fixed-term contract cannot be turned into a full-time contract by an extension;
**c5:** a conversion requires either the $c\_type$ or the $c\_flag$ to be changed (or both).

The data quality of the labour archive considered is very poor, several events are missing while several communications are recorded twice.

## 5.2   The Healthcare Database

The health services of the considered area are provided to all citizens and residents by a mixed public-private system. According to the law, specific drug sales and healthcare service provisioning require a general practitioner prescription, which is handled by a public information system. The policy makers and civil servants can access (anonymized) data concerning the prescriptions that the citizens have received. The dataset considered in this paper covers a period from 2007 until 2011. For our purposes we consider only records (1) about drug prescriptions having at least an active principle concerning antidepressant activities and (2) the patient is present in the Labour Dataset (i.e., we are able to analyse its working career). In this setting, the analysed database is composed by 3,243,560 prescriptions related to 323,806 patients. A prescription is composed by the following attributes of interest:

**r_id:** it represents the id identifying the region involved;
**w_id:** it represents the id identifying the patient involved;
**w_birth:** the patient's date of birth;
**d_q:** the number of drug units;
**d_ap:** the drug active principle;

Clearly, a prescription record can be considered as an *event* while an event sequence models the patient drug prescription history. The archive data quality has been investigated, some *duplicate* and *null value* issues have been identified in a first inspection.

## 6   Combined Cleansing and Integration

The existence of a mutual relationship (if any) between unemployment and the abuse of antidepressants should be carefully verified in all its key elements, which may range from medical to statistical, considering also the data quality perspective. The data cleansing procedures may strongly affect such investigation, therefore a framework for evaluating the cleansing effects is required.

In this paper, the authors describe an extension to an existing cleansing framework [132] that can be used to rapidly design and implement data integration and cleansing procedures. The proposed framework simplifies the development of cleansing and integration procedures, the proposed cleansing and integration process is described in Fig. 2. According to this, the several source archives undergo a preliminary data quality preprocessing addressing trivial (local) issues (e.g. duplicate detection and elimination). The resulting datasets then undergo a model based cleansing and integration process.

The cleansing and integration output can be easily modified by changing the cleansing policy and/or the consistency (and synthesis) model as well. Hence, the analysts can easily experiment and evaluate several cleansing options. An example is detailed in the following.

Let's suppose we would like to integrate the information stored in the labour and the healthcare database. We assume that the design of an integrated schema has already been performed and we focus on the data (contents) integration, also called *data fusion* or *data extensional integration*. The integrated archive model is described in table 3 and is aimed to support a specific analysis that is detailed next. Each record describes a time interval, a new record is created whenever the *employment status* of a person changes. The status is reflected into the *employment status* field which may assume the boolean values {*True*, *False*}.

The *antidepressant consumption* field describes the quantity of antidepressant drugs received as prescription (expressed as milligrams of active ingredient). For the sake of simplicity we do not distinguish among the several drugs and active ingredients. The work described in the paper can be easily extended to separately manage them.

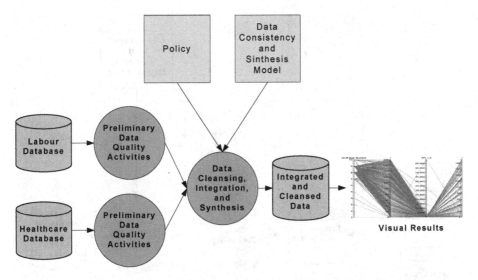

**Fig. 2.** An overview of the proposed data integration, cleansing, and synthesis framework

**Table 3.** The synthetic data derived from the labour and the healthcare database

| Person ID | Start Date | End Date | Employ-ment Status | Drug Con-sumpt. |
|---|---|---|---|---|
| ... | ... | ... | ... | ... |

The archives data quality is very poor, and the data quality and integration issues cannot be addressed in a complete independent way as previously showed in section 1. The choice on when to date a missing event may affect the timeslot drug attribution e.g., in case of a missing job cessation event, a drug prescription may be associated either to the working period or to the subsequent unemployment one. Managing these issues for large datasets where the magnitude of errors can be very high is a very complex task that calls for tools and procedures to support people activities.

## 6.1   Model Based Data Cleansing and Integration

In the Universal Cleanser approach described in section 4.1 a Finite State System (FSS) is used to describe a consistency model from which a cleanser can be derived. Our proposal is to enrich the FSS and turn it into a Finite State Transducer (FST) that can be used for both data integration and cleansing. An FST can be defined as a finite state automaton which maps between two sets of symbols [133]. The FST can be used for two purposes: 1) to synthesize the Universal Cleanser, and 2) to describe the data integration semantic, so that the data integration can be automatically performed.

The *Data Cleansing, Integration, and Synthesis* process is achieved through the following steps:

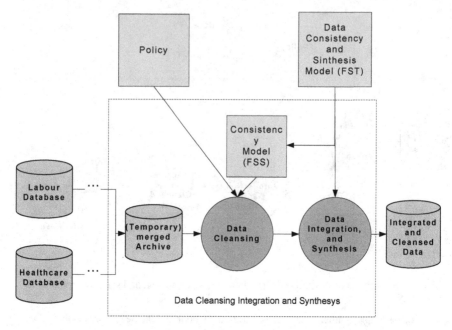

**Fig. 3.** An expansion of the Data Cleansing, Integration, and Synthesis activities of Figure 2

1. the data from the data sources are merged *as is* in a temporary archive. For this purpose, a temporary data structure is used, whose attributes are the union of the attributes of the source archives plus a flag stating from which source the record content comes, the two archives records are merged and ordered with respect to the date since both sources are longitudinal datasets;
2. the temporary data structure is fed into a cleanser built upon the Universal Cleanser and drove by the given policy;
3. the cleanser output is fed into the transducer that integrates the data.

A representation of the process is shown in Figure 3.

The Figure 4 represents a finite state transducer (FST hereafter) which can be used to produce the integrated dataset showed in table 3 from the two databases described in section 5. The FST described in figure 4 is derived from the automaton described in [132] which was designed for cleansing purposes only. According to our proposal, the FST contains the knowledge to perform both the data integration and data cleansing. The cleanser generation process, described in section 4.1, starts from an FSS that can be derived from the FST of Figure 4 by suppressing the output related parts. From now on we will refer to the FST and the FSS as if they were distinct automata, although the FSS is contained into the FST. Both automata have three state variables at a given time point: the list of companies for which the worker has an active contract ($C[]$), the list of modalities (part-time, full-time) for each contract ($M[]$) and the list of contract types ($T[]$). To give an example, $C[0] = 12$, $M[0] = PT$, $T[0] = unlimited$ models a worker having an active unlimited part-time contract with company 12.

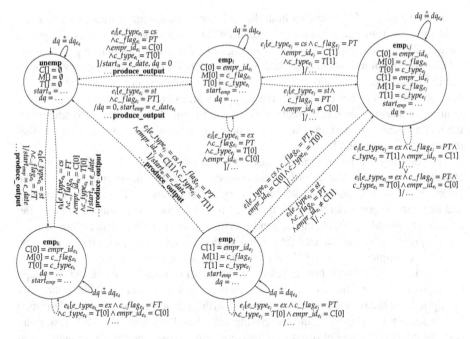

**Fig. 4.** A graphical representation of the labour and healthcare FST where $st = start$, $cs = cessation$, $cn = conversion$, and $ex = extension$. The $e_i$, $e_j$, $e_k$ refers to labour events, while the $e_d$ refers to drug prescription events. The comments on the edges are structured as follows: trigger [guard] /effect. A "..." in the edge description means that some state value assignments were moved to the node to improve readability. Dashed edges refer to events from the labour dataset whilst solid ones refer to the events from the healthcare dataset. To improve readability, some of the FST output values have been summarized by the **produce_output** label. Specifically, the latter is a placeholder for the *start* variable value, the *e_date* last event value, the *dq* variable value, and the *employment_status* (unemployed or employed).

The differences between the FST and the FSS are:

- edges and state variables dealing with drug consumption events;
  - state variables are introduced to manage the drug consumption information: 1) the period start and end date, 2) a variable to count the consumption quantity
  - self edges used to manage drug consumption events. These edges increment the counter when a drug consumption event happens;
  - counter variable resettability is added: when a labour event makes the automaton to enter or exit the *unemp* state, the drug counter is set to 0;
  - when the person enter or exit an employment or unemployment state (respectively $emp_i$, $emp_j$, $emp_{i,j}$, $emp_k$ for the former and *unemp* for the latter), the start and end dates are updated accordingly.
- the output part of the transducer, i.e. when an event makes the automaton to change the employment state, the edge specifies the information to be written as output. The information written in output is: the period start and end date, the drug consumption quantity, and of course the Person ID, and Employment Status.

Since the same FST describes both the cleansing and the integration process at the same time, the transducer can take the cleansed data as input and produce an integrated dataset. We now closely look at the cleansing task. The process of deriving an Universal Cleanser from an FSS is described in section 4.1. When an inconsistency is found the UC based cleanser scans the UC looking for a feasible correction. Since the UC may provide more than one corrective action for the same inconsistency, a *policy* is required to select a suitable correction. Once a correction has been properly identified, the inconsistency is fixed and the new sequence is verified iteratively until no further inconsistencies are found.

The resulting instrument (the UC based cleanser plus the transducer) can be used to cleanse and integrate data according to the models described through the FSS and the policy. It is worth to note that the output vary as the policy varies (i.e., the cleansing and integration results depend upon the given policy). Since the cleansing policies can be easily replaced, several behavior can be designed, implemented, and evaluated.

Two policies that can be used for evaluating the cleansing impact on the data will be shown as examples. The policy details are outlined in the next section.

A further discussion on how to select a suitable set of policies falls out of the scope of this work. Nevertheless, once the UC has been synthesised any kind of policy can be applied and the results evaluated. A person wishing to use the architecture described in this section for cleansing and integrating data, has 1) to build the FST describing both the consistency model (used for cleansing) and the data integration semantic; and 2) to select a policy. This gives into the hands of the analysts a rapid prototyping tool to manage the data cleansing and integration tasks. Knowledge on data cleansing and integration can be derived by iterating the following steps: designing the FST and the policy, executing the cleansing and integration process, analyzing the results by making use of visualization techniques as showed in the next section. The knowledge can be used to improve the overall cleansing process.

# 7   Experimental Results

The data cleansing and integration framework described in section 6 has been used on the databases described in section 5. A Universal cleanser has been generated from the FST described in figure 4 (specifically, an FSS has been extracted from the FST, an Universal Cleanser has been built and used to cleanse the data), then the cleansed data have been given in input to the FST which produced the integrated dataset. Two policies have been used for cleansing the data, their details are outlined in the following: both policies select the corrective action that minimizes the interventions on the data in terms of tuples to be inserted. E.g., if after a full time job cessation ($e_a$) a part-time cessation is recorded ($e_b$), two corrective actions could be used: 1) to insert a part-time job start in between, or 2) to insert a part-time job start, then a part-time job cessation, then a part-time job start again. The option 1) minimizes the interventions on the data, therefore it is chosen. If several actions satisfy the minimality criterion, one is selected with the aid of a domain expert. The policy should also estimate the parameters e.g., the event date. In the just introduced example, the date of the events to be added, should be chosen between the $e_a$ date and the $e_b$ date. The first policy (called $P1$ hereafter) will choose the day after the $e_a$ event while the second policy (called P2 hereafter) will choose the day before $e_b$. Two different datasets are derived by cleansing and integrating the data using the two policies. The two cleansed datasets can be used to evaluate how cleansing affects the data. Of course, several policies can be used and their impact can be evaluated as described next.

To analyse the results produced by the two policies on the drug consumption allocation, we used a well-suited multidimensional visualisation technique, namely the *parallel-coordinates* (abbrv: ‖-coord see [134]). Informally speaking, ‖-coord allow one to represent an $n$-dimensional datum $(x_1, \ldots, x_n)$ as a polyline, by connecting each $x_i$ point in $n$ parallel $y$-axes.

We used the ‖-coord to plot a dataset in figure 5(a) and 5(b) showing, for each worker: the average duration of the working timeslots cleansed using policy P1 minus the average duration of the working timeslots corrected using policy P2 (*avg_plus_days* axis); the average consumption of drugs in the working timeslots, cleansed using policy P1, minus the average consumption of drugs in the working timeslots, cleansed using policy P2 (*pharma_increment* axis);

Generally, ‖-coord tools show their powerfulness when used interactively (i.e., by selecting ranges from the y-axes, by emphasising the lines traversing through specific ranges, etc). For the sake of completeness, two snapshots are showed in figure 5. The figure 5(a) shows the plot where no axes is filtered, while figure 5(b) shows a plot where a filter has been applied (on the *pharma_increment* axis). The filter is aimed at identifying the people that have a *remarkable gap* in the *timeslot average drug consumption* computed according policy P1 and policy P2.

The examples of figure 5(a) and 5(b) are not showed for the purpose of going into detailed analysis but to outline the capabilities of visualization techniques. The ‖-coord allows the analysts to finely identify the people whose average drug consumption per time slot is strongly affected by the data cleansing. Although only a small subset of the people analyzed has a remarkable gap (we assumed *pharma_increment* > 5 as a criterion), the results is a valuable information for the analysts, furthermore the people subset is clearly identified and further analysis can be performed. The knowledge extracted on the subsets of the population identified can be used to validate or invalidate the analysis on the overall population.

Our results show that the combined use of 1) model-based approaches for data cleansing and integration and 2) visualisation techniques, give the users the instruments to tackle the complexities of managing huge masses of data extracted from several sources. The analysts can evaluate several cleansing policies and select the best one for their specific analysis purposes. Furthermore, the knowledge gained during the model design and the policy selection process will be useful also when performing the subsequent analysis. We also presented a real-world scenario in the labour market and healthcare domain where the cleansing, integration, and visualisation techniques have been successfully used.

## 8  Open Problems

In this section a list of open problems in the field of data quality and data integration is presented.

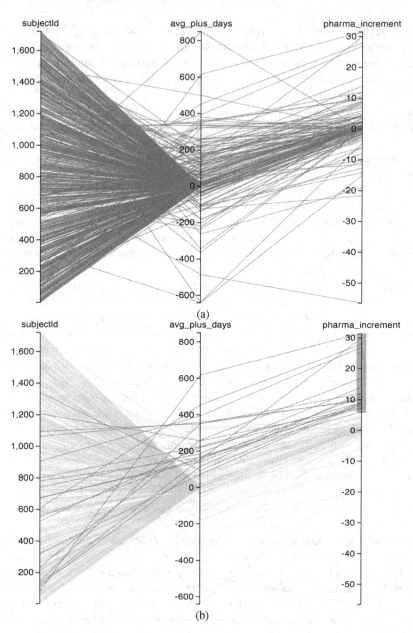

**Fig. 5.** A dataset plotted in ‖-coord showing, for each worker (the *subjectid* axes): the average duration of the timeslots (in days) cleansed using policy *P*1 minus the average duration of the timeslots corrected using policy *P*2 (the *avg_plus_days* axis); the average consumption of drugs in the timeslots (expressed in milligrams of active principle), cleansed using policy *P*1 minus the average consumption of drugs in the timeslots, cleansed using policy *P*2 (the *pharma_increment* axis). Figure 5(a) has no filters, while figure 5(b) shows a plot where a filter has been applied on the *pharma_increment* axis. The plot shows 1700 people data, the subjects were randomly selected.

- *Open Problem 1.* Choosing the right combination of technologies and tools to perform data integration is a critical challenge, experience with several integration projects suggests that a broader framework is required, perhaps even a theory, which explicitly takes into account the requirements on the result and considers the entire end-to-end integration process [58]. Furthermore, there is little support for iteration between schema-level and data-level tasks in the integration process, an integration engine seamlessly working with both data mappings and schema mappings is required [61].
- *Open Problem 2.* Despite some tools incorporating the latest results of the data quality research have been made available (e.g. NADEEF [97], LLUNATIC [98], Orchestra [135], and BIO-AJAX [106]), there is still a huge gap between the research findings and the data quality effectively performed, even in research laboratories. In the authors opinion, this gap is only the tip of an iceberg. Data quality is frequently a (neglected) step of a larger knowledge discovery process. The theoretical intersection between data quality and other research fields should be further explored, including knowledge discovery from data (KDD). E.g., as the authors of [136] state, data quality is loosely encompassed by the general term *noise* in data mining research, but the latter does not consider any linkage between data quality dimensions and noise.
- *Open Problem 3.* The data quality and integration challenges have been mostly addressed in isolation, although some works pointed out the benefit of addressing the two issues in a combined way [58]. Incorporating the notions of data quality and data integration into a formal framework [22] is still an open issue at the present time.

## 9  Future Outlook

Some research perspectives will be outlined for the open problems previously described.

Considering the *open problem 1*, an interesting research scenario are the works on dataspaces or on lightweight information integration approaches (those where base functionalities are provided, while the labor intensive aspects of data integration are postponed until needed [26]). Logging and studying the users' activities while they interact with a dataspace (or with linked data) can be used to infer semantic about the relationships between the data sources [26]. The research fields of data visualization and Human-Computer Interaction have to be investigated for achieving the aforementioned goal.

Considering the *open problem 2*, a research perspective is to investigate the data quality and analysis requirements for specific groups of people. The need for effective analysis of data is widely recognized today and many tools aim to support professional data scientists from industry and science, however, there are several growing groups of users who need to analyze data [137]: from users having no formal training in data science (called Data Enthusiasts in [138]) to people who have a limited background on data analysis and that only recently started performing data investigations in their activities. Such users require tools, paradigms, and methodologies to master their data analysis needs. Both he scenarios where professional data scientists and data enthusiasts are involved, are a fertile ground for combining two areas which bring ideal pre-conditions to solve data-centric problems: Human-Computer Interaction (HCI) and Knowledge Discovery and Data Mining (KDD) [139].

Considering the *open problem 3*, weakly structured data (i.e. data that resemble a random walk on a graph [115]) represent an interesting field where data integration and cleansing can be investigated in a combined way. Indeed, the graph information and topology of weakly structured data can be used to support the data integration, quality assessment, and even cleansing tasks, as outlined in the work presented in this paper. Furthermore, the boundaries between effective cleansing and signal destruction are still to be explored in weakly structured data cleansing.

**Acknowledgments.** This work is partially supported within a Research Project granted by the CRISP Research Centre (Interuniversity Research Centre on Public Services - http://www.crisp-org.it) and Arifl (Regional Agency for Education and Labour - http://www.arifl.regione.lombardia.it).

# References

1. Fayyad, U.M., Piatetsky-Shapiro, G., Uthurusamy, R.: Summary from the kdd-03 panel. ACM SIGKDD Explorations Newsletter 5(2), 191–196 (2003)
2. Mezzanzanica, M., Boselli, R., Cesarini, M., Mercorio, F.: Data quality sensitivity analysis on aggregate indicators. In: International Conference on Data Technologies and Applications (DATA), pp. 97–108. SciTePress (2012)
3. Tee, S., Bowen, P., Doyle, P., Rohde, F.: Data quality initiatives: Striving for continuous improvements. International Journal of Information Quality 1(4), 347–367 (2007)
4. Redman, T.C.: The impact of poor data quality on the typical enterprise. Commun. ACM 41, 79–82 (1998)
5. Batini, C., Scannapieco, M.: Data Quality: Concepts, Methodologies and Techniques. Data-Centric Systems and Applications. Springer (2006)
6. Fayyad, U., Piatetsky-Shapiro, G., Smyth, P.: The kdd process for extracting useful knowledge from volumes of data. Communications of the ACM 39(11), 27–34 (1996)
7. Sadiq, S.: Handbook of Data Quality. Springer (2013)
8. Fisher, C., Lauría, E., Chengalur-Smith, S., Wang, R.: Introduction to information quality. AuthorHouse (2012)
9. Holzinger, A., Yildirim, P., Geier, M., Simonic, K.M.: Quality-based knowledge discovery from medical text on the web. In: [142], pp. 145–158
10. Pasi, G., Bordogna, G., Jain, L.C.: An introduction to quality issues in the management of web information. In: [142], pp. 1–3
11. Herrera-Viedma, E., Peis, E.: Evaluating the informative quality of documents in sgml format from judgements by means of fuzzy linguistic techniques based on computing with words. Information Processing & Management 39(2), 233–249 (2003)
12. Boselli, R., Cesarini, M., Mercorio, F., Mezzanzanica, M.: Inconsistency knowledge discovery for longitudinal data management: A model-based approach. In: Holzinger, A., Pasi, G. (eds.) HCI-KDD 2013. LNCS, vol. 7947, pp. 183–194. Springer, Heidelberg (2013)
13. Widom, J., Ceri, S.: Active database systems: Triggers and rules for advanced database processing. Morgan Kaufmann (1996)
14. Xu, H., Jin, Y.: Biorl: An xml-based active rule language for biological database constraint management. In: International Conference on BioMedical Engineering and Informatics, BMEI 2008, vol. 1, pp. 883–887. IEEE (2008)

15. Calvanese, D., De Giacomo, G., Montali, M.: Foundations of data-aware process analysis: A database theory perspective. In: Proceedings of the 32nd Symposium on Principles of Database Systems, PODS 2013, pp. 1–12. ACM, New York (2013)

16. Shapiro, S.C.: Artificial Intelligence. In: Encyclopedia of Artificial Intelligence, vol. 2, John Wiley & Sons, Inc., New York (1992)

17. Turing, A.M.: Computing machinery and intelligence. Mind 59(236), 433–460 (1950)

18. Morgan, T.: Business Rules and Information Systems: Aligning IT with Business Goals. Pearson Education (2002)

19. Han, J., Kamber, M., Pei, J.: Data mining: Concepts and techniques. Morgan kaufmann (2006)

20. Naumann, F., Bilke, A., Bleiholder, J., Weis, M.: Data fusion in three steps: Resolving schema, tuple, and value inconsistencies. IEEE Data Eng. Bull. 29(2), 21–31 (2006)

21. Arens, Y., Chee, C.Y., Hsu, C.N., Knoblock, C.A.: Retrieving and integrating data from multiple information sources. International Journal of Intelligent and Cooperative Information Systems 2(02), 127–158 (1993)

22. Lenzerini, M.: Data integration: A theoretical perspective. In: Proceedings of the Twenty-First ACM SIGMOD-SIGACT-SIGART Symposium on Principles of Database Systems, pp. 233–246. ACM (2002)

23. Halevy, A.Y.: Answering queries using views: A survey. The VLDB Journal 10(4), 270–294 (2001)

24. Hull, R.: Managing semantic heterogeneity in databases: a theoretical prospective. In: Proceedings of the Sixteenth ACM SIGACT-SIGMOD-SIGART Symposium on Principles of Database Systems, pp. 51–61. ACM (1997)

25. Ullman, J.D.: Information integration using logical views. In: Afrati, F.N., Kolaitis, P.G. (eds.) ICDT 1997. LNCS, vol. 1186, pp. 19–40. Springer, Heidelberg (1996)

26. Halevy, A., Franklin, M., Maier, D.: Principles of dataspace systems. In: Proceedings of the Twenty-Fifth ACM SIGMOD-SIGACT-SIGART Symposium on Principles of Database Systems, pp. 1–9. ACM (2006)

27. Bizer, C., Heath, T., Berners-Lee, T.: Linked data-the story so far. International Journal on Semantic Web and Information Systems 5(3), 1–22 (2009)

28. Wang, R.Y.: A product perspective on total data quality management. Commun. ACM 41, 58–65 (1998)

29. Scannapieco, M., Missier, P., Batini, C.: Data Quality at a Glance. Datenbank-Spektrum 14, 6–14 (2005)

30. Wang, Y.R., Madnick, S.E.: The inter-database instance identification problem in integrating autonomous systems. In: Proceedings of the Fifth International Conference on Data Engineering, pp. 46–55. IEEE (1989)

31. Vassiliadis, P., Simitsis, A., Skiadopoulos, S.: Conceptual modeling for etl processes. In: Proceedings of the 5th ACM International Workshop on Data Warehousing and OLAP, DOLAP 2002, pp. 14–21. ACM, New York (2002)

32. Codd, E.F.: Further normalization of the data base relational model. Data Base Systems 6, 33–64 (1972)

33. Bohannon, P., Fan, W., Geerts, F., Jia, X., Kementsietsidis, A.: Conditional functional dependencies for data cleaning. In: IEEE 23rd International Conference on Data Engineering (ICDE 2007), pp. 746–755. IEEE (2007)

34. Fan, W., Geerts, F., Li, J., Xiong, M.: Discovering conditional functional dependencies. IEEE Transactions on Knowledge and Data Engineering 23(5), 683–698 (2011)

35. Wiederhold, G.: Mediators in the architecture of future information systems. Computer 25(3), 38–49 (1992)

36. Garcia-Molina, H., Papakonstantinou, Y., Quass, D., Rajaraman, A., Sagiv, Y., Ullman, J., Vassalos, V., Widom, J.: The tsimmis approach to mediation: Data models and languages. Journal of intelligent information systems 8(2), 117–132 (1997)
37. Welty, C.: Guest editorial: Ontology research. AI Mag. 24(3), 11–12 (2003)
38. Noy, N.F.: Semantic integration: a survey of ontology-based approaches. ACM Sigmod Record 33(4), 65–70 (2004)
39. Batini, C., Lenzerini, M., Navathe, S.B.: A comparative analysis of methodologies for database schema integration. ACM Comput. Surv. 18, 323–364 (1986)
40. Miller, R.J., Haas, L.M., Hernández, M.A.: Schema mapping as query discovery. In: VLDB, vol. 2000, pp. 77–88 (2000)
41. Bouzeghoub, M., Lenzerini, M.: Introduction to: data extraction, cleaning, and reconciliation a special issue of information systems, an international journal. Information Systems 26(8), 535–536 (2001)
42. Fox, C., Levitin, A., Redman, T.: The notion of data and its quality dimensions. Information Processing & Management 30(1), 9–19 (1994)
43. Levitin, A., Redman, T.: Quality dimensions of a conceptual view. Information Processing & Management 31(1), 81–88 (1995)
44. Ballou, D.P., Tayi, G.K.: Enhancing data quality in data warehouse environments. Communications of the ACM 42(1), 73–78 (1999)
45. Hipp, J., Güntzer, U., Grimmer, U.: Data quality mining-making a virute of necessity. In: DMKD (2001)
46. Haug, A., Zachariassen, F., Van Liempd, D.: The costs of poor data quality. Journal of Industrial Engineering and Management 4(2), 168–193 (2011)
47. Dasu, T.: Data glitches: Monsters in your data. In: Handbook of Data Quality, pp. 163–178. Springer (2013)
48. Delen, D., Walker, G., Kadam, A.: Predicting breast cancer survivability: a comparison of three data mining methods. Artificial Intelligence in Medicine 34(2), 113–127 (2005)
49. Lavrač, N.: Selected techniques for data mining in medicine. Artificial Intelligence in Medicine 16(1), 3–23 (1999); Data Mining Techniques and Applications in Medicine
50. Kriegel, H.P., Borgwardt, K.M., Kröger, P., Pryakhin, A., Schubert, M., Zimek, A.: Future trends in data mining. Data Mining and Knowledge Discovery 15(1), 87–97 (2007)
51. Yan, X., Zhang, C., Zhang, S.: Toward databases mining: Pre-processing collected data. Applied Artificial Intelligence 17(5-6), 545–561 (2003)
52. Espinosa, R., Zubcoff, J., Mazón, J.-N.: A set of experiments to consider data quality criteria in classification techniques for data mining. In: Murgante, B., Gervasi, O., Iglesias, A., Taniar, D., Apduhan, B.O. (eds.) ICCSA 2011, Part II. LNCS, vol. 6783, pp. 680–694. Springer, Heidelberg (2011)
53. Zhang, S., Zhang, C., Yang, Q.: Data preparation for data mining. Applied Artificial Intelligence 17(5-6), 375–381 (2003)
54. Rajagopalan, B., Isken, M.W.: Exploiting data preparation to enhance mining and knowledge discovery. IEEE Transactions on Systems, Man, and Cybernetics, Part C: Applications and Reviews 31(4), 460–467 (2001)
55. Zhu, X., Wu, X.: Class noise vs. attribute noise: A quantitative study. Artificial Intelligence Review 22(3), 177–210 (2004)
56. Troyanskaya, O., Cantor, M., Sherlock, G., Brown, P., Hastie, T., Tibshirani, R., Botstein, D., Altman, R.B.: Missing value estimation methods for dna microarrays. Bioinformatics 17(6), 520–525 (2001)
57. Halevy, A.Y.: Data integration: A status report. In: Proc. BTW 2003 (2003)
58. Haas, L.: Beauty and the beast: The theory and practice of information integration. In: Schwentick, T., Suciu, D. (eds.) ICDT 2007. LNCS, vol. 4353, pp. 28–43. Springer, Heidelberg (2006)

59. Huang, S.S., Green, T.J., Loo, B.T.: Datalog and emerging applications: An interactive tutorial. In: Proceedings of the 2011 ACM SIGMOD International Conference on Management of Data, SIGMOD 2011, pp. 1213–1216. ACM, New York (2011)

60. Halevy, A., Rajaraman, A., Ordille, J.: Data integration: the teenage years. In: Proceedings of the 32nd International Conference on Very Large Data Bases, pp. 9–16. VLDB Endowment (2006)

61. Haas, L.M., Hentschel, M., Kossmann, D., Miller, R.J.: Schema AND data: A holistic approach to mapping, resolution and fusion in information integration. In: Laender, A.H.F., Castano, S., Dayal, U., Casati, F., de Oliveira, J.P.M. (eds.) ER 2009. LNCS, vol. 5829, pp. 27–40. Springer, Heidelberg (2009)

62. Bleiholder, J., Naumann, F.: Data fusion. ACM Computing Surveys (CSUR) 41(1), 1 (2008)

63. Sattler, K.U., Conrad, S., Saake, G.: Adding conflict resolution features to a query language for database federations. In: Roantree, M., Hasselbring, W., Conrad, S. (eds.) International Workshop on Engineering Federated Information Systems (EFIS), pp. 41–52 (2000)

64. Schallehn, H., Saltler, K.U.: Using similarity-based operations for resolving data-level conflicts. In: James, A., Younas, M., Lings, B. (eds.) BNCOD 2003. LNCS, vol. 2712, pp. 172–189. Springer, Heidelberg (2003)

65. Schallehn, E., Sattler, K.U., Saake, G.: Efficient similarity-based operations for data integration. Data & Knowledge Engineering 48(3), 361–387 (2004)

66. Franklin, M., Halevy, A., Maier, D.: From databases to dataspaces: A new abstraction for information management. SIGMOD Rec. 34(4), 27–33 (2005)

67. Zobel, J., Moffat, A.: Inverted files for text search engines. ACM Computing Surveys (CSUR) 38(2), 6 (2006)

68. Meng, W., Yu, C., Liu, K.L.: Building efficient and effective metasearch engines. ACM Computing Surveys (CSUR) 34(1), 48–89 (2002)

69. Uschold, M., Gruninger, M.: Ontologies and semantics for seamless connectivity. SIGMOD Rec. 33(4), 58–64 (2004)

70. Calvanese, D., De Giacomo, G.: Data integration: A logic-based perspective. AI Magazine 26(1), 59 (2005)

71. Abello, J., Pardalos, P.M., Resende, M.G.: Handbook of massive data sets, vol. 4. Springer (2002)

72. Mayfield, C., Neville, J., Prabhakar, S.: Eracer: a database approach for statistical inference and data cleaning. In: Proceedings of the 2010 ACM SIGMOD International Conference on Management of Data, pp. 75–86. ACM (2010)

73. Winkler, W.E.: Editing discrete data. Bureau of the Census (1997)

74. Fellegi, I., Holt, D.: A systematic approach to automatic edit and inputation. Journal of the American Statistical Association 71(353), 17–35 (1976)

75. Winkler, W.E.: Machine learning, information retrieval and record linkage. In: Proc. Section on Survey Research Methods, American Statistical Association, pp. 20–29 (2000)

76. Fellegi, I., Sunter, A.: A theory for record linkage. Journal of the American Statistical Association 64(328), 1183–1210 (1969)

77. Newcombe, H.B., Kennedy, J.M.: Record linkage: making maximum use of the discriminating power of identifying information. Communications of the ACM 5(11), 563–566 (1962)

78. Elmagarmid, A., Ipeirotis, P., Verykios, V.: Duplicate record detection: A survey. IEEE Transactions on Knowledge and Data Engineering 19(1), 1–16 (2007)

79. Winkler, W.: Methods for evaluating and creating data quality. Information Systems 29(7), 531–550 (2004)

80. Holzinger, A., Bruschi, M., Eder, W.: On interactive data visualization of physiological low-cost-sensor data with focus on mental stress. In: Cuzzocrea, A., Kittl, C., Simos, D.E., Weippl, E., Xu, L. (eds.) CD-ARES 2013. LNCS, vol. 8127, pp. 469–480. Springer, Heidelberg (2013)

81. Ferreira de Oliveira, M.C., Levkowitz, H.: From visual data exploration to visual data mining: A survey. IEEE Trans. Vis. Comput. Graph. 9(3), 378–394 (2003)
82. Clemente, P., Kaba, B., Rouzaud-Cornabas, J., Alexandre, M., Aujay, G.: SPTrack: Visual analysis of information flows within sELinux policies and attack logs. In: Huang, R., Ghorbani, A.A., Pasi, G., Yamaguchi, T., Yen, N.Y., Jin, B. (eds.) AMT 2012. LNCS, vol. 7669, pp. 596–605. Springer, Heidelberg (2012)
83. Bertossi, L.: Consistent query answering in databases. ACM Sigmod Record 35(2), 68–76 (2006)
84. Chomicki, J., Marcinkowski, J.: On the computational complexity of minimal-change integrity maintenance in relational databases. In: Bertossi, L., Hunter, A., Schaub, T. (eds.) Inconsistency Tolerance. LNCS, vol. 3300, pp. 119–150. Springer, Heidelberg (2005)
85. Yu, L., Wang, S., Lai, K.K.: An integrated data preparation scheme for neural network data analysis. IEEE Transactions on Knowledge and Data Engineering 18(2), 217–230 (2006)
86. Wang, H., Wang, S.: Discovering patterns of missing data in survey databases: an application of rough sets. Expert Systems with Applications 36(3), 6256–6260 (2009)
87. Chomicki, J., Marcinkowski, J.: Minimal-change integrity maintenance using tuple deletions. Information and Computation 197(1), 90–121 (2005)
88. Greco, G., Greco, S., Zumpano, E.: A logic programming approach to the integration, repairing and querying of inconsistent databases. In: Codognet, P. (ed.) ICLP 2001. LNCS, vol. 2237, pp. 348–364. Springer, Heidelberg (2001)
89. Arenas, M., Bertossi, L.E., Chomicki, J.: Consistent query answers in inconsistent databases. In: ACM Symp. on Principles of Database Systems, pp. 68–79. ACM Press (1999)
90. Yakout, M., Berti-Équille, L., Elmagarmid, A.K.: Don't be scared: use scalable automatic repairing with maximal likelihood and bounded changes. In: Proceedings of the 2013 International Conference on Management of Data, pp. 553–564. ACM (2013)
91. Cong, G., Fan, W., Geerts, F., Jia, X., Ma, S.: Improving data quality: Consistency and accuracy. In: Proceedings of the 33rd International Conference on Very Large Data Bases, pp. 315–326. VLDB Endowment (2007)
92. Kolahi, S., Lakshmanan, L.V.: On approximating optimum repairs for functional dependency violations. In: Proceedings of the 12th International Conference on Database Theory, pp. 53–62. ACM (2009)
93. Vardi, M.: Fundamentals of dependency theory. In: Trends in Theoretical Computer Science, pp. 171–224 (1987)
94. Chomicki, J.: Efficient checking of temporal integrity constraints using bounded history encoding. ACM Transactions on Database Systems (TODS) 20(2), 149–186 (1995)
95. Fan, W.: Dependencies revisited for improving data quality. In: Proceedings of the Twenty-Seventh ACM SIGMOD-SIGACT-SIGART Symposium on Principles of Database Systems, pp. 159–170 (2008)
96. Fan, W., Li, J., Ma, S., Tang, N., Yu, W.: Towards certain fixes with editing rules and master data. Proceedings of the VLDB Endowment 3(1-2), 173–184 (2010)
97. Dallachiesa, M., Ebaid, A., Eldawy, A., Elmagarmid, A.K., Ilyas, I.F., Ouzzani, M., Tang, N.: Nadeef: a commodity data cleaning system. In: Ross, K.A., Srivastava, D., Papadias, D. (eds.) SIGMOD Conference, pp. 541–552. ACM (2013)
98. Geerts, F., Mecca, G., Papotti, P., Santoro, D.: The llunatic data-cleaning framework. PVLDB 6(9), 625–636 (2013)
99. Boselli, R., Cesarini, M., Mercorio, F., Mezzanzanica, M.: Towards data cleansing via planning. Intelligenza Artificiale 8(1) (2014)
100. Choi, E.H., Tsuchiya, T., Kikuno, T.: Model checking active database rules under various rule processing strategies. IPSJ Digital Courier 2, 826–839 (2006)

101. Ray, I., Ray, I.: Detecting termination of active database rules using symbolic model checking. In: Caplinskas, A., Eder, J. (eds.) ADBIS 2001. LNCS, vol. 2151, pp. 266–279. Springer, Heidelberg (2001)
102. Neven, F.: Automata theory for xml researchers. SIGMOD Rec. 31, 39–46 (2002)
103. Dovier, A., Quintarelli, E.: Model-checking based data retrieval. In: Ghelli, G., Grahne, G. (eds.) DBPL 2001. LNCS, vol. 2397, pp. 62–77. Springer, Heidelberg (2002)
104. Dovier, A., Quintarelli, E.: Applying Model-checking to solve Queries on semistructured Data. Computer Languages, Systems & Structures 35(2), 143–172 (2009)
105. Afanasiev, L., Franceschet, M., Marx, M., de Rijke, M.: Ctl model checking for processing simple xpath queries. In: TIME, pp. 117–124 (2004)
106. Herbert, K.G., Gehani, N.H., Piel, W.H., Wang, J.T., Wu, C.H.: Bio-ajax: an extensible framework for biological data cleaning. ACM SIGMOD Record 33(2), 51–57 (2004)
107. Chen, J.Y., Carlis, J.V., Gao, N.: A complex biological database querying method. In: Proceedings of the 2005 ACM Symposium on Applied Computing, pp. 110–114. ACM, New York (2005)
108. Apiletti, D., Bruno, G., Ficarra, E., Baralis, E.: Data cleaning and semantic improvement in biological databases. Journal of Integrative Bioinformatics 3(2), 1–11 (2006)
109. Chellamuthu, S., Punithavalli, D.M.: Detecting redundancy in biological databases? an efficient approach. Global Journal of Computer Science and Technology 9(4) (2009)
110. Shui, W.M., Wong, R.K.: Application of xml schema and active rules system in management and integration of heterogeneous biological data. In: Proceedings of the Third IEEE Symposium on Bioinformatics and Bioengineering, pp. 367–374. IEEE (2003)
111. Wong, B.L.W., Xu, K., Holzinger, A.: Interactive visualization for information analysis in medical diagnosis. In: Holzinger, A., Simonic, K.-M. (eds.) USAB 2011. LNCS, vol. 7058, pp. 109–120. Springer, Heidelberg (2011)
112. Parsaye, K., Chignell, M.: Intelligent Database Tools and Applications: Hyperinformation access, data quality, visualization, automatic discovery. John Wiley (1993)
113. Simonic, K.-M., Holzinger, A., Bloice, M., Hermann, J.: Optimizing long-term treatment of rheumatoid arthritis with systematic documentation. In: International Conference on Pervasive Computing Technologies for Healthcare, PervasiveHealth, pp. 550–554. IEEE (2011)
114. Holzinger, A., Zupan, M.: Knodwat: A scientific framework application for testing knowledge discovery methods for the biomedical domain. BMC Bioinformatics 14, 191 (2013)
115. Holzinger, A.: On knowledge discovery and interactive intelligent visualization of biomedical data - challenges in human-computer interaction & biomedical informatics. In: Helfert, M., Francalanci, C., Filipe, J. (eds.) DATA. SciTePress (2012)
116. Holzinger, A.: Weakly structured data in health-informatics: the challenge for human-computer-interaction. In: Proceedings of INTERACT 2011 Workshop: Promoting and Supporting Healthy Living by Desing, IFIP, pp. 5–7 (2011)
117. Wong, B.L.W., Xu, K., Holzinger, A.: Interactive visualization for information analysis in medical diagnosis. In: Holzinger, A., Simonic, K.-M. (eds.) USAB 2011. LNCS, vol. 7058, pp. 109–120. Springer, Heidelberg (2011)
118. Lovaglio, P.G., Mezzanzanica, M.: Classification of longitudinal career paths. Quality & Quantity 47(2), 989–1008 (2013)
119. Hansen, P., Järvelin, K.: Collaborative information retrieval in an information-intensive domain. Information Processing & Management 41(5), 1101–1119 (2005)
120. Prinzie, A., Van den Poel, D.: Modeling complex longitudinal consumer behavior with dynamic bayesian networks: an acquisition pattern analysis application. Journal of Intelligent Information Systems 36(3), 283–304 (2011)
121. Devaraj, S., Kohli, R.: Information technology payoff in the health-care industry: a longitudinal study. Journal of Management Information Systems 16(4), 41–68 (2000)

122. Mezzanzanica, M., Boselli, R., Cesarini, M., Mercorio, F.: Data quality through model checking techniques. In: Gama, J., Bradley, E., Hollmén, J. (eds.) IDA 2011. LNCS, vol. 7014, pp. 270–281. Springer, Heidelberg (2011)

123. Della Penna, G., Intrigila, B., Magazzeni, D., Mercorio, F.: UPMurphi: a tool for universal planning on PDDL+ problems. In: ICAPS, pp. 106–113. AAAI Press (2009)

124. Fox, M., Long, D., Magazzeni, D.: Plan-based policies for efficient multiple battery load management. J. Artif. Intell. Res. (JAIR) 44, 335–382 (2012)

125. Fox, M., Long, D., Magazzeni, D.: Automatic construction of efficient multiple battery usage policies. In: Walsh, T. (ed.) IJCAI, IJCAI/AAAI, pp. 2620–2625 (2011)

126. Della Penna, G., Intrigila, B., Magazzeni, D., Mercorio, F., Tronci, E.: Cost-optimal strong planning in non-deterministic domains. In: Proceedings of the 8th International Conference on Informatics in Control, Automation and Robotics (ICINCO), pp. 56–66. SciTePress (2011)

127. Della Penna, G., Intrigila, B., Magazzeni, D., Mercorio, F.: A PDDL+ benchmark problem: The batch chemical plant. In: Proceedings of ICAPS 2010, pp. 222–224. AAAI Press (2010)

128. Della Penna, G., Magazzeni, D., Mercorio, F.: A universal planning system for hybrid domains. Applied Intelligence 36(4), 932–959 (2012)

129. Della Penna, G., Intrigila, B., Magazzeni, D., Melatti, I., Tronci, E.: Cgmurphi: Automatic synthesis of numerical controllers for nonlinear hybrid systems. European Journal of Control (2013)

130. Mercorio, F.: Model checking for universal planning in deterministic and non-deterministic domains. AI Communications 26(2), 257–259 (2013)

131. Boselli, R., Mezzanzanica, M., Cesarini, M., Mercorio, F.: Planning meets data cleansing. In: 24th International Conference on Automated Planning and Scheduling, ICAPS (2014)

132. Mezzanzanica, M., Boselli, R., Cesarini, M., Mercorio, F.: Automatic synthesis of data cleansing activities. In: DATA 2013 - Proceedings of the International Conference on Data Technologies and Applications. SciTePress (2013)

133. Jurafsky, D., James, H.: Speech and Language Processing An Introduction to Natural Language Processing, Computational Linguistics, and Speech. Pearson Education (2000)

134. Inselberg, A.: The plane with parallel coordinates. The Visual Computer 1(2), 69–91 (1985)

135. Ives, Z.G., Green, T.J., Karvounarakis, G., Taylor, N.E., Tannen, V., Talukdar, P.P., Jacob, M., Pereira, F.: The orchestra collaborative data sharing system. ACM SIGMOD Record 37(3), 26–32 (2008)

136. Blake, R., Mangiameli, P.: The effects and interactions of data quality and problem complexity on classification. J. Data and Information Quality 2(2), 8:1–8:28 (2011)

137. Morton, K., Balazinska, M., Grossman, D., Mackinlay, J.: Support the data enthusiast: Challenges for next-generation data-analysis systems. Proceedings of the VLDB Endowment 7(6) (2014)

138. Hanrahan, P.: Analytic database technologies for a new kind of user: the data enthusiast. In: Proceedings of the 2012 ACM SIGMOD International Conference on Management of Data, pp. 577–578. ACM (2012)

139. Holzinger, A.: Human-computer interaction and knowledge discovery (HCI-KDD): What is the benefit of bringing those two fields to work together? In: Cuzzocrea, A., Kittl, C., Simos, D.E., Weippl, E., Xu, L. (eds.) CD-ARES 2013. LNCS, vol. 8127, pp. 319–328. Springer, Heidelberg (2013)

140. Pasi, G., Bordogna, G., Jain, L.C. (eds.): Qual. Issues in the Management of Web Information. ISRL, vol. 50. Springer, Heidelberg (2013)

# Interactive Data Exploration
# Using Pattern Mining

Matthijs van Leeuwen

Machine Learning group
KU Leuven, Leuven, Belgium
matthijs.vanleeuwen@cs.kuleuven.be

**Abstract.** We live in the era of data and need tools to discover valuable information in large amounts of data. The goal of exploratory data mining is to provide as much insight in given data as possible. Within this field, pattern set mining aims at revealing structure in the form of sets of patterns. Although pattern set mining has shown to be an effective solution to the infamous pattern explosion, important challenges remain.

One of the key challenges is to develop principled methods that allow user- and task-specific information to be taken into account, by directly involving the user in the discovery process. This way, the resulting patterns will be more relevant and interesting to the user. To achieve this, pattern mining algorithms will need to be combined with techniques from both visualisation and human-computer interaction. Another challenge is to establish techniques that perform well under constrained resources, as existing methods are usually computationally intensive. Consequently, they are only applied to relatively small datasets and on fast computers.

The ultimate goal is to make pattern mining practically more useful, by enabling the user to interactively explore the data and identify interesting structure. In this paper we describe the state-of-the-art, discuss open problems, and outline promising future directions.

**Keywords:** Interactive Data Exploration, Pattern Mining, Data Mining.

## 1   Introduction

We live in the era of data. Last year it was estimated that 297 exabytes of data had been stored, and this amount increases every year. Making sense of this data is one of the fundamental challenges that we are currently facing, with applications in virtually any discipline. Manually sifting through large amounts of data is infeasible, in particular because it is often unknown what one is looking for exactly. Therefore, appropriate tools are required to digest data and reveal the valuable information it contains.

Although data is everywhere, it is not unusual that the domain experts who have access to the data have no idea what information is contained in it. KDD, which stands for *Knowledge Discovery in Data*, aims to extract knowledge from data. In particular, the goal of the field of *exploratory data mining* is to provide

A. Holzinger, I. Jurisica (Eds.): Knowledge Discovery and Data Mining, LNCS 8401, pp. 169–182, 2014.

a domain expert as much insight in given data as possible. Although inherently vague and ill-defined, it aims to provide a positive answer to the question: *Can you tell me something interesting about my data?*

As such, its high-level aim is similar to that of *visual analytics*, but the approach is rather different. Whereas visual analytics focuses on visualization in combination with human-computer interaction to improve a user's understanding of the data, exploratory data mining focuses on finding models and patterns that explain the data. This results in (typically hard) combinatorial search problems for which efficient algorithms need to be developed. Depending on the problem and the size of the data, exact or heuristic search is used.

**Pattern Mining.** Within exploratory data mining, *pattern mining* aims to enable the discovery of patterns from data. A *pattern* is a description of some structure that occurs locally in the data, i.e., it describes part of the data. The best-known instance is probably frequent itemset mining [1], which discovers combinations of 'items' that frequently occur together in the data. For example, a bioinformatician could use frequent itemset mining to discover treatments and symptoms that often co-occur in a dataset containing patient information.

A pattern-based approach to data mining has clear advantages, in particular in an exploratory setting. One advantage is that patterns are interpretable representations and can thus provide explanations. This is a very desirable property, and is in stark contrast to 'black-box' approaches with which it is often unclear why certain outcomes are obtained. A second large advantage is that patterns can be used for many well-known data mining tasks.

Unfortunately, obtaining interesting results with traditional pattern mining methods can be a tough and time-consuming job. The two main problems are that: 1) humongous amounts of patterns are found, of which many are redundant, and 2) background knowledge of the domain expert is not taken into account. To remedy these issues, careful tuning of the algorithm parameters and manual filtering of the results is necessary. This requires considerable effort and expertise from the data analyst. That is, the data analyst needs be both a domain expert and a data mining expert, which makes the job extremely challenging.

**Pattern Set Mining.** As a solution to the redundancy problem in pattern mining, a recent trend is to mine pattern *sets* instead of individual patterns. The difference is that apart from constraints on individual patterns, additional constraints and/or an optimisation criterion are imposed on the complete set of patterns. Although *pattern set mining* [2] is a promising and expanding line of research, it is not yet widely adopted in practice because, like pattern mining, directly applying it to real-world applications is often not trivial.

One of the main issues is that the second problem of pattern mining has not yet been addressed: background knowledge of the domain expert is not taken into account. Because of this, algorithms still need to be tuned by running the algorithm, waiting for the final results, changing the parameters, re-running, waiting for the new results, etc. Most existing methods can only deal with interestingness measures that are completely *objective*, i.e., interestingness of a pattern or pattern set is computed from the data only.

**Related Approaches.** To tackle the problems of tuning and uninteresting results, Guns et al. [3] advocate an approach based on *declarative modelling*. The analyst can specify the desired results by means of constraints and, optionally, an optimisation criterion. The idea is that constraints are intuitive, and can be iteratively added to the declarative model. A downside is that modelling background knowledge and the task at hand can be tough and still requires substantial skills from the analyst. Furthermore, the constraints need to constructed manually, while interactive approaches could learn these automatically.

Only very few existing exploratory data mining methods use *visualisation* and/or *human-computer interaction* (HCI). To spark attention to the potential synergy of combining these fields with data mining, a recent workshop [4] brought together researchers from all these fields. When visualisation is used in data mining, this is often done after the search [5,6]. MIME [7] is an interactive tool that allows a user to explore itemsets, but only using traditional interestingness measures, which makes it still hard to find something that is subjectively interesting. Although data mining suites like RapidMiner[1] and KNIME[2] have graphical user interfaces that make data analysis relatively accessible, one needs to construct a workflow and tune parameters.

The importance of taking user knowledge and goals into account was first emphasised by Tuzhilin [8]. More recently De Bie et al. [9,10] argued that traditional objective quality measures are of limited practical use and proposed a general framework that models background knowledge. This work strongly focuses on *modelling* subjective interestingness, and using the resulting measure for mining is not always straightforward.

**Aims and Roadmap.** The purpose of this paper is to discuss the current state-of-the-art in interactive data exploration using pattern mining, and to point out open problems and promising future directions. In the end, the overall goal is to make pattern set mining a more useful tool for exploratory data mining: to enable efficient pattern-based data exploration and identify interesting structure in data, where interestingness is both user- and task-specific.

For this, we argue that it is essential to *actively involve the user in the discovery process*. After all, interestingness is both user- and task-specific. To achieve this, close collaboration between data mining and both human-computer interaction and visualisation will be needed, as Holzinger [11] recently also argued. By integrating efficient pattern mining algorithms into the visual analytics loop [12], and combining these with sophisticated and adaptive subjective interestingness measures, pattern-based data exploration will be able to tell you something interesting about your data.

After providing an introduction to pattern mining and pattern set mining in Section 2, Section 3 describes the current state-of-the-art in interactive pattern mining. After that, Section 4 illustrates the potential of interactive pattern mining with a case study in sports analytics. Section 5 discusses open problems and potential directions for future research, after which we conclude in Section 6.

---

[1] www.rapidminer.com

[2] www.knime.org

# 2    Background and Glossary

This section provides an introduction to pattern mining and pattern set mining, which can be safely skipped by readers already familiar with these areas.

## 2.1    Pattern Mining

*Pattern mining* aims to reveal structure in data in the form of patterns. A pattern is an element of a specified pattern language $\mathcal{P}$ that describes a subset in a dataset $D$; a pattern can be regarded as a description of some *local structure*. The commonly used formalisation of pattern mining is called theory mining, where the goal is to find the theory $Th(\mathcal{P}; D; q) = \{p \in \mathcal{P} \mid q(p, D) = \texttt{true}\}$, with $q$ a selection predicate that returns true iff $p$ satisfies the imposed constraints on $D$.

Many instances of this task exist, with different algorithms for each of them. For example, frequent itemsets [1] are combinations of items that occur more often than a given threshold. In this context, a database $D$ is a bag of transactions over a set of items $I$, where a transaction $t$ is a subset of $I$, i.e., $t \subseteq I$. Furthermore, a pattern $p$ is an itemset, $p \subseteq I$, and pattern language $\mathcal{P}$ is the set of all such possible patterns, $\mathcal{P} = 2^I$. An itemset $p$ occurs in a transaction $t$ iff $p \subseteq t$, and its support is defined as the number of transactions in $D$ which it occurs, i.e., $supp(p, D) = |\{t \subseteq D \mid p \subseteq t\}|$. A pattern $p$ is said to be frequent iff its support exceeds the minimum support threshold *minsup*. That is, $q$ returns true iff $supp(p, D) > minsup$, and the theory consists of all itemsets satisfying $q$. Frequent itemsets can be mined efficiently due to monotonicity of the frequency constraint. Other types of frequent patterns exist for e.g., sequences and graphs.

*Subgroup discovery* [13, 14] is another example of pattern mining. It is concerned with finding subsets of a dataset for which a target property of interest deviates substantially when compared to the entire dataset. In the context of a bank providing loans, for example, we could find that 16% of all loans with *purpose = used car* are not repaid, whereas for the entire population this proportion is only 5%. Subgroup discovery algorithms can cope with a wide range of data types, from simple binary data to numerical attributes and structured data. Subgroup interestingness measures generally compute a combination of the degree of deviation and the size of the subset.

All pattern mining techniques have the disadvantage that the selection predicate $q$ considers only individual patterns. Consequently, vast amounts of similar and hence redundant patterns are found – the infamous *pattern explosion*. Suppose a supermarket that sells $n$ different products. In this case, there are $2^n$ combinations of products that each form an itemset $p$. If an itemset $p$ frequently occurs in the data, all $r \subseteq p$ are automatically also frequent. In practice this means that $Th(\mathcal{P}; D; q)$ contains an enormous amount of patterns, of which many are very similar to each other.

An initial attempt to solve this problem was the notion of condensed representations. Closed frequent itemsets [15], for example, are those itemsets $p$ for which no $r \subset p$ exists that describes the same subset of the data. From the set of closed itemsets, the full set of frequent itemsets can be reconstructed and the condensed representation is, hence, lossless. Unfortunately, most condensed representations result in pattern collections that are still too large to be practically useful or interpretable by domain experts.

Also making this observation, Han wrote in 2007 [16]:

> We feel the bottleneck of frequent pattern mining is not on whether we can derive the complete set of frequent patterns under certain constraints efficiently but on whether we can derive a compact but high quality set of patterns that are most useful in applications.

## 2.2    Pattern Set Mining

A recent trend that alleviates the pattern explosion is pattern set mining [2], by imposing constraints on the complete result set in addition to those on individual patterns. From a theory mining perspective, this results in the following formalisation: $Th(\mathcal{P}; D; q) = \{S \subseteq \mathcal{P} \mid q(S, D) = \texttt{true}\}$.

Depending on the constraints, in practice this can still result in a gigantic set of results, but now consisting of pattern sets instead of patterns. Mining all pattern sets satisfying the constraints is therefore both undesirable and infeasible, and it is common practice to mine just one. For this purpose, some optimisation criterion is often added. Due to the large search space this can still be quite challenging and heuristic search is commonly employed.

While a pattern describes only local structure, a pattern set is expected to provide a global perspective on the data. Hence, it can be regarded as a (global) model consisting of (local) patterns, and a criterion is needed to perform model selection. Depending on the objective, such criteria are based on e.g. mutual information [17] or the Minimum Description Length (MDL) principle [18]. In all cases, the task can be paraphrased as: *Find the best set of patterns.*

As an example, KRIMP [18] uses the MDL principle to induce itemset-based descriptions of binary data. Informally, the MDL principle states that the best model is the one that compresses the data best, and the goal of KRIMP is to find a set of patterns that best compresses the data. It was already mentioned that one of the advantages of pattern-based approaches is that patterns can be used for many other data mining tasks. This is particularly true for the compression approach to pattern-based modelling: successful applications include, e.g., classification [19], clustering [20], and difference characterisation [21].

## 2.3    Glossary

**Pattern Mining.** Discovering local structure from data through algorithmic search, where structure is represented by interpretable elements from a pattern language.

**Frequent Pattern Mining.** Includes frequent itemset mining, but also methods for mining frequent sequences, (sub)graphs, and other pattern types.

**Subgroup Discovery.** Subgroup discovery can be seen as an instance of *supervised descriptive rule discovery* [22]. It aims at discovering descriptions of data subsets that deviate with respect to a specified target.

**Top-K Pattern Mining.** Search for the $k$ best patterns with regard to an interestingness measure. Does not solve the pattern explosion, because of the redundancy in the used pattern languages and correlations in the data.

**Pattern Set Mining.** Mine *sets of patterns* instead of individual patterns. The large advantage of imposing global constraints and/or having an optimisation criteria is that redundancy can be eliminated.

**Descriptive Pattern Set Mining.** One of the main classes that can be distinguished in pattern set mining, which aims to provide compact and interpretable descriptions of the data.

**Supervised Pattern Set Mining.** A second main class, used when there is a specific target property of interest. Subgroup discovery is an example of a supervised pattern mining task, and pattern set mining variants also exist.

**Objective Interestingness.** Almost all interestingness measures for pattern (set) mining up to date are unable to deal with background knowledge or user feedback provided by a domain expert, and are therefore called objective.

**Subjective Interestingness.** Interestingness is inherently subjective and should take into account the goals and background knowledge of the current user.

## 3    State-of-the-Art

For the sake of brevity, in this section we restrict ourselves to recent pattern mining techniques that go *beyond objective interestingness* and enable *user interaction*. We consider both descriptive and supervised techniques. See Kontonasios et al. [9] for a discussion of interestingness measures based on *unexpectedness*.

### 3.1    Integrating Interaction into Search

Subjective interestingness can be attained in several ways, and one high-level approach is to exploit user feedback to directly influence search.

Bhuiyan et al. [23] proposed a technique that is based on Markov Chain Monte Carlo (MCMC) sampling of frequent patterns. By sampling individual patterns from a specified distribution, the pattern explosion can be avoided while still ensuring a representative sample of the complete set of patterns. While sampling patterns, the user is allowed to provide feedback by *liking* or *disliking* them. This feedback is used to update the sampling distribution, so that new patterns are mined from the updated distribution. For the distribution, a scoring function is assumed in which each individual item has a weight and all items are independent of each other. By updating the weights, the scores of the itemsets and thus the sampling distribution change. Initially all weights are set to 1, so that the initial sampling distribution is the uniform distribution over all patterns.

In similar spirit, Dzyuba & Van Leeuwen [24] recently proposed Interactive Diverse Subgroup Discovery (IDSD), an interactive algorithm that allows a user to provide feedback with respect to provisional results and steer the search away from regions that she finds uninteresting. The intuition behind the approach is that the 'best' subgroups often correspond to common knowledge, which is usually uninteresting to a domain expert.

IDSD builds upon Diverse Subgroup Set Discovery (DSSD) [25]. DSSD was proposed in an attempt to eliminate redundancy by using a *diverse* beam search. For IDSD we augmented it by making the beam selection strategy interactive: on each level of the search, users are allowed to influence the beam by *liking* and *disliking* subgroups, as with the previous method. This affects the interestingness measure, which effectively becomes subjective. IDSD uses a naive scheme to influence the search and, as a result, does not always provide the desired results. However, as we will see in the next section, even a simple method like this can vastly improve the results by exploiting user feedback.

Galbrun and Miettinen [26] introduced SIREN, a system for visual and interactive mining of geospatial redescriptions. Geospatial redescription mining aims to discover pairs of descriptions for the same region, with each description over a different set of features. The system visualises the regions described by the discovered patterns, and allows the user to influence the search in ways similar to those used by IDSD; SIREN is also based on beam search. Although its specialisation to the geospatial setting is both an advantage and a disadvantage, it is another proof-of-concept demonstrating the potential of user interaction.

### 3.2 Learning User- and Task-Specific Interestingness

Although the methods in the previous subsection use interaction to influence the results, their ability to 'capture' subjective interestingness is limited. This is due both to the type of feedback and the mechanisms used to process this feedback.

Taking these aspects one step further, one can *learn* subjective interestingness from feedback given to patterns. This idea was recently investigated independently by both Boley et al. [27] and Dzyuba et al. [28]. The central idea is to *alternate between mining and learning*: the system mines an initial batch of patterns, a user is given the opportunity to provide feedback, the system learns the user's preferences, a new collection of patterns is mined using these updated preferences, etc. For learning the preferences of the user, standard machine learning techniques can be used, e.g., preference learning. Although the two approaches have a lot in common, there are also some important differences.

The *One Click Mining* system presented by Boley et al. can use any combination of pattern mining algorithms and learns two types of preferences at the same time. One one hand, it uses a multi-armed bandit strategy to learn which pattern mining algorithms produce the results that are most appreciated by the user. This is used to allocate the available computation time to the different algorithms. On the other hand and at the same time, co-active learning is used to learn a utility function over a feature representation of patterns. This utility function is used to compute a ranking over all mined patterns, which is used to determine which patterns are presented, and in what order, to the user. Both learning algorithms completely rely on input provided by means of *implicit user feedback*. Mined patterns are presented in a graphical user interface and the user can freely inspect and store them, or move them to the thrash.

Dzyuba et al. focus on a narrower research question: is it possible to learn a subjective ranking, i.e., a total order, over the space of all possible patterns, from a limited number of small 'queries' that are ranked by a user? For this, they partly build on the work by Rueping [29]. The assumption is that a user has an implicit preference between any pair of patterns, but cannot express this preference relation for all possible pairs. The proposed approach gives the user a small number of patterns (subgroups) and asks her to rank these patterns. RankSVM is then used to learn a preference relation over a feature representation of the patterns, and the resulting utility function can be used to mine subjectively more interesting patterns. An important difference with the approach by Boley et al. is that the learnt utility function is used as optimization criterion in the mining phase, and not only to rank the patterns returned by mining algorithms using objective interestingness measures. Also, query selection strategies inspired by active learning and information retrieval are used to select queries that minimise the effort required from the user.

### 3.3   Formalising Subjective Interestingness

All methods discussed so far focus on learning and mining subjectively interesting patterns based on user feedback, but by using a specific learning algorithm they all potentially introduce a strong learning bias. To avoid this, one should first *formalise* subjective interestingness with a principled approach, and then develop the machinery required for using this formalisation.

De Bie [10] has developed a formal framework for exploratory data mining that formalises subjective interestingness using information theoretical principles. The general strategy is to consider prior beliefs, e.g., background information, as constraints on a probabilistic model representing the uncertainty of the data. To avoid introducing any bias, the Maximum Entropy distribution given the prior beliefs is used as model for the data. Given such a 'MaxEnt model', any pattern can be scored against it: one can compute how informative a pattern is given the current model. To avoid overly specific patterns from getting very high scores, the scores are normalised by the complexities of the pattern descriptions.

This framework lends itself well to *iterative data mining*: starting from a MaxEnt model based on prior beliefs, one can look for the subjectively most interesting pattern, which can then be added to the model, after which one can start looking for the next pattern, etc. Because the model is updated after the discovery of each high-scoring pattern, redundancy is avoided. A disadvantage is that the exact implementation of the 'MaxEnt approach' heavily relies on the specific data and pattern types at hand, but instances have been proposed for a variety of data types, e.g. for binary data [30] and multi-relational-data [31].

### 3.4   Advantages and Disadvantages

Some advantages of pattern-based approaches to exploratory data mining have already been discussed, i.e., patterns are not only interpretable, they can also be

**Table 1.** Subgroups discovered from the NBA dataset, (a) without and (b) with interaction. Given for each subgroup are its description, its size (number of tuples for which the description holds), and its (objective) interestingness. Taken from [24].

| Description | Size | Interestingness |
|---|---|---|
| $opp\_def\_reb = F \wedge opponent \neq ATL \wedge thabeet = F$ | 219 | 0.0692 |
| $opp\_def\_reb = F \wedge opponent \neq ATL$ | 222 | 0.0689 |
| $opp\_def\_reb = F \wedge opponent \neq ATL \wedge ajohnson = F$ | 222 | 0.0689 |
| $opp\_def\_reb = F \wedge thabeet = F \wedge opponent \neq PHI$ | 225 | 0.0685 |
| $opp\_def\_reb = F \wedge opponent \neq PHI$ | 228 | 0.0682 |

(a) Without interaction – DSSD.

| Description | Size | Interestingness |
|---|---|---|
| $crawford = F \wedge matthews = T$ | 96 | 0.0328 |
| $hickson = T$ | 143 | 0.0219 |
| $crawford = F \wedge hickson = T$ | 63 | 0.0211 |
| $matthews = T \wedge hickson = T$ | 99 | 0.0163 |
| $matthews = T \wedge pace < 88.518$ | 303 | 0.0221 |

(b) With interaction – IDSD.

used for many other data mining tasks. Another advantage is that pattern languages are generally very expressive, which makes it possible to discover almost any local structure that is present in the data. This is, however, also one of the major disadvantages: because the languages are so expressive, in practice many patterns describe highly similar or even equivalent parts of the data.

Specific advantages of the methods presented in this section are that they allow the user to interactively find subjectively interesting patterns, at least to some extent. The methods in the first two subsections are limited when it comes to modelling interestingness, while the MaxEnt approach primarily focuses on scoring patterns and cannot be (straightforwardly) used for interactive learning and/or mining. All methods focus primarily on mining individual patterns rather than pattern sets, although the MaxEnt framework partially solves this by making iterative mining possible. Additional limitations and disadvantages of existing methods are discussed in Section 5.

## 4   Case Study: Sports Analytics

Let us illustrate the potential of interactive pattern mining with an example taken from Dzyuba et al. [24]. The example concerns a case study on basketball games played in the NBA. More specifically, experiments were performed on a categorical dataset containing information about games played by the Portland Trail Blazers in the 2011/12 season. Each tuple corresponds to a game segment and the attributes represent presence of individual players and standard game statistics. Please refer to [24] for further details.

Table 1 presents the results obtained on this data with two different subgroup discovery methods: one with and one without interaction. As target property of interest, offensive rating was used, i.e., the average number of points per shot. This means that subgroups with high interestingness describe game situations with a high average number of points per shot, which obviously makes it more likely for the team to win the game. The results were evaluated by a domain expert, i.e., a basketball journalist.

For the setting without interaction, DSSD [25] was used with its default parameter settings (Table 1(a)). The results suffer from two severe problems. First, the results are clearly redundant, i.e., diversity could not be attained with the default parameter settings. In fact, the subgroups together describe only 231 of 923 game segments (25.3%). Second, none of the discovered subgroups are interesting to the domain expert, as the descriptions contain no surprising and/or actionable information. For example, it is a trivial fact for experts that poor defensive rebounding by an opponent ($opp\_def\_reb = F$) makes scoring easier, while *absence of reserve players* Thabeet and A. Johnson is not informative either – they more often than not are on the bench anyway.

For the interactive setting, the basketball journalist was asked to use IDSD [24] and evaluate its results (Table 1(b)). With limited effort, he was able to find subgroups that he considered more interesting and actionable: Crawford, Matthews, and Hickson were key players and they often played for the team. So although *objective* interestingness of the subgroups was clearly lower, *subjective* interestingness was substantially higher. In addition, the five subgroups together cover 512 game segments (55.5% of the dataset), implying that the interactive results are also more diverse than the non-interactive. A disadvantage of this particular approach is that not all sessions resulted in interesting results, but this is due to the (ad hoc) way in which feedback is elicited and processed.

## 5   Open Problems and Future Outlook

We now discuss a number of open problems that we believe need to be solved in order to achieve the overall goal of interactive, pattern-based data exploration.

**1. Discovery of Pattern-Based Models for Specific Users and/or Tasks.** We have argued that purely objective interestingness measures that cannot be influenced are inherently problematic, since interestingness depends on the specific user and task at hand. Hence, adaptivity and subjective interestingness are required. For this, we need an iterative approach to pattern-based modelling that learns what models are interesting during the discovery process, as illustrated in Figure 1. By learning user- and/or task-specific interestingness based on intermediate results, the system can gradually refine and improve its results.

This could be achieved through interaction with a domain expert, but another approach would be to automatically learn task-specific utility, e.g. by having some (automated) feedback procedure as to how useful intermediate results are in an online setting. In such situations an important challenge might be to deal with concept drift, i.e., interestingness must be adaptive and change when needed.

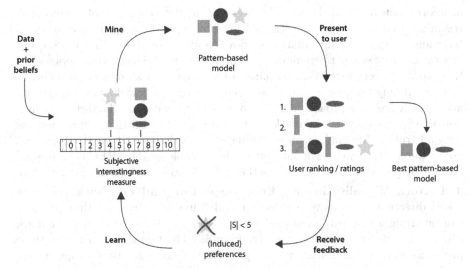

**Fig. 1.** General approach to learning subjective interestingness for pattern sets

The methods described in the previous section are a good start in this direction, but they all have their limitations. We need more principled solutions that incorporate both 1) *learning and modelling of interestingness*, and 2) *mining of subjectively interesting pattern-based models*. In particular, most existing interactive pattern mining techniques consider only the subjective interestingness of individual patterns, not that of pattern sets.

**2. Resource-Constrained Pattern Set Mining through Sampling.** Even on modern desktop computers and dedicated computing servers, existing pattern set mining methods require at least minutes and sometimes hours to compute a result. This makes it hard to apply these methods in a realistic environment, e.g., for purposes of interactive mining, in settings where resources are constrained, or when there is ample of data. Interactive data mining can only become successful if results can be computed and presented to the user virtually instantly.

Pattern (set) sampling according to some subjective, learnt interestingness measure could provide a solution to this problem. Due to extensive redundancy in the solution space, it is sufficient to identify good solutions rather than the optimal solution. These can be presented to, and evaluated by, the user or system, so that feedback can be given and the subjective interestingness can be updated.

**3. Principled Evaluation of Exploratory Data Mining Results.** Over the past years we have witnessed the publication of a large number of novel algorithms for exploratory data mining. Despite this, there is still a lack of principled methods for the qualitative evaluation of these techniques. Consequently, it is not always clear which methods perform well and under what circumstances.

Although this problem is partly due to the nature of the area, i.e., *exploratory* data mining, the field would greatly benefit from principled evaluation methods. One approach would be to do (possibly large-scale) user studies, as is also done in information retrieval. It could be argued that the evaluation of pattern sets resembles that of documents retrieved for queries, and therefore measures and techniques inspired by information retrieval could be used. For that reason, collaborations between pattern mining and information retrieval researchers on this topic could be very valuable. A disadvantage is that user studies are complex to conduct, if only because in many cases only one or very few domain experts are available. Another approach might be to construct benchmark datasets for which domain experts know what knowledge they contain. If this can be represented as 'ground truth', this might help to evaluate both existing and novel algorithms. For example, the benchmark datasets made available by the TREC conferences[3] have helped substantially to advance the state-of-the-art in information retrieval.

**4. Pattern Visualisation for Easy Inspection and Feedback.** The proposed directions to solving problems 1 and 3 implicitly assume that patterns can be straightforwardly presented to the user, and that the desired feedback can be elicited, but these are non-trivial problems by themselves. To solve these problems, close collaboration with experts from fields like visualisation, visual analytics, and human-computer interaction will be essential.

One problem concerns the *visualisation of patterns together with the data.* Although the descriptions of patterns can be easily presented to a user, interpretation takes time. In particular when a set of patterns is to be evaluated by a user, it would help to visualise the structure in the data that it represents. Even for itemsets and binary data, this can already be quite complex: a single itemset can be visualised as a square in the matrix, but multiple itemsets do not need to be contiguous and may overlap.

A second problem concerns the *interaction between the user and patterns.* Different types of feedback can be used for inducing subjective interestingness, either implicit (inspect, thrash, ignore, etc.) or explicit (ratings, ranking patterns, etc.). But what is the best way to let a user interact with patterns? In the context of pattern mining this question is currently completely unexplored.

# 6   Conclusions

We argued that it is essential to actively involve the user in the exploratory data mining process in order to discover more interesting results. The state-of-the-art in interactive pattern mining demonstrates that even simple techniques can already vastly improve the results. Still, four important challenges remain.

The first key challenge is to develop principled methods for *learning and modelling user- and task-specific interestingness.* The second challenge is tightly connected to this and is to enable *resource-constrained mining of subjectively interesting pattern-based models.* Once solved, the solutions to these challenges will together form a firm foundation for interactive data mining, but to make this successful the last two challenges will need to be addressed as well.

That is, the third challenge concerns the *principled evaluation of exploratory data mining results,* which is important to be able to compare methods. In particular

---

[3] http://trec.nist.gov/

for interactive data mining, solid evaluation methodologies are required, because results are likely to be deemed too subjective otherwise. The fourth and final challenge is to establish *visualisation and interaction designs for pattern-based models*, to enable effective presentation and feedback elicitation.

The ultimate goal is to make pattern mining practically more useful, by enabling the user to interactively explore the data and identify interesting structure through pattern-based models that can be visualised and interacted with.

**Acknowledgments.** The author is supported by a Postdoctoral Fellowship of the Research Foundation Flanders (FWO). He would like to thank Vladimir Dzyuba for providing useful comments on an early version of this paper.

# References

1. Agrawal, R., Imielinksi, T., Swami, A.: Mining association rules between sets of items in large databases. In: Proceedings of the SIGMOD 1993, pp. 207–216. ACM (1993)
2. Bringmann, B., Nijssen, S., Tatti, N., Vreeken, J., Zimmermann, A.: Mining sets of patterns: Next generation pattern mining. In: Tutorial at ICDM 2011(2011)
3. Guns, T., Nijssen, S., Raedt, L.D.: Itemset mining: A constraint programming perspective. Artif. Intell. 175(12-13), 1951–1983 (2011)
4. Chau, D.H., Vreeken, J., van Leeuwen, M., Faloutsos, C. (eds.): Proceedings of the ACM SIGKDD Workshop on Interactive Data Exploration and Analytics, IDEA 2013. ACM, New York (2013)
5. Atzmüller, M., Puppe, F.: Semi-automatic visual subgroup mining using vikamine. Journal of Universal Computer Science 11(11), 1752–1765 (2005)
6. Lucas, J.P., Jorge, A.M., Pereira, F., Pernas, A.M., Machado, A.A.: A tool for interactive subgroup discovery using distribution rules. In: Neves, J., Santos, M.F., Machado, J.M. (eds.) EPIA 2007. LNCS (LNAI), vol. 4874, pp. 426–436. Springer, Heidelberg (2007)
7. Goethals, B., Moens, S., Vreeken, J.: MIME: A framework for interactive visual pattern mining. In: Gunopulos, D., Hofmann, T., Malerba, D., Vazirgiannis, M. (eds.) ECML PKDD 2011, Part III. LNCS (LNAI), vol. 6913, pp. 634–637. Springer, Heidelberg (2011)
8. Tuzhilin, A.: On subjective measures of interestingness in knowledge discovery. In: Proceedings of KDD 1995, pp. 275–281 (1995)
9. Kontonasios, K.N., Spyropoulou, E., De Bie, T.: Knowledge discovery interestingness measures based on unexpectedness. Wiley Int. Rev. Data Min. and Knowl. Disc. 2(5), 386–399 (2012)
10. De Bie, T.: An information theoretic framework for data mining. In: Proceedings of KDD 2011, pp. 564–572 (2011)
11. Holzinger, A.: Human-computer interaction and knowledge discovery (hci-kdd): What is the benefit of bringing those two fields to work together? In: Cuzzocrea, A., Kittl, C., Simos, D.E., Weippl, E., Xu, L. (eds.) CD-ARES 2013. LNCS, vol. 8127, pp. 319–328. Springer, Heidelberg (2013)
12. Keim, D.A., Andrienko, G., Fekete, J.-D., Görg, C., Kohlhammer, J., Melançon, G.: Visual analytics: Definition, process, and challenges. In: Kerren, A., Stasko, J.T., Fekete, J.-D., North, C. (eds.) Information Visualization. LNCS, vol. 4950, pp. 154–175. Springer, Heidelberg (2008)

13. Klösgen, W.: Explora: A Multipattern and Multistrategy Discovery Assistant. In: Advances in Knowledge Discovery and Data Mining, pp. 249–271 (1996)
14. Wrobel, S.: An algorithm for multi-relational discovery of subgroups. In: Komorowski, J., Żytkow, J. (eds.) PKDD 1997. LNCS, vol. 1263, pp. 78–87. Springer, Heidelberg (1997)
15. Pasquier, N., Bastide, Y., Taouil, R., Lakhal, L.: Discovering frequent closed itemsets for association rules. In: Beeri, C., Bruneman, P. (eds.) ICDT 1999. LNCS, vol. 1540, pp. 398–416. Springer, Heidelberg (1998)
16. Han, J., Cheng, H., Xin, D., Yan, X.: Frequent pattern mining: Current status and future directions. Data Mining and Knowledge Discovery 15(1), 55–86 (2007)
17. Peng, H., Long, F., Ding, C.: Feature selection based on mutual information: Criteria of max-dependency, max-relevance, and min-redundancy. IEEE Transactions on Pattern Analysis and Machine Intelligence 27(8), 1226–1238 (2005)
18. Vreeken, J., van Leeuwen, M., Siebes, A.: Krimp: mining itemsets that compress. Data Mining and Knowledge Discovery 23(1), 169–214 (2011)
19. van Leeuwen, M., Vreeken, J., Siebes, A.: Compression picks item sets that matter. In: Fürnkranz, J., Scheffer, T., Spiliopoulou, M. (eds.) PKDD 2006. LNCS (LNAI), vol. 4213, pp. 585–592. Springer, Heidelberg (2006)
20. van Leeuwen, M., Vreeken, J., Siebes, A.: Identifying the components. Data Min. Knowl. Discov. 19(2), 173–292 (2009)
21. Vreeken, J., van Leeuwen, M., Siebes, A.: Characterising the difference. In: Proceedings of the KDD 2007, pp. 765–774 (2007)
22. Kralj Novak, P., Lavrač, N., Webb, G.: Supervised descriptive rule discovery: A unifying survey of contrast set, emerging pattern and subgroup mining. Journal of Machine Learning Research 10, 377–403 (2009)
23. Bhuiyan, M., Mukhopadhyay, S., Hasan, M.A.: Interactive pattern mining on hidden data: A sampling-based solution. In: Proceedings of CIKM 2012, pp. 95–104. ACM, New York (2012)
24. Dzyuba, V., van Leeuwen, M.: Interactive discovery of interesting subgroup sets. In: Tucker, A., Höppner, F., Siebes, A., Swift, S. (eds.) IDA 2013. LNCS, vol. 8207, pp. 150–161. Springer, Heidelberg (2013)
25. van Leeuwen, M., Knobbe, A.: Diverse subgroup set discovery. Data Mining and Knowledge Discovery 25, 208–242 (2012)
26. Galbrun, E., Miettinen, P.: A Case of Visual and Interactive Data Analysis: Geospatial Redescription Mining. In: Instant Interactive Data Mining Workshop at ECML-PKDD 2012 (2012)
27. Boley, M., Mampaey, M., Kang, B., Tokmakov, P., Wrobel, S.: One Click Mining — Interactive Local Pattern Discovery through Implicit Preference and Performance Learning. In: Interactive Data Exploration and Analytics (IDEA) workshop at KDD 2013, pp. 28–36 (2013)
28. Dzyuba, V., van Leeuwen, M., Nijssen, S., Raedt, L.D.: Active preference learning for ranking patterns. In: Proceedings of ICTAI 2013, pp. 532–539 (2013)
29. Rüping, S.: Ranking interesting subgroups. In: Proceedings of ICML 2009, pp. 913–920 (2009)
30. Bie, T.D.: Maximum entropy models and subjective interestingness: an application to tiles in binary databases. Data Min. Knowl. Discov. 23(3), 407–446 (2011)
31. Spyropoulou, E., Bie, T.D., Boley, M.: Interesting pattern mining in multi-relational data. Data Min. Knowl. Discov. 28(3), 808–849 (2014)

# Resources for Studying Statistical Analysis of Biomedical Data and R

Mei Kobayashi

IBM Research-Tokyo, 5-6-52 Toyosu, Koto-ku, Tokyo 135-8511 Japan
MeiKobayashi@acm.org

**Abstract.** The past decade has seen explosive growth in digitized medical data. This trend offers medical practitioners an unparalleled opportunity to identify effectiveness of treatments for patients using summary statistics and to offer patients more personalized medical treatments based on predictive analytics. To exploit this opportunity, statisticians and computer scientists need to work and communicate effectively with medical practitioners to ensure proper measurement data, collection of sufficient volumes of heterogeneous data to ensure patient privacy, and understanding of probabilities and sources of errors associated with data sampling. Interdisciplinary collaborations between scientists are likely to lead to the development of more effective methods for explaining probabilities, possible errors, and risks associated with treatment options to patients. This chapter introduces some online resources to help medical practitioners with little or no background in summary and predictive statistics learn basic statistical concepts and implement data analysis on their personal computers using R, a high-level computer language that requires relatively little training. Readers who are only interested in understanding basic statistical concepts may want to skip the subsection on R.

**Keywords:** big data, data mining, knowledge discovery, KDD, KDDM, medical informatics, genomics, P4 medicine, privacy preserving data mining, PPDM, summary statistics, inferential statistics, R programming language.

## 1 Introduction

The past decade has seen an explosive growth in digitized medical data. A 2010 survey of healthcare providers found 41% of respondents expected 25% annual increases in data volume, and 18.1% of respondents expected annual increases between 25% and 50% [1]. The main drivers of data growth cited by the report were: digital imaging files, electronic personal records, electronic health records, and scanned documents. A follow-up survey in 2012 found that the healthcare industry was generating roughly 30% of worldwide data, and the volume was increasing daily [2]. Moreover, 80% of medical data is unstructured and clinically relevant [3]. In the United States, the trend towards digitization of medical data was accelerated in 2009 following the enactment of the electronic health record mandate within the American Recovery and Reinvestment Act of 2009 (President Obama's economic stimulus bill) [4, 5]. Ideas in the legislation, which promotes the use of electronic medical records,

A. Holzinger, I. Jurisica (Eds.): Knowledge Discovery and Data Mining, LNCS 8401, pp. 183–195, 2014.
© Springer-Verlag Berlin Heidelberg 2014

were supported as far back as 2004 when President Bush called for digitization of medical records in his State of the Union address.

Until recently, digitized medical data sets were relatively small, and the high cost of computing limited most analyses of the output to summary statistics (e.g., mean, median, mode, standard deviation, kurtosis, skewness, and correlation coefficients). Evaluation of treatments required long-term studies, and conditions under which data were measured were variable due to inevitable changes that were beyond the control of parties conducting the measurements. Examples of these changes include: seasonal flux of the weather, changes in medical staff, repair or replacement of equipment, and changes in patient treatments due to advances in science and technology.

The advent of relatively inexpensive storage media (including clouds), high performance PCs, and a new generation of sophisticated medical equipment are igniting a digital revolution in medical data acquisition and storage. Vast new repositories of more accurate and complete, digitized data offer medical practitioners an unparalleled opportunity to develop predictive, probabilistic models of patient outcomes for treatments. However, analysis of medical data poses a completely new set of restrictions and challenges.

Although scientists have made major advances in mining massive datasets – both static and dynamic (i.e., data streams and data in motion), medical data analysis can be constrained by additional factors, such as:

- *Dearth of high quality data from consistent, reliable sources* – For rare medical conditions, combining data sets from different sources may be necessary to obtain a sufficient volume of data to enable meaningful analysis. Fusion of data sets from multiple sources is often complicated by variations in measurement methodologies, conditions under which data are collected, and different types of inherent and human-induced errors.
- *Limited means for data collection* – Usually only people in ill health undergo extensive testing. Sometimes data on normal, healthy people are needed to serve as baseline data. However, large volumes of data on healthy people may not be available for some types of tests due to the high cost (e.g., MRI) or health and safety concerns restricting their use (e.g., radiation or hazardous chemical exposure).
- *Patient privacy concerns and laws* – Restrictions on data access may be necessary if mining of the data can pinpoint patient identities. Since the data will not be accessible, analysis to verify claims of research scientists cannot be carried out. Verification may be further complicated when highly specific biological samples are needed to reproduce research experiments.
- *Contamination of samples or high errors in data* – Detection and confirmation of inherent experimental errors or contamination of experimental equipment and samples may be difficult from reading a research paper or experimental report.

In a survey paper presenting a broad overview detailing the evolution of medical data analytics [6], the authors note a fundamental difference between medical informatics and traditional data mining application scenarios (e.g., market basket analysis, recommendation systems, sales campaign design, change point and anomaly detection). Analysis of medical data for knowledge discovery requires the intervention of highly skilled human experts, while many traditional data mining problems can be solved through the design and implementation of automated solutions that are based on statistical analysis, pattern matching, and machine learning. Higher rates of error (including those involving outliers) can be tolerated for many non-medical applications. Interpretation of patient data can be regarded as a form of art, requiring a deep understanding of the medical field as well as a keen sense of intuition based on hands-on clinical experience. Often there is no clear-cut, "correct solution" that is guaranteed to lead to a happy outcome. Two medical experts may reach different (but not necessarily incompatible) conclusions and recommendations, and the final choice may be up to the patient.

To summarize, the long-term goal of medical data analytics is to identify several candidate treatments for patients using their genomic data and predictive analytics applied to relevant data retrieved from massive repositories of historical medical data. Dubbed, "*P4 Medicine*" – shorthand for predictive, preventive, participatory, and personalized medical care [7] – medical professionals and statisticians will work with patients to enable them to choose from a menu of personalized treatment options [8], each of which will have possible benefits, as well as risks and costs.

To exploit the opportunity to develop personalized medical treatments, statisticians and computer scientists will need to work and communicate effectively with medical practitioners to: ensure proper measurement data; collect and process sufficient volumes of heterogeneous data to ensure patient privacy; and help medical personnel understand probabilities and sources of errors associated with data sampling [9]. This chapter introduces some online resources to help medical practitioners with little or no statistical background, quickly learn basic statistical concepts (associated with both summary and inferential statistics) and implement data analysis on their personal computers using *R* [10].

*R* is a new, high-level computer language and environment that is particularly well suited for statistical computing and graphics. Use of *R* is free. Its primary advantage over more traditional languages (such as FORTRAN, C, C++ and java) is its simplicity and ease in use. *R* was designed to free users from cumbersome punctuation rules and detailed coding of common mathematical operations. The popularity of the language has led to a large, international community of users who contribute computational routines for use by others. Readers who are only interested in understanding basic statistical concepts may want to skip the sections on *R*.

The remainder of this chapter is organized as follows. The next section presents our intended definitions of technical terms that appear in this chapter. Section 3 presents useful resources for quickly learning basic statistical concepts, guides for installation of *R*, and resources for learning the basics of *R*. Section 4 presents open problems for researchers, and the final section is a discussion of the future outlook for medical studies involving statistical analysis.

## 2        Glossary and Key Terms

This section presents definitions for important terms used in this chapter to ensure a common understanding for the material.

- *Medical informatics* is a relatively new, interdisciplinary field that seeks to improve human health through the study, understanding, and effective use of biomedical data. One of the practical goals is to analyze patient data, and summarize results in a manner that facilitates understanding by doctors and patients to enable them to actively discuss treatment options and actively participate in the decision making process [11]. The term *biomedical informatics* is used to emphasize use of biomedical (especially genomic) data.

- *Cloud computing* is involves the coordinated use of a large number of (possibly distributed) computers "connected through a communication network, such as the Internet ... (with) the ability to run a program or application on (the) many connected computers at the same time. ... The phrase *"in the cloud"* refers to software, platforms and infrastructure that are sold 'as a service', i.e. remotely through the Internet" [12]. Currently, computer security of public clouds is considered inadequate and unsuitable for analysis of medical data.

- *MOOC* is an acronym for *Massive Open Online Course*, i.e., an online course whose aim is to permit open, unlimited participation by Internet users through the web [13]. Most MOOCs are free for auditors. Some charge a relatively small fee for certification for having completed problem sets, assignments, and exams. In addition to traditional course materials such as videos, readings, and problem sets, some MOOCs provide wikis and discussion forums to help build an online community to emulate the interactive classroom experience for students.

- *Statistics* is a branch of mathematics that is concerned with the collection, analysis, and interpretation of very large sets of data [14]. Note: in the context of medical informatics, we intentionally delete the adjective *numerical* for *data* since patient demographics may involve categories, such as, gender, blood type, and ethnicity.

- *Descriptive statistics* is used to describe major features of a data set either quantitatively as summary statistics (e.g., mean, median, mode, standard deviation, kurtosis, skew-ness, and correlation coefficients), or visually (e.g., graphs and images) [15].

- *Inferential Statistics* uses samples of data to learn about the population, and uses the acquired information to develop propositions about populations. The propositions are tested through further sampling of the data [16].

- *Correlation* "is the degree of association between two random variables. (For example), the correlation between the graphs of two data sets is the degree to which they resemble each other. However, correlation is not the same as causation, and even a very close correlation may be no more than a coincidence. Mathematically, a correlation is expressed by a correlation coefficient that ranges from -1 (never occur together), through 0 (absolutely independent), to 1 (always occur together)" [17].

- *Probability* is a "branch of mathematics that studies the possible outcomes of events together with the outcomes' relative likelihoods and distributions. There are several competing interpretations. *Frequentists* view probability as a measure of the frequency of outcomes, while *Bayesians* (view) probability as a statistical procedure that endeavors to estimate parameters of an underlying distribution based on the observed distribution." [18].

- *R* is a very simple to program, high-level computer language specifically developed for statistical computing. More formally, it is a "free (no cost) software environment for statistical computing and graphics (that) compiles and runs on UNIX platforms, Windows and MacOS" [10].

- *Privacy preserving data mining (PPDM)*: focuses on the development of data mining techniques that support the protection of sensitive information from unsolicited or unsanctioned disclosure. "Most traditional data mining techniques analyze and model the data set statistically, in aggregation, while privacy preservation is primarily concerned with protecting against disclosure individual data records" [19]. Other excellent surveys on PPDM include [20-22].

# 3    State-of-the-Art

This section points to some useful resources for medical professionals with little or no background in statistics to get started and learn at their own pace through relatively inexpensive or free on-line resources. The first subsection presents resources for learning statistics – both descriptive and inferential. The second subsection begins with a brief review of commercial software for mining medical data before discussing the *R* programming language and resources for learning how to use *R*.

## 3.1    Statistical Analysis - Resources

Statistical analysis – particularly summary statistics – of medical data has been an important tool for understanding demographics of diseases. An example of a useful summary statistic is the median age of people who die from a serious condition, e.g., cancer or heart disease. This summary statistic has led to routine testing of overweight people in vulnerable age groups, with unhealthy lifestyles. The goal is to detect disorders during very early stages when changes in lifestyle can dramatically reduce the risk of mortality, and increase quality of life. The successful use of summary statistics in medicine is inspiring statisticians and medical practitioners to extend their collaborative work to include inferential statistics, correlational analysis, and predictive analytics.

Inferential statistics is a particularly effective tool well for medical informatics since the data available for analysis comes from patients who happen to undergo testing. We cannot designate patients that will become ill and patients that will stay healthy within the duration of a study. The limited availability of medical data available for inferential statistical analysis was a bottleneck to research until quite recently. The development of massive medical databases in the past few years, and the development of ever more sophisticated privacy preserving data mining (PPDM) algorithms are expected to contribute towards the resolution of data scarcity and lead to more reliable prediction of outcomes for candidate treatments for patients.

To exploit the opportunity to understand relationships between diseases and patient demographics and lifestyles, medical practitioners need to equip themselves with a solid understanding of statistics and (whenever possible) simple software tools to aid in data analysis. Likewise, statisticians and computer scientists who seek to work with the medical community need to study basic concepts and learn basic medical terminology and jargon. We present some pointers to help medical practitioners get started on learning statistics.

Most people find theoretical material, such as mathematics, probability, and statistics difficult to study in isolation, using only a textbook. A combination of lectures, reading, homework, and discussions with others are helpful. Fortunately, a variety of courses have become available through *massive online open courses* (MOOCs), such as: Coursera™ [23], MIT OpenCourseWare™ [24], Open Learning Initiative™ of Carnegie Mellon University (CMU) [25], and Udacity™ [26]. Course offerings change over time so the best way to find a course at an appropriate level to fill one's learning needs is to go to a MOOC website and conduct a keyword search, using search terms such as: *"statistics"* or *"elementary statistics"* or *"introduction to statistics"*. A list of courses will appear. Many of the courses available through Coursera and Udacity have trailers that introduce the lecturer, who describes the content, pre-requisites, policies, pace, etc. of the course.

Coursera's *Statistics One* by Andrew Conway of Princeton University is an excellent introductory statistics course for students majoring in the soft sciences. It eases listeners into understanding basic statistical concepts through real-world examples. Professor Conway points out common errors or misunderstandings to make sure students stay on the right track. This gentle and friendly introduction is mostly self-contained so purchase of a textbook is not necessary. The material stays faithful to the summary given in the trailer. Professor Conway speaks slowly and enunciates using standard American English, which may be particularly helpful for students are not native English speakers.

Udacity's *The Science of Decisions* by Sean Karaway and Ronald Rogers, both of San Jose State University, offers a friendly introduction to statistics through applications in every day life. An attractive feature of the course is a free, downloadable textbook that is posted on the website. Material covered in this course is more elementary than that in Coursera's *Statistics One*. A trailer for *The Science of Decisions* is available on the website.

*Probability & Statistics* of CMU's Open Leaning Initiative covers more material than the two MOOCs mentioned above. Students can choose between two versions, "each with a different emphasis": *Probability and Statistics* and *Statistical Reasoning*. The CMU offering has several drawbacks, such as: a higher level of difficulty; absence of an instructor; no videos; and need for Microsoft Excel™. The website posts the comment: *"This course was designed to be used as a stand alone (with no instruction in the background) however studies have shown that it is best and most effectively used in the hybrid mode together with face to face instruction."*

For readers interested in supplementing on-line courses with a traditional textbook, *General Statistics* by Chase and Bown [27] is replete with illustrations and examples to guide readers with little background in the subject. *Introduction to Probability and Statistics Using R* by G. Jay Kerns [28] is a relevant and inexpensive text. Kerns has made a rough draft of the book available online for free. Since a comprehensive list of excellent texts would be impossible and impractical to compile and list, a good way for prospective students to find a text at an appropriate level is to browse through textbooks at a local university store or library.

## 3.2    The R Computing Language and Environment for Statistical Analysis

The idea of using computers as a tool for processing medical data to expedite the understanding medical data has been contemplated for many years. However, until recently computing power and equipment were relatively expensive, so only well-to-do research institutions or large corporations could afford high quality commercial packages to generate summary statistics of medical data. Examples of these packages include: SAS™ [29], IBM SPSS™ [30], StatSoft™ STATISTICA™ [31], and Athena Health™ EMR [32]. Recent versions of many commercial packages have been enhanced with routines for predictive analytics. Although the input and output interfaces for commercial software can accommodate many types of commonly used file formats, and options for graphical output of results are beautiful, these packages are expensive. Furthermore, some packages require a solid background and understanding of statistics and significant training, such as one-week courses to learn how to use the software for various applications.

User-friendly open-source software for statistical analysis was not available until the release of *R*, version 1.0.0 in 2000. *R* is based on a programming language named *S*, which was designed and developed by John Chambers et al. at Bell Labs™ to be a simple language that would enable users to "turn ideas into software, quickly and faithfully" [33, 34]. Early versions of *R* were easy to learn and use, but were still not as sophisticated at most commercial packages. However, version 3.0.2, released in December of 2013, put *R* in the top league of software tools for statistical and predictive analysis. The latest version remains user friendly, and its price tag (free) is highly compelling. The open source community has embraced its use, and many researchers believe that it will become the software of choice for research institutions. Interestingly, many researchers who have studied computer science alongside their main discipline of study are contributing their software code in R for use by their colleagues who may not be as adept at programming.

There are many free, on-line resources for studying *R* for users at various levels of programming experience. A quick test drive of R that demonstrates the simplicity of the language is *Try R* [35] by Code School™ [36], sponsored by O'Reilly™ [37]. *Try R* is a good litmus test to determine whether a user will be capable of quickly picking up the programming language since it is gently introduces only a few of the most basic features of the languages. If completion of the chapters and quizzes for *Try R* proceeds smoothly, then on-line MOOCs for in-depth study of *R* is a realistic option.

Coursera's *Computing for Data Analysis*, with Roger Peng of Johns Hopkins Bloomberg School of Public Health™ is a fast-paced introductory course on statistical analysis using R specifically intended for first year graduate students in medical statistics [38]. The first few modules of the course walk students through the process of installing *R* on various operating systems, debugging programs, and asking for help from the *R* user community. The prerequisite for the course is an understanding of basic statistical reasoning. Although understanding of basic programming concepts is listed as "helpful", it should probably listed as a prerequisite for people intending to enroll and complete the material in 4 weeks. The popularity of the course inspired Professor Peng to post the video lectures on *YouTube*™ so interested students who do not want to be pressured by deadlines can access the material for study at their own pace. We note that the *YouTube* lectures do not have the simple quizzes to help check understanding of terminology and basic concepts introduced in the module. A word of warning: Professor Peng speaks standard American English, but he speaks extremely quickly. Students whose native language is not English may have difficulty following. Since videos can be replayed, the language barrier may be less of an issue than in a conventional classroom course. The slides for the lectures are available for download, which is helpful. A short trailer/video with a self-intro of the instructor and explanation of targets and features of the course is available on the website.

Two other Coursera MOOCs with slightly different target audiences are: *Data Analysis* by Jeff Leek of Johns Hopkins Bloomberg School of Public Health[TM] [39], and *Core Concepts in Data Analysis* by Boris Mirkin of National Research University's Higher School of Economics in Russia [40]. The former is intended for first year graduate students in biostatistics, and uses *R* for implementation studies. The latter covers the theory and practice of data analysis. It recommends use of MatLab[TM] or *R*, but accommodates the use of commonly used languages, with which the student may have familiarity, such as java[TM]. Both courses have a short video trailer on their respective websites.

Just as with textbooks, a good way to find a MOOC at an appropriate level and pace is to browse through MOOC sites and watch the trailer/video or the first few lectures.

# 4    Open Problems

Research in medical informatics is still in its infancy, and many interesting and important problems are just beginning to come to light. We present some below as starting points for discussion. Given the tremendous pace of innovation, it is likely that completely new, yet-to-be-discovered areas for research will emerge in the near future.

*Data Fusion and Privacy Preserving Data Mining (PPDM) Algorithms:* For some relatively rare diseases, the dearth of sufficiently large data sets presents patient confidentiality and privacy issues. Fusion of data is one approach towards resolving this problem, but many medical institutions are reluctant to contribute their data to externally monitored data pools due to legal issues regarding security and privacy. In addition, data fusion is not always simple since the personnel, environment and equipment used to collect data from multiple sources may be so different that they will introduce unacceptably large errors. Customized data pre-processing algorithms may be needed to resolve inconsistencies in the data collection processes. Another approach to resolving problems associated with small data sets is to develop new types of PPDM algorithms. Development of new PPDM algorithms that introduce ever-smaller errors, while guaranteeing patient anonymity will continue to be in high demand in the foreseeable future.

*High Speed Medical Data Analysis:* Currently, medical teams in intensive care units (ICUs) are overwhelmed by too much high-speed data from too many different sources being processed at very low precision. On a typical day, equipment monitoring a typical ICU patient produces 300 to 400 false alarms. Many times, several alarms ring in unison, making it difficult for medical staff to identify which are ringing and which require immediate attention. The problem, known as *alarm fatigue,* is begging for a solution. Currently, it is not known whether patient genomic data and patient history will help computers sift through the mountain of alarm data to accurately identify alarms that have a high probability of being critical and requiring immediate attention.

*International Sharing of Medical Data:* Different countries have different policies on permissible uses of personal data, including medical patient data. Medical data from minority groups in the United States or immigrant groups in other nations may be too small for PPDM. However, if data across many countries could be merged for small demographic groups, PPDM might become possible. Resolution to this problem can only come through coordinated work by international governments. However, the medical and statistical research communities need to bring this issue to the attention of government officials and citizens to expedite passing of new laws. International sharing of medical data could also be used to study cultural differences in patient treatments and their effectiveness.

*Computer System and Network Security*: Security of computer systems and networks is a major topic of concern for all businesses, institutions, and the general public. It is particularly important in the case of medical data since patients with diseases that require expensive treatments may experience discrimination when seeking employment. Information about a serious disease plaguing a high-ranking executive may also affect the stock price of a company. For example, speculation over the health of Steve Jobs, the late founder and CEO of Apple™ [41] affected the company's stock price over the years [42]. More recently, "Bezos's health mishap (kidney stone attack in January of 2014) is a reminder to Amazon stockholders of the CEO's value to the company" [43].

## 5    Future Outlook

Speculating on the long-term of outlook at a scientific field is difficult, and particularly so for an emerging, interdisciplinary field, such as medical informatics. The fast pace of technological advances introduces an additional layer of complexity. However, speculation requires deep thought and imagination, which may lead to discussion and debate, which may in turn inspire creativity and innovation. Below are four questions, which we hope will serve as starting points for friendly debate and discussion.

*Q1: Can big databases replace clinical trials?* This question was raised at a 2013 December Forbes Healthcare Summit [44]. Among the participants was Jonathan Bush, the founder and chief executive of Athena Health™, whose business is to "deliver cloud-based services for EHR (electronic health records), practice management and care coordination" [45]. His reply was an unequivocal, "yes", as truly massive medical datasets come into existence in the future. Another participant expressed some reservations. Susan Desmond-Hellman, the chancellor of UCSF, and future chief executive officer of the Bill and Melinda Gates Foundation, also agreed, but only in some cases.

*Q2: Will R become the dominant software environment and tool for statistical analysis of biomedical data? And if so, which organization or government will maintain the repository for programs and publications for R?* The idea is not without precedent. The wide adoption of FORTRAN by the scientific community led to the establishment of *Netlib* [46], a repository for FORTRAN-based programs and libraries and related publications [47]. R is currently being maintained by the *R Foundation*.

*Q3: Will access to large datasets enable timely detection of fraudulent data used to claim major findings in research studies?* In 2009, Hwang Woo-suk, a South Korean Scientist was found guilty of fraudulent claims on stem cell research work that was published in a major journal [48]. Fraudulent data and practices remain a problem in scientific research. As recently as January of 2014, the Japanese government started an investigation regarding the possibly fraudulent claims of major medical findings based on possibly falsified data in an Alzheimer study involving 11 drug firms and almost 40 Japanese hospitals [49, 50]. The J-ADNI project (Japan Alzheimer Disease Neuroimaging Initiative) started in 2007 [51].

*Q4: In the future, will the average person willingly participate in long-term-studies to monitor their vital organs in exchange for personalized advice on lifestyle changes to improve their overall well-being and health?* The Leroy Hood of the Institute of Systems Biology in Seattle, embarked on *The Hundred Person Wellness Project*, a nine-month study to "monitor healthy people in detail – and encourage them to respond to the results" [8]. Research scientists recruited 100 healthy people to wear digital devices 24-7 to monitor various aspects of vital organs (e.g., the brain, heart, liver, colon, lungs, lymphatic system, insulin sensitivity, chromosomes). Based on the data, "patients" will receive counseling on making lifestyle changes to improve overall health. The effectiveness of the lifestyle changes will in turn be monitored to determine the speed and extent of the impact on the patient's health. The President of the Institute, Leroy Hood recognizes that "The study violates many rules of trial design: it dispenses with blinding and randomization, and will not even have a control group. But Hood is confident in its power to disrupt the conventional practice of medicine." [8].

**Acknowledgements.** The author would like to thank Andreas Holzinger for organizing a multidisciplinary group of scientists to share ideas and thoughts on medical bioinformatics and for the invitation to participate in the publication of this book.

# References

1. Report on BridgeHead's 2010 Data Management Healthcheck Survey Results, http://www.bridgeheadsoftware.com/resources/category/reports/ (accessed February 19, 2014)

2. The BridgeHead Software 2011 International Healthcheck Data Management Survey, http://www.bridgeheadsoftware.com/resources/category/reports/ (accessed February 19, 2014)

3. IBM Big Data Website, http://www-01.ibm.com/software/data/bigdata/ industry-healthcare.html#2 (accessed February 19, 2014)

4. Creswell, J.: A digital shift on health data swells profits in an industry. NY Times on-line, http://ww.nytimes.com/2013/02/20/business/a-digital-shift-on-health-data-swells-profits.html?pagewanted=all&_r=0 (February 19, 2013)

5. Kerr, W., Lau, E., Owens, G., Trefler, A.: The future of medical diagnostics: large digitized databases. Yale Journal of Biology and Medicine 85(3), 363–377 (2012), http://www.ncbi.nlm.nih.gov/pmc/articles/PMC3447200/

6. Holzinger, A., Dehmer, M., Jurisica, I.: Knowledge discovery and interactive data mining in bioinformatics – state-of-the-art, future challenges and research directions. BMC Bioinformatics 15(suppl. 6) (2014)

7. Hood, L., Rowen, L., Galas, D., Aitchison, J.: Systems biology at the Institute of Systems Biology. Briefings in Functional Genomics and Proteomics 7(4), 239–248 (2008)

8. Gibbs, W.: Medicine gets up close and personal. Nature, http://www.nature.com/news/medicine-gets-up-close-and-personal-1.14702 (accessed February 11, 2014)

9. Holzinger, A.: Human-computer interaction and knowledge discovery (HCI-KDD): What is the benefit of bringing those two fields to work together? In: Cuzzocrea, A., Kittl, C., Simos, D.E., Weippl, E., Xu, L. (eds.) CD-ARES 2013. LNCS, vol. 8127, pp. 319–328. Springer, Heidelberg (2013)

10. The R project for statistical computing, http://www.r-project.org/ (accessed February 11, 2014)

11. Holzinger, A.: Biomedical Informatics: Computational Sciences meets Life Sciences. BoD, Norderstedt (2012)

12. Wikipedia, http://en.wikipedia.org/wiki/Cloud_computing (February 11, 2014)

13. Wikipedia, http://en.wikipedia.org/wiki/Massive_Open_Online_Course (February 11, 2014)

14. Merriam-Webster on-line, http://www.merriam-webster.com/dictionary/ statistics

15. Wikipedia, http://en.wikipedia.org/wiki/Summary_statistics (February 11, 2014)

16. Wikipedia, http://en.wikipedia.org/wiki/Statistical_inference (February 11, 2014)

17. Merriam-Webster, http://www.merriam-webster.com/dictionary/ correlation (February 11, 2014)

18. Wolfram MathWorldTM, http://mathworld.wolfram.com/Probability.html

19. Evfimievski, A., Grandison, T.: Privacy-preserving data mining. In: Ferraggine, V., Doorn, J., Rivero, L. (eds.) Handbook of Research on Innovations in Database Technologies and Applications, pp. 527–536. IGI Global, Hershey (2009)

20. Aggarwal, C., Yu, P.: A general survey of privacy-preserving data mining models and algorithms. In: Aggarwal, C. Yu, P. (eds.), pp. 11–52. Springer, New York (2008)

21. Pasierb, K., Kajdanowicz, T., Kazienko, P.: Privacy-preserving data mining, sharing and publishing. Journal of Medical Informatics and Technologies 18, 69–76 (2011)

22. Vaidya, J., Clifton, C., Zhu, M.: Privacy and data mining. In: Vaidya, J., Clifton, C., Zhu, M. (eds.) Privacy Preserving Data Mining, ch. 1. Springer, NY (2006)

23. Coursera website, http://www.coursera.org

24. MIT OpenCourseware website, http://ocw.mit.edu/index.htm

25. CMU's Open Learning Initiative, http://oli.cmu.edu

26. Udacity website, http://www.udacity.com

27. Chase, W., Bown, F.: General Statistics, 3rd edn. John Wiley and Sons, NY (1997)

28. Kerns, G.: Introduction to Probability and Statistics Using R. G. Jay Kerns publisher (2010), http://www.amazon.com, incomplete, rough draft available on-line, http://cran.r-project.org/web/packages/IPSUR/vignettes/IPSUR.pdf (accessed February 19, 2014)

29. Der, G., Everitt, J.: Applied Medical Statistics using SAS. CRC Press, Boca Raton (2013)

30. IBM SPSS, http://www.ibm.com/software/analytics/spss/products/modeler/

31. StatSoft STATISTICA, http://www.statsoft.com/Solutions/Healthcare

32. Athena Health Electronic Medical Record (EMR), http://www.athenahealth.com/Clinicals

33. Wikipedia entry for S, http://en.wikipedia.org/wiki/S_%28programming_language%29

34. Becker, R.: A brief history of S, http://kabah.lcg.unam.mx/~lcollado/R/resources/history_of_S.pdf (accessed February 20, 2014)

35. Try R, http://tryr.codeschool.com/

36. Code School, http://www.codeschool.com/

37. O'Reilly, http://oreilly.com/

38. Computing for Data Analysis, Coursera, http://www.coursera.org/course/compdata

39. Data Analysis, Coursera, http://www.coursera.org/course/dataanalysis

40. Core Concepts in Data Analysis, Coursera, http://www.coursera.org/course/datan

41. Apple, http://www.apple.com

42. Prinzel, Y.: How Steve Jobs' health problems have impacted Applestock over the years. Covestor.com (January 11, 2011), http://investing.covestor.com/2011/01/how-steve-jobs-health-problems-have-impacted-apple-stock-over-the-years-aapl

43. Ovide, S.: Amazon CEO Jeff Bezos evacuated for kidney stone attack. Wall Street Jour. (January 11, 2011), http://blogs.wsj.com/digits/2014/01/04/amazon-ceo-gives-kidney-stones-zero-stars/

44. Herper, M.: From fitbits to clinical studies: how big data could change medicine. Forbes on-line (December 16, 2013), http://www.forbes.com/sites/matthewherper/2013/12/16/from-fitbits-to-clinical-studies-how-big-data-could-change-medicine/

45. Athena Health website, `http://www.athenahealth.com/our-company/about-us/medical-practice-management.php`
46. Netlib, `http://www.netlib.org/`
47. Dongarra, J., Grosse, E.: Distribution of mathematical software via electronic mail. Comm. of the ACM 30(5), 403–407 (1987)
48. Sang-Hun, C.: Disgraced cloning expert convicted in South Korea. NY Times (October 26, 2009), `http://www.nytimes.com/2009/10/27/world/asia/27clone.html?ref=hwangwoosuk&_r=0`
49. Agence France-Presse, Tokyo: Japan looks into claim 'falsified' data was used in Alzheimer's drug study (January 10, 2014), `http://www.scmp.com/news/asia/article/1402542/japan-looks-claim-falsified-data-was-used-alzheimers-drug-study`
50. Takenaka, K., Kelland, K.: Japanese scientist urges withdrawal of own 'breakthrough' stem cell research. InterAksyon.com (March 11, 2014), `http://www.interaksyon.com/article/82452/japanese-scientist-urges-withdrawal-of-own-breakthrough-stem-cell-research`
51. J-ADNI homepage, `http://www.j-adni.org/etop.html`

# A Kernel-Based Framework for Medical Big-Data Analytics

David Windridge and Miroslaw Bober

Centre for Vision, Speech and Signal Processing
University of Surrey, Guildford, GU2 7XH, UK
{d.windridge,m.bober}@surrey.ac.uk

**Abstract.** The recent trend towards standardization of Electronic Health Records (EHRs) represents a significant opportunity and challenge for medical big-data analytics. The challenge typically arises from the nature of the data which may be heterogeneous, sparse, very high-dimensional, incomplete and inaccurate. Of these, standard pattern recognition methods can typically address issues of high-dimensionality, sparsity and inaccuracy. The remaining issues of incompleteness and heterogeneity however are problematic; data can be as diverse as handwritten notes, blood-pressure readings and MR scans, and typically very little of this data will be co-present for each patient at any given time interval.

We therefore advocate a kernel-based framework as being most appropriate for handling these issues, using the neutral point substitution method to accommodate missing inter-modal data. For pre-processing of image-based MR data we advocate a Deep Learning solution for contextual areal segmentation, with edit-distance based kernel measurement then used to characterize relevant morphology.

**Keywords:** Knowledge Discovery, Kernel-Based Methods, Medical Analytics.

## 1 Introduction

The introduction of electronic health records as a means of standardizing the recording and storage of healthcare information has been significantly accelerating in recent years, resulting in massive volumes of patient data being stored online in a manner readily accessible to clinicians and health-care professionals [1, 2]. Clinicians routinely support patient diagnosis and the selection of the individual treatment by analysis of symptoms in conjunction with the longitudinal patterns evident in physiological data, past clinical events, family history, genetic tests, etc. The availability of this online data resource, covering large cross-sections of the population, offers an unrivaled opportunity to employ big data analytics to spot trends, relations and patterns that may escape the eye of even most experienced clinicians. The results will support personalized medicine, where decisions, practices, and treatments are tailored to the individual patient [3]. (Decision support in particular is a key topic in biomedical

A. Holzinger, I. Jurisica (Eds.): Knowledge Discovery and Data Mining, LNCS 8401, pp. 197–208, 2014.
© Springer-Verlag Berlin Heidelberg 2014

informatics; it will likely prove essential in clinical practice for human intelligence to be supported by machine intelligence: HumanComputer Interaction and Knowledge Discovery will thus be critical areas of endeavor [4]).

However, analysis of medical records poses several serious challenges due to the nature of the data which is typically heterogeneous, sparse, high-dimensional and often both uncertain and incomplete [5]. Furthermore, image and video data may contain not only the organs/regions of interest but also neighboring areas with little relevance to the diagnosis.

In this paper we propose a kernel-based framework for medical big data analytics to address the issue of heterogeneous data, which employs a *neutral point substitution* method to address the missing data problem presented by patients with sparse or absent data modalities. In addition, since medical records contain many images (X-ray, MRI, etc) we propose to employ a deep-learning approach to address the problem of progressive areal segmentation, in order to improve analysis and classification of key organs or regions.

In the following section we present the kernel-based framework for medical big data analytics. Section 3 presents our arguments for the use of deep learning in medical image segmentation. Final remarks and conclusions are presented in Section 4.

## 1.1    Glossary and Key Terms

*Kernel-Methods:* Kernel-Methods constitute a complete machine learning paradigm wherein data is mapped into a (typically) high-dimensional linear feature-space in which classification and regression operations can take place (the support vector machine being the most commonplace). The great advantage of kernel-methods is that, by employing the kernel-trick, the coordinates of the implicitly constructed embedding space need never be directly computed; only the *kernel matrix* of intra-object comparisons are required.

*Kernel:* A kernel is defined as a symmetric function of arity-2 which forms a positive semidefinite matrix for each finite collection of objects in which pairwise comparison is possible. Critically, this matrix defines a *linear* space such that, in particular, a maximum-margin classifier can be constructed in this embedding space using the (kernelized) support vector machine. The convex optimization problem is solved via the Lagrangian dual, with the decision hyperplane defined by the set of support objects (those with non-zero Lagrangian multipliers).

*Neutral Point Substitution:* Kernel matrices can be linearly combined while retaining their kernel properties. This makes them ideal for the combination of very heterogeneous data modalities (in multiple-kernel learning the coefficients of this combination are explicitly optimized over). However, the absence of data in any given modality presents significant difficulties in constructing the embedding space. The neutral point substitution method attempts to overcome these in an SVM context by utilizing an appropriate mathematical substitute to allow embedding-space construction while minimally biasing the classification outcome.

*Deep-learning:* Deep-learning is the strategy of building multi-layered artificial neural networks (ANNs) via a greedy layer-on-layer process in order to avoid problems with standard back-propagation training. Hinton and Salakhutdinov demonstrated that the greedy layering of unsupervised restricted Boltzmann machines (see below) with a final supervised back-propagation step overcomes many of the problems associated with the deep-layering of tradition ANNs, enabling the building of networks with a distributed, progressively-abstracted representational structure.

*Boltzmann machines:* A Boltzmann machine consists in a network of units equipped with weighted connection-strengths to other units along with a bias offset. Activation of units is governed stochastically (in contrast to the otherwise similar Hopfield Network) according to the Boltzmann distribution; each unit thus contributes an 'energy' when activated to the overall global energy of the network which derives from the weighted sum of its activations from other units plus the bias. The activation likelihood is itself dependant on the thermodynamic temperature multiplied by this energy magnitude (in accordance with the Boltzmann distribution). Units are themselves split into hidden and visible categories, with the training process consisting in a gradient descent over weights such that the Kullback-Leibler divergence between the thermal equilibrium solution of the network marginalized over the hidden units (obtained via simulated annealing with respect to the temperature) and the distribution over the training set is minimized.

Restricted Boltzmann machines are a special class of the above in which a layering of units is apparent, i.e. such that there are no intra-layer connections between hidden units. These can thus be 'stacked' by carrying out layer-wise training in the manner above, with hidden units from the layer beneath providing the training-data distributions for the layer above.

## 2    A Kernel-Based Framework for Medical Big Data

Kernel methods [6–8] incorporate important distinctions from traditional statistical pattern recognition approaches, which typically involve an analysis of object clustering within a measurement space. Rather, kernel-based approaches implicitly construct an *embedding space* via similarity measurements between objects, within which the classification (e.g. via an SVM) or regression takes place. The dimensionality of the space is dictated by number of objects and the choice of kernel rather than the underlying feature dimensionality.

Kernel methods thus provide an ideal basis for combining heterogeneous medical information for the purposes of regression and classification, where data can range from hand-written medical notes to MR scans to genomic micro array data. Under standard pattern recognition, pre-processing of individual medical data modalities would be required to render this data combination problem tractable (i.e. representable in a real vector space), and such representation would invariably involve a loss of information when the data is in a non-vector (e.g graph-based) format.

## 2.1  Dealing with Heterogeneous Data

Kernel methods provide an excellent framework for combination of heterogeneous data for two principle reasons:

### 1. Mercer Kernels Are Now for All Data Types

A kernel obeying Mercer's properties (i.e one which leads to a positive definite kernel matrix) can now be built for almost all data formats, for instance:

- **text** (via NLP parse-tree kernels/LSA kernels [9, 10])
- **graphs and sequences**  (via string kernels, random walk kernels [11, 12])
- **shapes** (via edit distance kernels [13])
- **real vectors** (via dot product kernels, polynomial kernels etc [14])
- **sets of pixels/voxels** (efficient match kernels, pyramid match kernels [15])
- **stochastic data** (Fisher kernels [8])

Almost all forms of medical data (hand-written medical notes, MR scans, micro array data, temporal blood pressure measurements etc) fall into one or other of these categories. This means that even the most heterogeneous medical data archive is potentially kernalizable.

### 2. The Linear Combination of a Set of Mercer Kernels Is Also a Mercer Kernel

This means that the combination of kernalizable heterogeneous medical data is straightforward; it is only required to solve the kernel weighting problem (i.e. the optimal coefficients of the linear combination). Fortunately, for the most typical classification context (SVM classification), this is straightforwardly soluble (if no longer convex). Since the sum of kernel matrices of equal size does not increase the summed matrix size we are free (within the limits of the above MKL problem) to add additional kernels indefinitely. This can be useful when multiple kernels are available for each modality, either of different types, or else due to a range a parametric settings available for individual kernels. We can thus capture an enormous range of problem representations - and, of course, we may also employ 'meta' kernels - for instance Gaussian/RBFs built in conjunction with the above kernels, further massively extending the range of possible representations (both individually and collectively). This can be advantageous e.g. for inducing linear separability in the data (Gaussian/RBF kernels are guaranteed to achieve this).

## 2.2  Dealing with Missing Data

While kernel methods thus, in general, make the problem of combining heterogeneous medical data much more tractable than would be the case for standard pattern recognition methods, there are certain caveats that are specific to them. The most critical of these is due to the *missing intermodal data problem*, e.g. where a person has incomplete data in a given modality (this is especially common in time-series data where e.g. blood pressure measurements or ECG measurements [16] may have been made irregularly over some interval of the patient's life). This is problematic in standard pattern recognition of course, but can be straightforwardly addressed by interpolating the existing data distribution over the feature space. However, this option is not immediately available for kernel methods, where the data itself *defines* the embedding space.

However, methods developed by the author (the 'neutral point substitution' method [17–19]) render this tractable. (Neutral point substitution involves the unbiased missing value substitution of a placeholder mathematical object in multi-modal SVM combination). We thus, in principle, have the expertise and tool sets required to address the big medical data challenge.

Because of the imaging-based aspect of certain of the data (MR scans in particular), we would anticipate that the kernelized framework for medical data combination would be employed in the context of other computer vision areas, in particular segmentation. Segmentation would be employed, in particular, to identify individual organs prior to kernelized shape characterization for incorporation into the above medical data combination framework.

This aspect of medical segmentation lend itself, in particular, to deep learning approaches, which we now explore.

## 3    Deep Learning for Medical Image Segmentation

We propose to leverage the hierarchical decompositional characteristics of deep belief networks to address the problem of medical imaging, specifically the aspects of progressive areal segmentation, in order to improve classification of key organs.

Historically, neural networks have been limited to single hidden-layers due to the constraints of back-propagation - specifically the limitations of back-propagation when faced with the parametric freedom and local minima characteristics of the optimization function generated by multiple hidden layers.

The recent development of Deep Networks [20–23] has addressed these issues through the use of a predominantly forward training based approach. Deep networks thus aim to form a generative model in which individual layers encode statistical relationships between units in the layer immediately beneath it in order to maximize the likelihood of the input training data. Thus, there is a greedy training of each layer, from the lowest level to the highest level using the previous layer's activations as inputs. A more recent advancement is the *convolutional deep belief network* [24] that explicitly aims to produce an efficient hierarchical generative model that supports both top-down and bottom-up probabilistic inference; it is these characteristics make it particularly applicable to image processing.

Typically, within a convolutional deep belief network, weights linking the hidden layers to visible layers are distributed over the entire lower layer e.g. an image pixel grid at the lower layer; in which case the second layer constitutes a bank of image *filters* (note that since higher-level representations are over-complete a sparsity constraint is enforced). However, while such weight learning is a forward-only, greedy, layer-wise procedure, the network's *representation* of an image is constrained by both top-down and bottom-up constraints. Thus, since the network is pyramidal in shape, with *pooling* units serving to enforce compression of representation throughout the network, there is necessarily a bias towards *compositionality* in the network's image representation, since maximizing compositionality and factorizability renders the network as a whole more efficient. Consequently, a convolutional deep belief network is particularly well-suited to capturing progressively higher level hierarchical grammars, with higher levels representing progressively greater abstractions of the data to the extent that the higher levels can embody notions of *categoricity*.

We might, in an ideal case, thus anticipate an encoding of a set of images to consist of the following layers; firstly, an input level of pixel grids; secondly, a set of wavelet-like orthonormal bases for maximal representational compactness over the entire image database; thirdly, a set of feature detectors built from these orthonormal bases but tuned to specific common patterns in the image database. Finally, at the highest levels, we might hope for encoding of broad object categories such as *organs*. Thus, the network as a whole can readily function as an organ segmenter. There is hence a strong continuity of mechanism across the whole representation process, unlike the standard image processing pipeline, in which feature representation and classification are typically separate processes, with attendant numerical mismatches that manifest themselves, for example, as curse-of-dimensionality problems.

All of the above characteristics make deep belief networks and their variants particularly well suited to the proposed application domain of medical imaging. (In particular, a clear hierarchy of image grammars is present; at the highest level there are the individual organs and their relative positional relationship. At the lower level are the organ subcomponents (typically where disease is most manifest). Thus, (in the generative approach) the deep belief network forms a hierarchical segmentation of images in an unsupervised manner, in which different levels of interpretation (i.e. respective conceptual or spatial coarse-grainings) of the data are apparent.

Relevant here are the recent developments by Socher et al. [25] in which a complete NLP grammatical parse tree is distributed across the hierarchy of a recursive deep belief network. In particular, a *syntactically untied recursive neural network* is employed to simultaneously characterize both the relevant phrase structure *and* its most appropriate representation (the system thus learns both the parse tree and a compositional vector representation [i.e a semantic vector space] at the same time). The use of *recursive neural tensor networks* extends this representation to allow more complex 'operator'-type word-classes to exist within the parse tree.

There is no distinction, in principle, between a generative top-down visual grammar of topological relations between segmented regions of a medical image and the generative (recursive) construction of grammatical units within a NLP parse-tree. Hence, we would anticipate, a recursive, grammatical approach such as the above would be immediately applicable in the medical domain.

We thus, in summary, propose the hierarchical segmentation of medical data by using a deep learning approach. This will require experimentation with the methodology of convolutional deep belief networks in order to optimize the approach for hierarchical image decomposition in a manner most useful to medical objectives. Following this segmentation, morphology and other textural characteristics of the segmented reagion can be treated via an appropriate kernel-characterization in order to allow integration of the deep-learning process into the overall kernel combination framework (using e.g. edit-distance based kernels for contour comparison).

## 4  Conclusions

In this paper we have outlined two novel research directions to address critical issues in big medical data analytics in a complementary manner: (1) a kernel-based framework for combining heterogeneous data with missing or uncertain elements and (2) a new approach to medical image segmentation built around hierarchical abstraction for later kernel-based characterization.

Kernelization is thus the key to addressing data-heterogeneity issues; the way in which missing 'intermodal' data is combined in within the kernel-based framework depends on the authors' *neutral point substitution method*. A neutral point is defined as a unique (not necessarily specified) instantiation of an object that contributes exactly zero information to the classification (where necessary to actuate this substitution explicitly -i.e. where missing data occurs in both test and training data- we can select the minimum norm solution)

This is therefore an ideal substitute for missing values in that it contributes no overall bias to the decision. Crucially, it can be used in multi-kernel learning problems, enabling us to combine modalities optimally with arbitrary missing data.

The calculation of the neutral points turns the $O(n^3)$ complexity of the SVM problem into a maximum $O(n^4)$ complexity problem if uniform intermodal weightings are used. Solving for arbitrary weights, in the general MKL optimization procedure, is inherently a non-convex problem and solved via iterative alternation between maximizing over Lagrangian multipliers and minimizing over the modality weights. Appropriate modality weightings can thus be learned in multimodal problems of arbitrary data completion; we hence have the ability to combine any multiple modality data irrespective of modal omission.

Together, the two approaches of kernel-based combination of heterogeneous data with neutral point substitution and deep-learning would thus, we argue, address the major outstanding big-data challenges associated with Electronic Health Record standardization, in particular incompleteness and heterogeneity. However, there remain certain outstanding issues to be addressed:

# 5   Open-Problems

While the proposed kernel-based framework is extremely generic, in that almost any form of data can be accommodated, there has typically been a historical bias in kernel research towards classification (particularly SVM-based classification), particularly in terms of the algorithms that have deployed for kernel-based analysis. Classification, however, accounts for only a fraction of the medical big-data activity that one would wish to carry-out (in particular, it corresponds to the activity of *disease diagnosis*, though perhaps classification could also be employed for the induction of key binary variables relating to health-care, such as determining whether a patient is likely to be a smoker given the available evidence). The first open problem that we can thus identify is that of the *1. Breadth of Problem Specification.*

A second issue that we would need to address in an extensive treatment of EHRs is that of *2. Data Mining/Unsupervised Clustering Analysis.* Here, we wish to utilize all the available data (in particular the exogenous variables) in order to suggest investigative possibilities, rather than explicitly model or classify patient data. This approach thus differs from standard modes of assessment in which one seeks to test a null hypothesis against the available data. Typically, data mining is thus a precursory stage to hypothesis evaluation; instead it belongs to the stage of *hypothesis generation.* We may thus envisage a 'virtuous circle' of activity with progressive problem specification arising from the iterative interaction between medical practitioners and machine-learning researchers, with medical hypothesis suggestions being following by the progressive formalization of diagnostic evaluation criteria. The hypothesis suggestions themselves would arise from unsupervised clustering analysis; significant multimodality would be suggestive of subpopulations within the data, in particular subpopulations that may not be recognized within existing disease taxonomies.

A third related open problem is that of *3. Longitudinal Data Analysis* for both patients and any identified subpopulations within the data. This would generally take the form of *prediction modelling*, in which we would attempt to determine to what extent it is possible to predict an individual patient's disease prognosis from the data. A sufficiently comprehensive data set that extends across the diverse range of medical measurement modalities would potentially enable novel forms of analysis; for instance, apparently exogenous variables could prove to affect outcomes in different ways.

One additional aspect of time-series data that would also potentially have to be addressed is that of on-line learning; patient data would, in general, be collected continuously, and therefore methods of classification and regression would preferably therefore have to be trainable incrementally i.e. with relatively little cost involved in retraining with small quantities of additional data.

The final open problem associated with our framework is that of *4. Utilizing Human-Computer Interaction* in the most effective way, particularly as regards decision support. Here, we would not attempt to to directly resolve problems of e.g. medical diagnosis/prognosis via regression/classification. Rather, the aim is to utilize the framework to maximally assist the medical profession in arriving at their own diagnosis/prognosis decision. This might take the form of data-representation i.e where machine learning is used to determine salient aspects of the data set with respect to the current decision to be made. This can be at both the high-level (determination of patient or population context) or at the low-level (segmentation of relevant structures within imaging data). Another possibility for HCI is explicit hybridization of the decision process [4], utilizing the most effective respective areas of processing in combination (for example, pattern-spotting in humans in conjunction with large data-base accessing in computers).

In the following section we outline some provisional solutions and research directions for addressing the most immediately tangible of these open issues consistent with the proposed framework.

# 6   Future Outlook

To address the first open problem, *Breadth of Problem Specification*, it will likely be necessary, in addition to carrying-out classification within a kernel context, to exploit the full range of algorithms to which kernel methods apply: *kernel-principal component analysis, ridge regression, kernel-linear discriminant analysis, Gaussian processes* etc (these are typically all convex optimization problems). The latter of these, Gaussian processes, ought particularly to be useful for prediction of patient outcomes [26], and would directly assist with the missing data problem by allowing both longitudinal data-interpolation and longitudinal data-extrapolation.

A Gaussian process might thus be deployed for modelling time-series data via Gaussian process regression (kriging), producing the best linear unbiased prediction of extrapolation points. Primary outcome variables in a medical context would thus be likely to be disease progression indicators such as tumor-size.

We therefore propose to explore a number of areas of kernel regression consistent with our framework to address the big-data analytics problem.

In terms of the second open problem *Data Mining/Unsupervised Clustering Analysis*, we might wish to explore rule-mining type approaches, since the resulting logical clauses most closely resemble the diagnostic criteria used by medical professionals in evaluation disease conditions.

Unsupervised clustering, in particular the problem of determining the presence of sub-populations within the data, might be addressed by addressed by model-fitting (Kernel regression [27], or perhaps K-means or Expectation Maximization with Gaussian Mixture Modelling in sufficiently low-dimensional vector spaces) in conjunction with an appropriate model-selection criterion (for example, the Akaike Information Criterion [28] or Bayesian Information Criterion). The latter is required to correctly penalize model-parameterization with respect to goodness-of-fit measurements such that the overfitting-risk is minimized. The means of such partitioned clusters would then correspond to *prototypes* within the data, which may be used for e.g. efficient indexing and kernel based characterization of novel data. Manifold learning might also be required in order to determine the number of active factors within a data-set; Gaussian Process Latent Variable Modelling [29] would be a good fit to the proposed framework.

More generally, regarding the use of such hypothesis generation methods within a medical context, it is possible can regard the iterative process of experimental feedback and problem refinement as one of *Active Learning* [30]. Active-learning addresses the problem of how to choose the most informative examples to train a machine learner; it does so by selecting those examples that most effectively differentiate between hypotheses, thereby minimizing the number of experimental surveys that need to be conducted in order to form a complete model. It thus represents a maximally-efficient interaction model for medical professions and machine-learning researchers.

Finally, addressing the third open problem, *Longitudinal Analysis*, within the proposed kernel-based framework would likely involve the aforementioned Gaussian processes given their ready incorporation within the kernel methodology. Another possibility would be Structured Output Learning [31], a variant of the Support Vector Machine that incorporates a loss-function capable of measuring the distance between two structured outputs (for example, two temporal series of labels). The Structured Output Learning problem, however, is generally not tractable with standard SVM solvers due to the additional parameter complexity and thus requires bespoke iterative cutting plane-algorithms to train in polynomial time.

In sum, it would appear that the proposed kernel framework has sufficient flexibility to address many of the open questions identified, and indeed implicitly sets out a programme of research to address these. However, it will invariably be the case that each novel EHR dataset will involve characteristics that are more suited to one particular form of machine learning approach over another -it is not generally the case that this can be specified *a priori*, thereby necessitating a flexible research programme with the potential to leverage the full range of available kernel-based machine-learning techniques.

# References

1. Holzinger, A.: Biomedical Informatics: Discovering Knowledge in Big Data. Springer, New York (2014)
2. Holzinger, A., Dehmer, M., Jurisica, I.: Knowledge discovery and interactive data mining in bioinformatics state-of-the-art, future challenges and research directions. BMC Bioinformatics 15(suppl. 6)(I1) (2014)
3. Simonic, K.M., Holzinger, A., Bloice, M., Hermann, J.: Optimizing long-term treatment of rheumatoid arthritis with systematic documentation. In: Proceedings of Pervasive Health - 5th International Conference on Pervasive Computing Technologies for Healthcare, pp. 550–554. IEEE (2011)
4. Holzinger, A.: Human–computer interaction & knowledge discovery (hci-kdd): What is the benefit of bringing those two fields to work together? In: Cuzzocrea, A., Kittl, C., Simos, D.E., Weippl, E., Xu, L. (eds.) CD-ARES 2013. LNCS, vol. 8127, pp. 319–328. Springer, Heidelberg (2013)

5. Marlin, B.M., Kale, D.C., Khemani, R.G., Wetzel, R.C.: Unsupervised pattern discovery in electronic health care data using probabilistic clustering models. In: Proceedings of the 2nd ACM SIGHIT International Health Informatics Symposium, IHI 2012, pp. 389–398. ACM, New York (2012)
6. Scholkopf, B., Smola, A.: MIT Press (2002)
7. Shawe-Taylor, J., Cristianini, N.: Cambridge University Press (2004)
8. Hofmann, T., Schlkopf, B., Smola, A.J.: A review of kernel methods in machine learning (2006)
9. Collins, M., Duffy, N.: Convolution kernels for natural language. In: Advances in Neural Information Processing Systems 14, pp. 625–632. MIT Press (2001)
10. Aseervatham, S.: A local latent semantic analysis-based kernel for document similarities. In: IJCNN, pp. 214–219. IEEE (2008)
11. Nicotra, L.: Fisher kernel for tree structured data. In: Proceedings of the IEEE International Joint Conference on Neural Networks IJCNN 2004. IEEE press (2004)
12. Borgwardt, K.M., Kriegel, H.P.: Shortest-path kernels on graphs. In: Proceedings of the Fifth IEEE International Conference on Data Mining (ICDM 2005), pp. 74–81. IEEE Computer Society, Washington, DC (2005)
13. Daliri, M.R., Torre, V.: Shape recognition based on kernel-edit distance. Computer Vision and Image Understanding 114(10), 1097–1103 (2010)
14. Smola, A.J., Ovri, Z.L., Williamson, R.C.: Regularization with dot-product kernels. In: Proc. of the Neural Information Processing Systems (NIPS), pp. 308–314. MIT Press (2000)
15. Grauman, K., Darrell, T.: The pyramid match kernel: Efficient learning with sets of features. J. Mach. Learn. Res. 8, 725–760 (2007)
16. Holzinger, A., Stocker, C., Bruschi, M., Auinger, A., Silva, H., Gamboa, H., Fred, A.: On applying approximate entropy to ecg signals for knowledge discovery on the example of big sensor data. In: Huang, R., Ghorbani, A.A., Pasi, G., Yamaguchi, T., Yen, N.Y., Jin, B. (eds.) AMT 2012. LNCS, vol. 7669, pp. 646–657. Springer, Heidelberg (2012)
17. Panov, M., Tatarchuk, A., Mottl, V., Windridge, D.: A modified neutral point method for kernel-based fusion of pattern-recognition modalities with incomplete data sets. In: Sansone, C., Kittler, J., Roli, F. (eds.) MCS 2011. LNCS, vol. 6713, pp. 126–136. Springer, Heidelberg (2011)
18. Poh, N., Windridge, D., Mottl, V., Tatarchuk, A., Eliseyev, A.: Addressing missing values in kernel-based multimodal biometric fusion using neutral point substitution. IEEE Transactions on Information Forensics and Security 5(3), 461–469 (2010)
19. Windridge, D., Mottl, V., Tatarchuk, A., Eliseyev, A.: The neutral point method for kernel-based combination of disjoint training data in multi-modal pattern recognition. In: Haindl, M., Kittler, J., Roli, F. (eds.) MCS 2007. LNCS, vol. 4472, pp. 13–21. Springer, Heidelberg (2007)
20. LeCun, Y., Boser, B., Denker, J.S., Henderson, D., Howard, R.E., Hubbard, W., Jackel, L.D.: Backpropagation applied to handwritten zip code recognition. Neural Computation 1, 541–551 (1989)
21. Bengio, Y., Lamblin, P., Popovici, D., Larochelle, H.: Greedy layer-wise training of deep networks. In: Schölkopf, B., Platt, J., Hoffman, T. (eds.) Advances in Neural Information Processing Systems 19, pp. 153–160. MIT Press, Cambridge (2007)
22. Ranzato, M., Huang, F.J., Boureau, Y.L., LeCun, Y.: Unsupervised learning of invariant feature hierarchies with applications to object recognition. In: CVPR. IEEE Computer Society (2007)

23. Hinton, G.E., Salakhutdinov, R.R.: Reducing the dimensionality of data with neural networks. Science 313(5786), 504–507 (2006)
24. Lee, H., Grosse, R., Ranganath, R., Ng, A.Y.: Convolutional deep belief networks for scalable unsupervised learning of hierarchical representations (2009)
25. Socher, R., Manning, C.D., Ng, A.Y.: Learning continuous phrase representations and syntactic parsing with recursive neural networks
26. Shen, Y., Jin, R., Dou, D., Chowdhury, N., Sun, J., Piniewski, B., Kil, D.: Socialized gaussian process model for human behavior prediction in a health social network. In: 2012 IEEE 12th International Conference on Data Mining (ICDM), pp. 1110–1115 (December 2012)
27. Song, C., Lin, X., Shen, X., Luo, H.: Kernel regression based encrypted images compression for e-healthcare systems. In: 2013 International Conference on Wireless Communications Signal Processing (WCSP), pp. 1–6 (October 2013)
28. Elnakib, A., Gimel'farb, G., Inanc, T., El-Baz, A.: Modified akaike information criterion for estimating the number of components in a probability mixture model. In: 2012 19th IEEE International Conference on Image Processing (ICIP), pp. 2497–2500 (September 2012)
29. Gao, X., Wang, X., Tao, D., Li, X.: Supervised gaussian process latent variable model for dimensionality reduction. IEEE Transactions on Systems, Man, and Cybernetics, Part B: Cybernetics 41(2), 425–434 (2011)
30. Cai, W., Zhang, Y., Zhou, J.: Maximizing expected model change for active learning in regression. In: 2013 IEEE 13th International Conference on Data Mining (ICDM), pp. 51–60 (December 2013)
31. Yan, J.F., Kittler, Mikolajczyk, K., Windridge, D.: Automatic annotation of court games with structured output learning. In: 2012 21st International Conference on Pattern Recognition (ICPR), pp. 3577–3580 (November 2012)

# On Entropy-Based Data Mining

Andreas Holzinger[1], Matthias Hörtenhuber[2], Christopher Mayer[2],
Martin Bachler[2], Siegfried Wassertheurer[2],
Armando J. Pinho[3], and David Koslicki[4]

[1] Medical University Graz, A-8036 Graz, Austria
Institute for Medical Informatics, Statistics & Documentation,
Research Unit Human–Computer Interaction
a.holzinger@hci4all.at

[2] AIT Austrian Institute of Technology GmbH, Health & Environment Department,
Biomedical Systems, Donau-City-Str. 1, A-1220 Vienna, Austria
{christopher.mayer,martin.bachler,matthias.hoertenhuber,siegfried.
wassertheurer}@ait.ac.at

[3] IEETA / Department of Electronics, Telecommunications and Informatics,
University of Aveiro, 3810-193 Aveiro, Portugal
ap@ua.pt

[4] Oregon State University, Mathematics Department, Corvallis, OR, USA
david.koslicki@math.oregonstate.edu

**Abstract.** In the real world, we are confronted not only with complex
and high-dimensional data sets, but usually with noisy, incomplete and
uncertain data, where the application of traditional methods of knowledge discovery and data mining always entail the danger of modeling
artifacts. Originally, information entropy was introduced by Shannon
(1949), as a measure of uncertainty in the data. But up to the present,
there have emerged many different types of entropy methods with a large
number of different purposes and possible application areas. In this paper, we briefly discuss the applicability of entropy methods for the use
in knowledge discovery and data mining, with particular emphasis on
biomedical data. We present a very short overview of the state-of-the-
art, with focus on four methods: Approximate Entropy (ApEn), Sample
Entropy (SampEn), Fuzzy Entropy (FuzzyEn), and Topological Entropy
(FiniteTopEn). Finally, we discuss some open problems and future research challenges.

**Keywords:** Entropy, Data Mining, Knowledge Discovery, Topological
Entropy, FiniteTopEn, Approximate Entropy, Fuzzy Entropy, Sample
Entropy, Biomedical Informatics.

## 1 Introduction

Entropy, originating from statistical physics (see Section 3), is a fascinating and
challenging concept with many diverse definitions and various applications.

Considering all the diverse meanings, entropy can be used as a measure for
disorder in the range between total order (structured) and total disorder (unstructured) [1], as long as by order we understand that objects are segregated by

A. Holzinger, I. Jurisica (Eds.): Knowledge Discovery and Data Mining, LNCS 8401, pp. 209–226, 2014.
© Springer-Verlag Berlin Heidelberg 2014

their properties or parameter values. States of lower entropy occur when objects become organized, and ideally when everything is in complete order the Entropy value is zero. These observations generated a colloquial meaning of entropy [2]. Following the concept of the mathematical theory of communication by Shannon & Weaver (1949) [3], entropy can be used as a measure for the *uncertainty in a data set*. The application of entropy became popular as a measure for system complexity with the paper by Steven Pincus (1991) [4]: He described Approximate Entropy (see Section 5.1) as a statistic quantifying regularity within a wide variety of relatively short (greater than 100 points) and noisy time series data. The development of this approach was initially motivated by data length constraints, which is commonly encountered in typical biomedical signals including: heart rate, electroencephalography (EEG), etc. but also in endocrine hormone secretion data sets [5].

This paper is organized as follows: To ensure a common understanding we start with providing a short glossary; then we provide some background information about the concept of entropy, the origins of entropy and a taxonomy of entropy methods in order to facilitate a "big picture". We continue in chapter 4 with the description of some application areas from the biomedical domain, ranging from the analysis of EEG signals to complexity measures of DNA sequences. In chapter 5 we provide more detailed information on four particular methods: Approximate Entropy (ApEn), Sample Entropy (SampEn), Fuzzy Entropy (FuzzyEn), and Topological Entropy (FiniteTopEn). In chapter 6 we discuss some open problems and we conclude in chapter 7 with a short future outlook.

## 2    Glossary and Key Terms

*Anomaly Detection:* is finding patterns in data, non compliant to expected behavior (anomalies aka outliers, discordant observations, exceptions, aberrations, surprises, peculiarities). A topic related to anomaly detection is novelty detection, aiming at detecting previously unobserved, emergent patterns in data [6].

*Artifact:* is any error, anomaly and/or undesired alteration in the perception or representation of information from data.

*Data Quality:* includes (physical) quality parameters including: Accuracy, Completeness, Update status, Relevance, Consistency, Reliability and Accessibility [7], not to confuse with Information quality [8].

*Dirty Data:* data which is incorrect, erroneous, misleading, incomplete, noisy, duplicate, uncertain, etc. [9].

*Dirty Time Oriented Data:* time (e.g. time points, time intervals) is an important data dimension with distinct characteristics affording special consideration in the context of dirty data [10].

*Dynamical System:* is a manifold $M$ called the phase-space and possess a family of evolution functions $\phi(t)$ so that for any element of $t \in T$, the time, maps a point of the phase-space back into the phase-space; If $T$ is real, the dynamical system is called a *flow*; if $T$ is restricted to the non-negative reals, it is a semi-flow; in case of integers, it is called a cascade or map; and a restriction to the non-negative integers results in a so-called semi-cascade [2];

*Hausdorff Space:* is a separated topological space in which distinct points have disjoint neighbourhoods.

*Hausdorff Measure:* is a type of outer measure that assigns a number in $[0, \infty]$ to each set in $\mathbb{R}^n$. The zero-dimensional Hausdorff measure is the number of points in the set, if the set is finite, or $\infty$ if the set is infinite. The one-dimensional Hausdorff measure of a simple curve in $\mathbb{R}^n$ is equal to the length of the curve. Likewise, the two dimensional Hausdorff measure of a measurable subset of $\mathbb{R}^2$ is proportional to the area of the set. The concept of the Hausdorff measure generalizes counting, length, and area. These measures are fundamental in geometric measure theory.

*Topological Entropy:* is a nonnegative real number that is a measure of the complexity of a dynamical system. TopEn was first introduced in 1965 by Adler, Konheim and McAndrew. Their definition was modeled after the definition of the Kolmogorov–Sinai, or metric entropy.

*Heart Rate Variability (HRV):* measured by the variation in the beat-to-beat interval of heart beats.

*HRV Artifact:* noise through errors in the location of the instantaneous heart beat, resulting in errors in the calculation of the HRV.

*Information Entropy:* is a measure of the uncertainty in a random variable. This refers to the Shannon entropy, which quantifies the expected value of the information contained in a message.

## 3    Background

### 3.1    Physical Concept of Entropy

It is nearly impossible to write any paper on any aspect of entropy, without referring back to classical physics: The concept of entropy was first introduced in thermodynamics [11], where it was used to provide a statement of the second law of thermodynamics on the irreversibility of the evolution, i.e. an isolated system cannot pass from a state of higher entropy to a state of lower entropy.

In classical physics any system can be seen as a set of objects, whose state is parameterized by measurable physical characteristics, e.g. temperature. Later, statistical mechanics provided a connection between the macroscopic property of entropy and the microscopic state of a system by Boltzmann.

Shannon (1948) was the first to re-define entropy and mutual information, for this purpose he used a thought experiment to propose a measure of uncertainty in a discrete distribution based on the Boltzmann entropy of classical statistical mechanics (see next section). For more details on the basic concepts of entropy refer to [12].

## 3.2   Origins of Information Entropy

The foundation of information entropy (see Fig. 1) can be traced back into two major origins, the older may be found in the work of Jakob Bernoulli (1713), describing the *principle of insufficient reason*: we are ignorant of the ways an event can occur, the event will occur equally likely in any way. Thomas Bayes (1763) and Pierre-Simon Laplace (1774) carried on with works on how to calculate the state of a system with a limited number of expectation values and Harold Jeffreys and David Cox solidified it in the Bayesian Statistics, also known as **statistical inference**.

The second path is leading to the classical Maximum Entropy, not quite correctly often called "Shannon Entropy", but indeed, Jaynes (1957) [13] makes it clear on page 622/623 that he is utilizing Shannon's Entropy to *derive* the Maximum Entropy Principle and that those are not synonym principles. Following the path backwards the roots can be identified with the work of James Clerk Maxwell (1859) and Ludwig Boltzmann (1871), continued by Willard Gibbs (1902) and finally reaching Claude Elwood Shannon (1948). This work is geared toward developing the mathematical tools for statistical modeling of problems in information. These two independent lines of research are relatively similar. The objective of the first line of research is to formulate a theory and methodology that allows understanding of the general characteristics (distribution) of a given system from partial and incomplete information. In the second route of research, the same objective is expressed as determining how to assign (initial) numerical values of probabilities when only some (theoretical) limited global quantities of the investigated system are known. Recognizing the common basic objectives of these two lines of research aided Jaynes (1957) in the development of his classical work, the Maximum Entropy formalism (see also Fig. 2). This formalism is based on the first line of research and the mathematics of the second line of research. The interrelationship between Information Theory, statistics and inference, and the Maximum Entropy (MaxEnt) principle became clear in the 1950s, and many different methods arose from these principles [14], see Fig. 2.For more details on information entropy refer to [2].

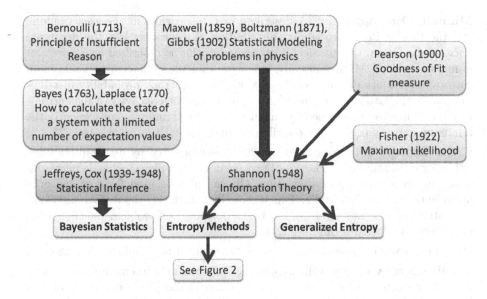

**Fig. 1.** The "big picture" in the developent of the concept of entropy [15]

### 3.3 Towards a Taxonomy of Entropy Methods

**Maximum Entropy** (MaxEn), described by [16], is used to estimate unknown parameters of a multinomial discrete choice problem, whereas the Generalized Maximum Entropy (GME) includes noise terms in the multinomial information constraints. Each noise term is modeled as the mean of a finite set of known points in the interval [-1,1] with unknown probabilities where no parametric assumptions about the error distribution are made. A GME model for the multinomial probabilities and for the distributions, associated with the noise terms is derived by maximizing the joint entropy of multinomial and noise distributions, under the assumption of independence [16].

**Graph Entropy** was described by [17] to measure structural information content of graphs, and a different definition, more focused on problems in information and coding theory, was introduced by Körner in [18]. Graph entropy is often used for the characterization of the structure of graph-based systems, e.g. in mathematical biochemistry, but also for any complex network [19]. In these applications the entropy of a graph is interpreted as its structural information content and serves as a complexity measure, and such a measure is associated with an equivalence relation defined on a finite graph; by application of Shannons Eq. 2.4 in [20] with the probability distribution we get a numerical value that serves as an index of the structural feature captured by the equivalence relation [20].

**Minimum Entropy** (MinEn), described by [21], provides us the least random, and the least uniform probability distribution of a data set, i.e. the minimum uncertainty. Often, the classical pattern recognition is described as a quest for minimum entropy. Mathematically, it is more difficult to determine a minimum entropy probability distribution than a maximum entropy probability distribution; while the latter has a global maximum due to the concavity of the entropy, the former has to be obtained by calculating all local minima, consequently the minimum entropy probability distribution may not exist in many cases [22].

**Cross Entropy** (CE), discussed by [23], was motivated by an adaptive algorithm for estimating probabilities of rare events in complex stochastic networks, which involves variance minimization. CE can also be used for combinatorial optimization problems (COP). This is done by translating the deterministic optimization problem into a related stochastic optimization problem and then using rare event simulation techniques [24].

**Rényi Entropy** is a generalization of the Shannon entropy (information theory).

**Tsallis Entropy** is a generalization of the BoltzmannGibbs entropy and was intended for statistical mechanics by Constantino Tsallis [25]; a decade ago it has been applied to computer science, see e.g. a pattern recognition example [26].

**Approximate Entropy** (ApEn), described by [4], is useable to quantify regularity in data without any a priori knowledge about the system.

**Sample Entropy** (SampEn), was used by [27] for a new related measure of time series regularity. SampEn was designed to reduce the bias of ApEn and is better suited for data sets with known probabilistic content.

**Fuzzy Entropy** (FuzzyEn), proposed by [28], replaces the Heaviside function to measure the similarity of two vectors as used in SampEn and ApEn by a fuzzy relationship function. This leads to a weaker impact of the threshold parameter choice.

**Fuzzy Measure Entropy** (FuzzyMEn), presented in [29], is an enhancement of FuzzyEn, by differentiating between local and global similarity.

**Topological Entropy** (TopEn), was introduced by [30] with the purpose to introduce the notion of entropy as an invariant for continuous mappings: Let $(X, T)$ be a topological dynamical system, i.e., let $X$ be a nonempty compact Hausdorff space and $T : X \rightarrow X$ a continuous map; the TopEn is a nonnegative number which measures the complexity of the system [31].

**Topological Entropy for Finite Sequences** (FiniteTopEn) was introduced in [32] by taking the definition of TopEn for symbolic dynamical systems and developing a finite approximation suitable for use with finite sequences.

**Algorithmic Entropy** or Kolmogorov Complexity was independently introduced by Solomonoff [33,34], Kolmogorov [35] and Chaitin [36]. The algorithmic entropy of a string is formally defined as the length of a shortest program for a universal computer that outputs the string and stops.

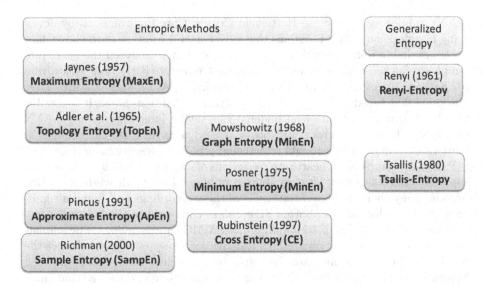

**Fig. 2.** A rough, incomplete overview on the most important entropy methods [15]

## 4    Application Areas

Entropy concepts found its way into many diverse fields of application within the biomedical domain:

Acharya et al. [37] proposed a methodology for the automatic detection of normal, pre-ictal, and ictal conditions from recorded EEG signals. Beside Approximate Entropy, they extracted three additional entropy variations from the EEG signals, namely Sample Entropy (SampEn), Phase Entropy 1 and Phase Entropy 2. They fed those features to seven different classifiers, and were able to show that the Fuzzy classifier was able to differentiate the three classes with an accuracy of 98.1 %. For this they took annotated recordings of five healthy subjects and five epilepsy patients. They showed that both ApEn and SampEn are higher in the case of normal signals, and lower for pre-ictal and ictal classes, indicating more self-similarity of the two later segments.

Hornero et al. [38] performed a complexity analysis of intracranial pressure dynamics during periods of severe intracranial hypertension. For that purpose they analyzed eleven episodes of intracranial hypertension from seven patients. They measured the changes in the intracranial pressure complexity by applying ApEn, as patients progressed from a state of normal intracranial pressure to intracranial hypertension, and found that a decreased complexity of intracranial pressure coincides with periods of intracranial hypertension in brain injury. Their approach is of particular interest to us, because they proposed classification based on ApEn tendencies instead of absolute values.

In the field of Electrocardiography analysis, Batchinsky et al. [39] recently performed a comprehensive analysis of the ECG and Artificial Neural Networks

(ANN) to improve care in the Battlefield Critical Care Environment, by developing new decision support systems that take better advantage of the large data stream available from casualties. For that purpose they analyzed the heart rate complexity of 800-beat sections of the R-to-R interval (RRI) time series from 262 patients by several groups of methods, including ApEn and SampEn. They concluded that based on ECG-derived noninvasive vital signs alone, it is possible to identify trauma patients who undergo Life-saving interventions using ANN with a high level of accuracy. Entropy was used to investigate the changes in heart rate complexity in patients undergoing post-burn resuscitation.

Pincus et al. took in [4] heart rate recordings of 45 healthy infants with recordings of an infant one week after an aborted sudden infant death syndrom (SIDS) episode. They then calculated the ApEn of these recordings and found a significant smaller value for the aborted SIDS infant compared to the healthy ones.

In [40] Sarlabous et al. used diaphragmatic MMG signals of dogs. The animals performed an inspiratory progressive resistive load respiratory test during the acquisition, in order to increase the respiratory muscular force. Afterwards the Approximate Entropy of these recordings were calculated and showed that these are able to quantify amplitude variations.

SampEn and ApEn were used in order to study gait data sets in [41]. For this purpose 26 healthy young adult and 24 healthy older adult subjects walked at least 200 steps on a treadmill. Their movement was tracked and step length, step width, and step time were calculated from the recordings. Both SampEn and ApEn showed significant differences between the younger and the older subjects in the step length and step width data sets.

In [42] Roerding et al. compared the postural sway of 22 stroke patients with 33 healthy also elderly subjects using different statistical tools including SampEn. All subjects were asked to do three trials while their sway was recorded. SampEn was significantly lower for the stroke patients.

The degree of randomness of a sequence is tightly related to its complexity, predictability, compressibility, repeatability and, ultimately, to the information theoretic notion of entropy. Most often, in genomics sequence analysis, information theoretic approaches are used (sometimes implicitly) to look for and to display information related to the degree of randomness of the sequences, aiming at finding meaningful structures. Early approaches include the sequence landscapes [43] and the sequence logos [44].

Pinho discusses some examples [45]: Some methods provide visual information of global properties of the DNA sequences. For example, the chaos game representation (CGR) [46] uses a distribution of points in an image to express the frequency of the Oligonucleotides that compose the sequence [47]. From these CGR images, other global representations can be derived, such as the entropic profiles [48], originally estimated using global histograms of the oligonucleotide frequencies, calculated using CGR images. Later, they have been generalized by Vinga et al. [49], based on the Rényi entropy, in order to calculate and visualize local entropic information. Other approaches for estimating the randomness along the sequence have also been proposed. For example, Crochemore *et al.* [50] used the number of different oligonucleotides that are found in a window of predefined size for estimating the entropy.

The idea of showing local information content while taking into account the global structure of the sequence was also addressed by Allison *et al.* [51]. Based on a statistical model, they have produced information sequences, which quantify the amount of surprise of having a given base at a given position (and, therefore, in some sense are estimates of the local entropy), knowing the remaining left (or right) part of the sequence. When plotted, these information sequences provide a quick overview of certain properties of the original symbolic sequence, allowing for example to easily identify zones of rich repetitive content [52,53,54].

The information sequences of Allison *et al.* [51] are tightly related to data compression and, consequently, to entropy estimation. In fact, the importance of data compression for pattern discovery in the context of DNA sequences was initially addressed by Grumbach *et al.* [55] and, since then, studied by others (e.g. [56,52]).

The existence of regularities in a sequence renders it algorithmically compressible. The algorithmic information content of a sequence is the size, in bits, of its shortest reversible description and hence an indication of its complexity and entropy. Complexity measures of DNA sequences have been explored by several researchers (e.g. [57,58,59]). In this case, the key concept is the algorithmic entropy. Let $x$ denote a binary string of finite length. Its algorithmic entropy, $K(x)$, is defined as the length of a shortest binary program $x^*$ that computes $x$ in a universal Turing machine and halts [60]. Therefore, $K(x) = |x^*|$, the length of $x^*$, represents the minimum number of bits of a program from which $x$ can be computationally retrieved [61]. Although conceptually quite different, the algorithmic entropy is closely related to Shannon's entropy [61].

Because the algorithmic entropy is non-computable [61], it is usually approximated, for example, by compression algorithms [62,54,63,45]. In fact, compression-related approaches have been used not only for estimating the entropy, but also for building DNA sequence signatures capable of supporting the construction of meaningful dendograms [64]. In this case, estimates of the entropy associated with each of the three bases of the DNA codons are used to construct entropy vectors. Compression has also been used for measuring distances, such as in [65], where a genome-wide, alignment-free genomic distance based on compressed maximal exact matches is proposed for comparing genome assemblies.

Holzinger et al. (2012) [66] experimented with point cloud data sets in the two dimensional space: They developed a model of handwriting, and evaluated the performance of entropy based slant and skew correction, and compared the results to other methods. This work is the basis for further entropy-based approaches, which are very relevant for advanced entropy-based data mining approaches.

# 5   Detailed Description of Selected Entropies

## 5.1   Approximate Entropy (ApEn)

Approximate Entropy measures the logarithmic likelihood that runs of patterns that are close on following incremental comparisons [4]. We state Pincus' definition [4,5], for the family of statistics ApEn$(m, r, N)$:

**Definition 1.** *Fix $m$, a positive integer and $r$, a positive real number. Given a regularly sampled time series $u(t)$, a sequence of vectors $x(1)^m, x^m(2), \ldots,$ $x^m(N - m + 1)$ in $\mathbb{R}^m$ is formed, defined by*

$$x^m(i) := [u(t_i), u(t_{i+1}), \ldots, u(t_{i+m-1})] \ . \tag{1}$$

*Define for each $i$, $1 \leq i \leq N - m + 1$,*

$$C_i^m(r) := \frac{\text{number of } j \text{ such that } d[x^m(i), x^m(j)] \leq r}{N - m + 1} \ , \tag{2}$$

*where $d[x(i), x(j)]$ is the Chebyshev distance given by:*

$$d[x^m(i), x^m(j)] := \max_{k=1,2,\ldots,m} \left( |u(t_{i+k-1}) - u(t_{j+k-1})| \right) \ . \tag{3}$$

*Furthermore, define*

$$\Phi^m(r) := (N - m + 1)^{-1} \sum_{i=1}^{N-m+1} \log C_i^m(r) \ , \tag{4}$$

*then the **Approximate Entropy** is defined as*

$$\text{ApEn}(m, r, N) := \Phi^m(r) - \Phi^{m+1}(r) \ . \tag{5}$$

## 5.2   Sample Entropy (SampEn)

Richman and Moorman showed in [27] that approximate entropy is biased towards regularity. Thus, they modified it to Sample Entropy. The main difference between the two is that sample entropy does not count self-matches, and only the first $N - m$ subsequences instead of all $N - m + 1$ are compared, for both $\phi^m$ and $\phi^{m+1}$ [27]. Similar to ApEn above, SampEn is defined as follows:

**Definition 2.** *Fix $m$, a positive integer and $r$, a positive real number. Given a regularly sampled time series $U(t)$, a sequence of vectors $x^m(1), x^m(2), \ldots,$ $x^m(N - m + 1) \in \mathbb{R}^m$ is formed, defined by Eq. (1). Define for each $i$, $1 \leq i \leq N - m + 1$ ,*

$$C_i^m = \frac{\text{number of } j \text{ such that } d[x^m(i), x^m(j)] \leq r \text{ and } i \neq j}{N - m + 1} \ , \tag{6}$$

where $d[(i),(j)]$ is the Chebyshev distance (see Eq. (3)). Furthermore, define

$$\Phi^m(r) := (N-m)^{-1} \sum_{i=1}^{N-m} C_i^m(r) \ , \tag{7}$$

then the **Sample Entropy** is defined as

$$\text{SampEn}(m,r,N) := \log(\Phi^m(r)) - \log(\Phi^{m+1}(r)) \ . \tag{8}$$

### 5.3 Fuzzy (Measure) Entropy (Fuzzy(M)En)

To soften the effects of the threshold value $r$, Chen et al. proposed in [28] Fuzzy Entropy, which uses a fuzzy membership function instead of the Heaviside function. FuzzEn is defined the following way:

**Definition 3.** *Fix* $m$, *a positive integer and* $r$, *a positive real number. Given a regularly sampled time series* $U(t)$, *a sequence of vectors* $\boldsymbol{x}^m(1), \boldsymbol{x}^m(2), \dots,$ $\boldsymbol{x}^m(N-m+1) \in \mathbb{R}^m$ *is formed, as defined by Eq. (1). This sequence is transformed into* $\overline{\boldsymbol{x}}^m(1), \overline{\boldsymbol{x}}^m(2), \dots, \overline{\boldsymbol{x}}^m(N-m+1)$, *with* $\overline{\boldsymbol{x}}^m(i) := \{u(t_i) - u0_i, \dots,$ $u(t_{i+m-1}) - u0_i\}$, *where* $u0_i$ *is the mean value of* $\boldsymbol{x}^m(i)$, *i.e.*

$$u0_i := \sum_{j=0}^{m-1} \frac{u_{i+j}}{m}. \tag{9}$$

*Next the fuzzy membership matrix is defined as:*

$$D_{i,j}^m := \mu(d(\overline{x}_i^m, \overline{x}_j^m), n, r) \ , \tag{10}$$

*with the Chebyshev distance* $d$ *(see Eq. (3)) and the fuzzy membership function*

$$\mu(\boldsymbol{x}, n, r) := e^{-(\boldsymbol{x}/r)^n} \ . \tag{11}$$

*Finally, with*

$$\phi^m := \frac{1}{N-m} \sum_{i=1}^{N-m} \sum_{j=1, j \neq i}^{N-m} \frac{D_{i,j}^m}{N-m-1} \ , \tag{12}$$

*the* **Fuzzy Entropy** *is defined as:*

$$\text{FuzzyEn}(m,r,n,N) := \ln \phi^m - \ln \phi^{m+1} \ . \tag{13}$$

Liu et al. proposed in [29] **Fuzzy Measure Entropy**, which introduces a distinction between local entropy and global entropy, based on FuzzyEn. It is defined as:

$$\text{FuzzyMEn}(m, r_L, r_F, n_L, n_F, N) := \ln \phi_L^m - \ln \phi_L^{m+1} + \ln \phi_F^m - \ln \phi_F^{m+1} \ , \tag{14}$$

where the local terms $\phi_L^m$ and $\phi_L^{m+1}$ are calculated as in Eq. (12) and the global terms $\phi_F^m$ and $\phi_F^{m+1}$ are calculated with Eq. (10) and Eq. (12), but with $\overline{\boldsymbol{x}}^m(i) :=$ $\{u(t_i) - u_{\text{mean}}, \dots, u(t_{i+m-1}) - u_{\text{mean}}\}$, where $u_{\text{mean}}$ is the mean value of the complete sequence $u(t)$.

## 5.4  Topological Entropy for Finite Sequences (FiniteTopEn)

As seen above, ApEn, SampEn, and Fuzzy(M)En all require the selection of a threshold value $r$ which can significantly change the value of the associated entropy. FiniteTopEn differs from these definitions in that no threshold selection is required. FiniteTopEn is defined in the following way. First, define the complexity function of a sequence (finite or infinite) to be the following:

**Definition 4.** *For a given sequence $w$, the complexity function $p_w : \mathbb{N} \to \mathbb{N}$ is defined as*

$$p_w(n) = |\{u : |u| = n \text{ and } u \text{ appears as a subword of } w\}|.$$

So $p_w(n)$ gives the number of distinct $n$-length subwords (with overlap) of $w$. Then FiniteTopEn is defined as follows.

**Definition 5.** *Let $w$ be a finite sequence of length $|w|$ constructed from an alphabet $\mathcal{A}$ of $m$ symbols. Let $n$ be the unique integer such that*

$$m^n + n - 1 \le |w| < m^{n+1} + n.$$

*Then for $v = w_1^{m^n + n - 1}$ the first $m^n + n - 1$ letters of $w$, the topological entropy of $w$ is defined to be*

$$FiniteTopEn(w) = \frac{1}{n} \log_m \left( P_v(n) \right).$$

FiniteTopEn is defined in this way primarily so that entropies of different length sequences and on possibly different alphabets can still be compared. Of course, if more is known about the process that generates a given sequence $w$, then the above definition can be modified as necessary (for example, by picking a smaller $n$ or else not truncating $w$). The definition given above makes the least amount of assumptions regarding $w$ (i.e. assumes that $w$ was generated via the full shift). It is not difficult to demonstrate that as $|w| \to \infty$, $FiniteTopEn(w)$ converges to $TopEn(w)$, that is, to the topoloical entropy of $w$ as originally defined in [30].

## 6  Open Problems

The main challenges in biomedical informatics today include [15], [67]:

- Heterogeneous data sources (need for data integration and data fusion)
- Complexity of the data (high-dimensionality)
- The discrepancy between data-information-knowledge (various definitions)
- Big data sets (which makes manual handling of the data nearly impossible)
- Noisy, uncertain data (challenge of pre-processing).

Particularly, on the last issue, dealing with noisy, uncertain data, entropy based methods might bring some benefits. However, in the application of entropy there are a lot of unsolved problems. We focus here on topological entropy, as this can be best used for data mining purposes.

*Problem 1.* **There is no universal method to calculate or estimate the topological entropy.** Zhou & Fang described in [68] topological entropy as one of the most important concepts in dynamical systems but they described also a number of open problems: TopEn describes the complexity of the motion in the underlying space caused by a continuous or differential action, i.e.: the bigger the topological entropy, the more complex the motion. Consequently, to obtain (calculate, measure, estimate) the topological entropy is an important research topic in dynamical systems. But as in the case of the Hausdorff measure, calculating the exact value of the topological entropy is, in general, very difficult, as to date there is no universal method. One might debate the clause *estimate* in the begin of this paragraph, since topological entropy can indeed be estimated (see Problem 2) for an arbitrary symbolic dynamical system. Then, a wide range of arbitrary dynamical systems can be approximated by an appropriate symbolic dynamical system.

*Problem 2.* A problem that has not been mentioned so far is the fact that to correctly estimate entropy (of any sort, and FiniteTopEnt in particular), one needs access to many data points. This is certainly not always the case, and so it would be beneficial to have something like a re-sampling/bootstrap regime. Since order matters to topological entropy, traditional bootstrapping cannot be used, which poses a big open problem.

*Problem 3.* How can sparse/infrequent data be re-sampled in a fashion appropriate to better estimate entropy.

*Problem 4.* For instance, for continuous mappings of the interval, the topological entropy being zero is equivalent to the period of any periodic point being a power of 2. For a general dynamical system, no similar equivalence condition has been obtained. A breakthrough regarding this depends upon a breakthrough in the investigation of the kernel problem of dynamical systems: the orbits topological structures or asymptotic behavior. An excellent source for this topic is [2].

*Problem 5.* The study of the topics mentioned in problem 4, is closely related to the ones in ergodic theory such as the invariant measure, the measure-theoretic entropy and the variational principle, as well as some fractal properties. Hence, the study of topological entropy has much potential in three fields: topology, ergodic theory and fractal geometry; albeit this will probably not unify these methods, topological entropy finds itself at the intersection of these subfields of mathematics.

*Problem 6.* In contrast to problem 5, FiniteTopEn is an approximation to topological entropy that is free from issues associated to choosing a threshold (problem 2). It was also shown in [32] that FiniteTopEn is computationally tractable, both theoretically (i.e its expected value) and practically (i.e. in computing entropy of DNA sequences). Applying this definition to the intron and exon regions of the human genome, it was observed that, as expected, the entropy of introns is significantly higher that that of exons. This example demonstrates that this parameter-free estimate of topological entropy is potentially well-suited to discern salient global features of weakly structured data.

*Problem 7.* How to select parameters for the entropy measures? Each entropy has a number of parameters to be selected before application. Thus, there are a large number of possible combinations of parameters. By now, this problem has not yet been solved especially for ApEn, SampEn, FuzzyEn and FuzzyMEn. There are different parameter sets published (e.g., [4,69,70,41,71]), but up to now not all possible combinations were tested and no consensus was reached. The parameter sets cover certain application areas, but are dependent on the data and its type. An example is the choice of the threshold value $r$ according to [69]. It is used only in the context of heart rate variability data and not applied to other data.

*Problem 8.* How to use entropy measures for classification of pathological and non-pathological data? In biomedical data, the goal is to discriminate between pathological and non-pathological measurements. There is still little evidence on how to use entropy measures for this classification problem and which data ranges to use. This is directly related to the parameter selection, since one of the hardest difficulties for ApEn, SampEn, FuzzyEn and FuzzyMEn lies in the choice of the threshold value $r$ due to the flip-flop effect, i.e., for some parameters one data set has a higher entropy compared to another, but this order is reversed for different parameter choices [70,72]. This can occur for simple signals, but also when analyzing heart rate variability data, as shown in [71]. This leads to difficulties with the interpretation of the entropy, i.e., the direct assignment of entropy values to pathological or non-pathological data without a given $r$.
Finally a few very short questions poses mega challenges in these area:

*Problem 9.* How to generally benchmark entropy measures?

*Problem 10.* How to select appropriate entropy measures and their parameters to solve a particular problem?

# 7    Conclusion and Future Outlook

Entropy measures have successfully been tested for analyzing short, sparse and noisy time series data. **However they have not yet been applied to weakly structured data in combination with techniques from computational topology.** Consequently, the inclusion of entropy measures for discovery of knowledge in high-dimensional biomedical data is a big future issue and there are a lot of promising research routes.

# References

1. Holzinger, A.: On knowledge discovery and interactive intelligent visualization of biomedical data - challenges in human computer interaction and biomedical informatics. In: DATA 2012, vol. 1, pp. 9–20. INSTICC (2012)
2. Downarowicz, T.: Entropy in dynamical systems, vol. 18. Cambridge University Press, Cambridge (2011)
3. Shannon, C.E., Weaver, W.: The Mathematical Theory of Communication. University of Illinois Press, Urbana (1949)
4. Pincus, S.M.: Approximate entropy as a measure of system complexity. Proceedings of the National Academy of Sciences 88(6), 2297–2301 (1991)
5. Pincus, S.: Approximate entropy (apen) as a complexity measure. Chaos: An Interdisciplinary Journal of Nonlinear Science 5(1), 110–117 (1995)
6. Chandola, V., Banerjee, A., Kumar, V.: Anomaly detection: A survey. ACM Comput. Surv. 41(3), 1–58 (2009)
7. Batini, C., Scannapieco, M.: Data Quality: Concepts, Methodologies and Techniques. Springer, Berlin (2006)
8. Holzinger, A., Simonic, K.-M. (eds.): Information Quality in e-Health. LNCS, vol. 7058. Springer, Heidelberg (2011)
9. Kim, W., Choi, B.J., Hong, E.K., Kim, S.K., Lee, D.: A taxonomy of dirty data. Data Mining and Knowledge Discovery 7(1), 81–99 (2003)
10. Gschwandtner, T., Gärtner, J., Aigner, W., Miksch, S.: A taxonomy of dirty time-oriented data. In: Quirchmayr, G., Basl, J., You, I., Xu, L., Weippl, E. (eds.) CD-ARES 2012. LNCS, vol. 7465, pp. 58–72. Springer, Heidelberg (2012)
11. Clausius, R.: On the motive power of heat, and on the laws which can be deduced from it for the theory of heat, poggendorff's annalen der physick, lxxix (1850)
12. Sethna, J.P.: Statistical mechanics: Entropy, order parameters, and complexity, vol. 14. Oxford University Press, New York (2006)
13. Jaynes, E.T.: Information theory and statistical mechanics. Physical Review 106(4), 620 (1957)
14. Golan, A.: Information and entropy econometrics: A review and synthesis. Now Publishers Inc. (2008)
15. Holzinger, A.: Biomedical Informatics: Discovering Knowledge in Big Data. Springer, New York (2014)
16. Jaynes, E.T.: Information theory and statistical mechanics. Physical Review 106(4), 620 (1957)
17. Mowshowitz, A.: Entropy and the complexity of graphs: I. an index of the relative complexity of a graph. The Bulletin of Mathematical Biophysics 30(1), 175–204 (1968)
18. Körner, J.: Coding of an information source having ambiguous alphabet and the entropy of graphs. In: 6th Prague Conference on Information Theory, pp. 411–425 (1973)
19. Holzinger, A., Ofner, B., Stocker, C., Calero Valdez, A., Schaar, A.K., Ziefle, M., Dehmer, M.: On graph entropy measures for knowledge discovery from publication network data. In: Cuzzocrea, A., Kittl, C., Simos, D.E., Weippl, E., Xu, L. (eds.) CD-ARES 2013. LNCS, vol. 8127, pp. 354–362. Springer, Heidelberg (2013)
20. Dehmer, M., Mowshowitz, A.: A history of graph entropy measures. Information Sciences 181(1), 57–78 (2011)
21. Posner, E.C.: Random coding strategies for minimum entropy. IEEE Transactions on Information Theory 21(4), 388–391 (1975)

22. Yuan, L., Kesavan, H.: Minimum entropy and information measure. IEEE Transactions on Systems, Man, and Cybernetics, Part C: Applications and Reviews 28(3), 488–491 (1998)
23. Rubinstein, R.Y.: Optimization of computer simulation models with rare events. European Journal of Operational Research 99(1), 89–112 (1997)
24. De Boer, P.T., Kroese, D.P., Mannor, S., Rubinstein, R.Y.: A tutorial on the cross-entropy method. Annals of Operations Research 134(1), 19–67 (2005)
25. Tsallis, C.: Possible generalization of boltzmann-gibbs statistics. Journal of Statistical Physics 52(1-2), 479–487 (1988)
26. de Albuquerque, M.P., Esquef, I.A., Mello, A.R.G., de Albuquerque, M.P.: Image thresholding using tsallis entropy. Pattern Recognition Letters 25(9), 1059–1065 (2004)
27. Richman, J.S., Moorman, J.R.: Physiological time-series analysis using approximate entropy and sample entropy. Am. J. Physiol. Heart Circ. Physiol. 278(6), H2039–H2049 (2000)
28. Chen, W., Wang, Z., Xie, H., Yu, W.: Characterization of surface emg signal based on fuzzy entropy. IEEE Transactions on Neural Systems and Rehabilitation Engineering 15(2), 266–272 (2007)
29. Liu, C., Li, K., Zhao, L., Liu, F., Zheng, D., Liu, C., Liu, S.: Analysis of heart rate variability using fuzzy measure entropy. Comput. Biol. Med. 43(2), 100–108 (2013)
30. Adler, R.L., Konheim, A.G., McAndrew, M.H.: Topological entropy. Transactions of the American Mathematical Society 114(2), 309–319 (1965)
31. Adler, R., Downarowicz, T., Misiurewicz, M.: Topological entropy. Scholarpedia 3(2), 2200 (2008)
32. Koslicki, D.: Topological entropy of dna sequences. Bioinformatics 27(8), 1061–1067 (2011)
33. Solomonoff, R.J.: A formal theory of inductive inference. Part I. Information and Control 7(1), 1–22 (1964)
34. Solomonoff, R.J.: A formal theory of inductive inference. Part II. Information and Control 7(2), 224–254 (1964)
35. Kolmogorov, A.N.: Three approaches to the quantitative definition of information. Problems of Information Transmission 1(1), 1–7 (1965)
36. Chaitin, G.J.: On the length of programs for computing finite binary sequences. Journal of the ACM 13, 547–569 (1966)
37. Acharya, U.R., Molinari, F., Sree, S.V., Chattopadhyay, S., Ng, K.-H., Suri, J.S.: Automated diagnosis of epileptic eeg using entropies. Biomedical Signal Processing and Control 7(4), 401–408 (2012)
38. Hornero, R., Aboy, M., Abasolo, D., McNames, J., Wakeland, W., Goldstein, B.: Complex analysis of intracranial hypertension using approximate entropy. Crit. Care. Med. 34(1), 87–95 (2006)
39. Batchinsky, A.I., Salinas, J., Cancio, L.C., Holcomb, J.: Assessment of the need to perform life-saving interventions using comprehensive analysis of the electrocardiogram and artificial neural networks. Use of Advanced Techologies and New Procedures in Medical Field Operations 39, 1–16 (2010)
40. Sarlabous, L., Torres, A., Fiz, J.A., Gea, J., Martínez-Llorens, J.M., Morera, J., Jané, R.: Interpretation of the approximate entropy using fixed tolerance values as a measure of amplitude variations in biomedical signals. In: 2010 Annual International Conference of the IEEE Engineering in Medicine and Biology Society (EMBC), pp. 5967–5970 (2010)

41. Yentes, J., Hunt, N., Schmid, K., Kaipust, J., McGrath, D., Stergiou, N.: The appropriate use of approximate entropy and sample entropy with short data sets. Annals of Biomedical Engineering 41(2), 349–365 (2013)
42. Roerdink, M., De Haart, M., Daffertshofer, A., Donker, S.F., Geurts, A.C., Beek, P.J.: Dynamical structure of center-of-pressure trajectories in patients recovering from stroke. Exp. Brain Res. 174(2), 256–269 (2006)
43. Clift, B., Haussler, D., McConnell, R., Schneider, T.D., Stormo, G.D.: Sequence landscapes. Nucleic Acids Research 14(1), 141–158 (1986)
44. Schneider, T.D., Stephens, R.M.: Sequence logos: A new way to display consensus sequences. Nucleic Acids Research 18(20), 6097–6100 (1990)
45. Pinho, A.J., Garcia, S.P., Pratas, D., Ferreira, P.J.S.G.: DNA sequences at a glance. PLoS ONE 8(11), e79922 (2013)
46. Jeffrey, H.J.: Chaos game representation of gene structure. Nucleic Acids Research 18(8), 2163–2170 (1990)
47. Goldman, N.: Nucleotide, dinucleotide and trinucleotide frequencies explain patterns observed in chaos game representations of DNA sequences. Nucleic Acids Research 21(10), 2487–2491 (1993)
48. Oliver, J.L., Bernaola-Galván, P., Guerrero-García, J., Román-Roldán, R.: Entropic profiles of DNA sequences through chaos-game-derived images. Journal of Theoretical Biology 160, 457–470 (1993)
49. Vinga, S., Almeida, J.S.: Local Renyi entropic profiles of DNA sequences. BMC Bioinformatics 8(393) (2007)
50. Crochemore, M., Vérin, R.: Zones of low entropy in genomic sequences. Computers & Chemistry, 275–282 (1999)
51. Allison, L., Stern, L., Edgoose, T., Dix, T.I.: Sequence complexity for biological sequence analysis. Computers & Chemistry 24, 43–55 (2000)
52. Stern, L., Allison, L., Coppel, R.L., Dix, T.I.: Discovering patterns in Plasmodium falciparum genomic DNA. Molecular & Biochemical Parasitology 118, 174–186 (2001)
53. Cao, M.D., Dix, T.I., Allison, L., Mears, C.: A simple statistical algorithm for biological sequence compression. In: Proc. of the Data Compression Conf., DCC 2007, Snowbird, Utah, pp. 43–52 (March 2007)
54. Dix, T.I., Powell, D.R., Allison, L., Bernal, J., Jaeger, S., Stern, L.: Comparative analysis of long DNA sequences by per element information content using different contexts. BMC Bioinformatics 8 (suppl. 2), S 10 (2007)
55. Grumbach, S., Tahi, F.: Compression of DNA sequences. In: Proc. of the Data Compression Conf., DCC 93, Snowbird, Utah, pp. 340–350 (1993)
56. Rivals, E., Delgrange, O., Delahaye, J.-P., Dauchet, M., Delorme, M.-O., Hénaut, A., Ollivier, E.: Detection of significant patterns by compression algorithms: The case of approximate tandem repeats in DNA sequences. Computer Applications in the Biosciences 13, 131–136 (1997)
57. Gusev, V.D., Nemytikova, L.A., Chuzhanova, N.A.: On the complexity measures of genetic sequences. Bioinformatics 15(12), 994–999 (1999)
58. Nan, F., Adjeroh, D.: On the complexity measures for biological sequences. In: Proc. of the IEEE Computational Systems Bioinformatics Conference, CSB-2004, Stanford, CA (August 2004 )
59. Pirhaji, L., Kargar, M., Sheari, A., Poormohammadi, H., Sadeghi, M., Pezeshk, H., Eslahchi, C.: The performances of the chi-square test and complexity measures for signal recognition in biological sequences. Journal of Theoretical Biology 251(2), 380–387 (2008)

60. Turing, A.: On computable numbers, with an application to the Entscheidungsproblem. Proceedings of the London Mathematical Society 42(2), 230–265 (1936)
61. Li, M., Vitányi, P.: An introduction to Kolmogorov complexity and its applications, 3rd edn. Springer (2008)
62. Chen, X., Kwong, S., Li, M.: A compression algorithm for DNA sequences and its applications in genome comparison. In: Asai, K., Miyano, S., Takagi, T. (eds.) Proc. of the 10th Workshop, Genome Informatics 1999, Tokyo, Japan, pp. 51–61 (1999)
63. Pinho, A.J., Ferreira, P.J.S.G., Neves, A.J.R., Bastos, C.A.C.: On the representability of complete genomes by multiple competing finite-context (Markov) models. PLoS ONE 6(6), e21588 (2011)
64. Pinho, A.J., Garcia, S.P., Ferreira, P.J.S.G., Afreixo, V., Bastos, C.A.C., Neves, A.J.R., Rodrigues, J.M.O.S.: Exploring homology using the concept of three-state entropy vector. In: Dijkstra, T.M.H., Tsivtsivadze, E., Marchiori, E., Heskes, T. (eds.) PRIB 2010. LNCS (LNBI), vol. 6282, pp. 161–170. Springer, Heidelberg (2010)
65. Garcia, S.P., Rodrigues, J.M.O.S., Santos, S., Pratas, D., Afreixo, V., Bastos, C.A.C., Ferreira, P.J.S.G., Pinho, A.J.: A genomic distance for assembly comparison based on compressed maximal exact matches. IEEE/ACM Trans. on Computational Biology and Bioinformatics 10(3), 793–798 (2013)
66. Holzinger, A., Stocker, C., Peischl, B., Simonic, K.M.: On using entropy for enhancing handwriting preprocessing. Entropy 14(11), 2324–2350 (2012)
67. Holzinger, A., Dehmer, M., Jurisica, I.: Knowledge discovery and interactive data mining in bioinformatics - state-of-the-art, future challenges and research directions. BMC Bioinformatics 15(suppl. 6), 11 (2014)
68. Zhou, Z., Feng, L.: Twelve open problems on the exact value of the hausdorff measure and on topological entropy: A brief survey of recent results. Nonlinearity 17(2), 493–502 (2004)
69. Chon, K., Scully, C.G., Lu, S.: Approximate entropy for all signals. IEEE Eng. Med. Biol. Mag. 28(6), 18–23 (2009)
70. Liu, C., Liu, C., Shao, P., Li, L., Sun, X., Wang, X., Liu, F.: Comparison of different threshold values r for approximate entropy: Application to investigate the heart rate variability between heart failure and healthy control groups. Physiol. Meas. 32(2), 167–180 (2011)
71. Mayer, C., Bachler, M., Hörtenhuber, M., Stocker, C., Holzinger, A., Wassertheurer, S.: Selection of entropy-measure parameters for knowledge discovery in heart rate variability data. BMC Bioinformatics 15
72. Boskovic, A., Loncar-Turukalo, T., Japundzic-Zigon, N., Bajic, D.: The flip-flop effect in entropy estimation, pp. 227–230 (2011)

# Sparse Inverse Covariance Estimation for Graph Representation of Feature Structure

Sangkyun Lee

Fakultät für Informatik, LS VIII
Technische Universität Dortmund, 44221 Dortmund, Germany
sangkyun.lee@tu-dortmund.de

**Abstract.** The access to more information provided by modern high-throughput measurement systems has made it possible to investigate finer details of complex systems. However, it also has increased the number of features, and thereby the dimensionality in data, to be processed in data analysis. Higher dimensionality makes it particularly challenging to understand complex systems, by blowing up the number of possible configurations of features we need to consider. Structure learning with the Gaussian Markov random field can provide a remedy, by identifying conditional independence structure of features in a form that is easy to visualize and understand. The learning is based on a convex optimization problem, called the sparse inverse covariance estimation, for which many efficient algorithms have been developed in the past few years. When dimensions are much larger than sample sizes, structure learning requires to consider statistical stability, in which connections to data mining arise in terms of discovering common or rare subgraphs as patterns. The outcome of structure learning can be visualized as graphs, represented accordingly to additional information if required, providing a perceivable way to investigate complex feature spaces.

**Keywords:** Structure Learning, Sparse Inverse Covariance Matrix, Gaussian Markov Random Fields, Sparsity.

## 1  Introduction

Advances in measurement technology have enabled us to explore greater details of complex systems. For instance, modern high-throughput genomic profiling platforms such as whole-transcript microarrays (e.g. http://www.affymetrix.com) or next generation sequencing (e.g. http://www.illumina.com) provide information on a few million subsequences of human DNA (or their molecular products). With rapid decrease in their cost [1, 2], these platforms become prominent in biology and related computer scientific and statistical research.

The primary goal in high-throughput genomic studies is to identify the key players (often referred to as biomarkers) from a large amount of features that contribute to the development of diseases, and furthermore, to understand the relations of biomarkers to controllable genes so to discover a possible cure for a

A. Holzinger, I. Jurisica (Eds.): Knowledge Discovery and Data Mining, LNCS 8401, pp. 227–240, 2014.

disease. Identification of biomarkers is typically achieved by *feature selection* [3], with respect to various measures on features (e.g. relevance to clinical outcome, independence amongst selected features, etc.) However, typical feature selection methods do not provide structural information of selected features, and therefore another (often costly bio-chemical) analysis typically follows to identify how the selected features contribute to a complex system.

Some structural information is available on genomic features, for instance, the Gene Ontology (`http://www.geneontology.org`) provides the hierarchical relation of genes in terms of their cellular locations, biological processes, and molecular functions, and the KEGG (`http://www.genome.jp`) database provides known biological pathways associated with gene products. However, these databases are often incomplete or inconsistent [4,5], providing unspecific or partial structural information on features. Therefore with the lack of full structural information on features, it is natural to consider high-throughput genomic profile data as weakly structured.

The purpose of learning structure in features is to improve the identification of feature relations from weakly structured data, by capturing relevant information in a way that is (i) statistically sound and (ii) easy to visualize and understand. Probabilistic graphical models in machine learning [6] fits well for the motive, where features are represented as nodes and relations among features are represented as edges in a graph. In these models, a random variable is associated with each node, and the joint probability distribution of all nodes is determined by the structure of an underlying graph. Conversely, the joint probability distribution can be used to identify the structure of an underlying graph so to maximize the likelihood of generating certain data from the distribution.

A classical choice of probabilistic graphical models in biomedical studies is the Bayesian network [7]. In a Bayesian network, edges are directional and the entire graph is required to contain no cycle (such graphs are referred to as DAGs, directed acyclic graphs.) Bayesian networks are capable of representing complex statistical dependency structures, and have been successfully applied for analyzing gene expression data [8], discovering signaling pathways from cellular data [9], and detecting disease outbreaks [10]. However, learning the structure of Bayesian networks has a major drawback that the search is essentially combinatorial and therefore computationally intractable [11,12]. For this reason, structure learning for Bayesian networks is not well suited for high-dimensional settings where graphs involve a large number of nodes and many different possible ways of connections.

For high-dimensional structure learning, a simpler probabilistic graphical model has been studied quite extensively recently [13–21], for which efficient convex optimization procedures exist to find the structure of the underlying graph. This model uses undirected connections between nodes and allows for cycles, and assumes that the random variable of each node follows the Gaussian distribution. The resulting graphical model is called the *Gaussian Markov random field* (GMRF), which have been applied in various areas including biostatistics [22–26] and image analysis [27–31]. The structure learning for GMRFs is often referred to as the *sparse inverse covariance estimation* or the *graph/graphical lasso*. The original idea of learning covariance structure goes back to covariance selection [22] and model selection for the Gaussian concentration graphs [32]. Greedy stepwise forward/backward selection algorithms have been used to solve the estimation problem, despite their computational and statistical weaknesses [33]. A more efficient selection method was proposed recently [13], but still parameter estimation and model selection steps were handled separately. The two steps were finally combined in a convex optimization problem [14], which became a focus of recent studies in machine learning, statistics, and optimization.

Structure learning of GMRFs provides sparse graphical representations of feature spaces, revealing conditional independence relations amongst features. Such graphs can provide decomposable views of a complex feature space in big data, by means of small connected components that can be easily visualized or understood. Moreover, such representation enables us to use tools from graph theory, so that a feature space can be analyzed in perspectives of node degree distributions, average shortest path lengths, and so on. Small subgraphs can also be considered as patterns consisting of a small set of features, for which data mining approaches will be essential to find prominent or rare patterns in a statistically robust fashion from collections of graphs obtained with subsamples of genomic profiles.

## 2  Glossary and Key Terms

**Undirected Graph:** A graph $G = (V, E)$ consists of a set of nodes (vertices) $V$ and a set of edges $E$ is undirected if the edges in $E$ does not contain any direction associated, and only a single undirected connection, if any, between two nodes is allowed.

**Gaussian Markov Random Field (GMRF):** A random vector $\mathbf{x} \in \Re^p$ following the Gaussian distribution $\mathcal{N}(\mu, \Sigma)$ with the probability density function,

$$p(\mathbf{x}) = (2\pi)^{-p/2} \det(\Sigma)^{-1/2} \exp\left(-\frac{1}{2}(\mathbf{x} - \mu)^T \Sigma^{-1} (\mathbf{x} - \mu)\right), \qquad (1)$$

is called the Gaussian Markov random field (GMRF) when for the elements of $\mathbf{x}$ represented as nodes in an undirected graph $G = (V, E)$, there is no edge between two nodes $i$ and $j$ if the associated random variables $\mathbf{x}_i$ and $\mathbf{x}_j$ are independent conditioned on all the other random variables in $\mathbf{x}$ [34].

**Inverse Covariance Matrix:** The inverse of the covariance matrix $\Sigma$ in Eq. (1) is also known as the precision or the concentration matrix [35]. The precision matrix $\Sigma^{-1}$ of a GMRF satisfies the property that $\Sigma_{ij}^{-1} = 0$ if and only if the nodes $i$ and $j$ are not connected (i.e. conditionally independent) in the associated graph $G$ [36].

**Structure Learning:**   For a GMRF, structure learning is equivalent to deducing the set of edges $E$ of the associated undirected graph $G = (V, E)$ using observed data. After a proper centering of data (so that $\mu = 0$), this corresponds to estimating the precision matrix $\Sigma^{-1}$ of the GMRF from data and identify its nonzero elements $\{(i, j) : \Sigma_{ij}^{-1} \neq 0\}$.

**Convex Optimization:**   In optimization, a problem to minimize a cost function $f(x)$ over points $x$ in a constraint set $C$ is written as

$$\min_x \ f(x) \ \text{subject to} \ x \in C.$$

If $f$ is a convex function and $C$ is a convex set, then the problem is called a convex optimization problem [37]. Efficient algorithms exist for convex optimization problems, especially when $f$ is smooth or the structure of $C$ is simple. Estimation of the sparse inverse covariance (precision) matrix, i.e. the structure learning of a GMRF, can be formulated as a convex optimization problem.

## 3   Sparse Inverse Covariance Estimation

The Gaussian Markov random field (GMRF) is built upon an assumption that features follow a multivariate Gaussian distribution $\mathcal{N}(\mu, \Sigma)$ (Eq. (1)) with a mean vector $\mu$ and a covariance matrix $\Sigma$. This assumption is suitable for gene expression measurements, given that the number of profiled patients is large enough (typically > 30.) It enables us to perform structure learning with efficient computation algorithms.

### 3.1   Gaussian Markov Random Field (GMRF)

The Markov random field (MRF) is a collection of $p$ random variables (we assume that they are collected in a vector $\mathbf{x} \in \Re^p$) represented as nodes in a graph, where the conditional dependency structure of nodes is represented by undirected edges between nodes. Such a graph is denoted by $G = (V, E)$, where $V$ is the set of all nodes (therefore $|V| = p$) and $E$ is the set of all edges. For such a graph to be an MRF, it has to satisfy the Markov properties [34] which enable us to compute the joint probability density function of the random variables efficiently in a factorized form.

The Gaussian MRF (GMRF) is a special type of MRFs, where the random variables follow the Gaussian distribution (Eq. (1)). In this particular setting the Markov properties simplify to the condition that if the $(i, j)$th entry of the inverse covariance matrix (also known as the precision matrix) $\Sigma_{ij}^{-1}$ is zero, then there is no edge connecting the two nodes $i$ and $j$ [34]. This means that the random variables $\mathbf{x}_i$ and $\mathbf{x}_j$ associated with the nodes $i$ and $j$ are *conditionally independent* given all the other nodes [36], that is,

$$\Sigma_{ij}^{-1} = 0 \ \Leftrightarrow \ \begin{aligned} &P(\mathbf{x}_i, \mathbf{x}_j | \{\mathbf{x}_k\}_{k \in \{1,2,\dots,p\} \setminus \{i,j\}}) \\ &= P(\mathbf{x}_i | \{\mathbf{x}_k\}_{k \in \{1,2,\dots,p\} \setminus \{i,j\}}) P(\mathbf{x}_j | \{\mathbf{x}_k\}_{k \in \{1,2,\dots,p\} \setminus \{i,j\}}). \end{aligned}$$

In other words, the graph $G$ of a GMRF represents the conditional independence structure of a feature space.

In fact, the entries of the precision matrix $\Sigma_{ij}^{-1}$ represent conditional correlation between the nodes $i$ and $j$ [36]. If $\Sigma_{ij}^{-1} \neq 0$, then we connect the two nodes $i$ and $j$ with an edge to represent their nonzero correlation. Since the zero correlation ($\Sigma_{ij}^{-1} = 0$) implies statistical independence for the case of Gaussian random variables, this result is consistent with our discussion above.

## 3.2   Structure Learning of GMRFs

The structure of a GMRF is determined by the inverse covariance matrix $\Sigma^{-1}$. A typical way to estimate this matrix is the maximum likelihood estimation (MLE) framework [38]. Suppose that $n$ observations of feature vectors $\mathbf{x}^1, \mathbf{x}^2, \ldots, \mathbf{x}^n$ are sampled independently and identically from a multivariate Gaussian distribution $\mathcal{N}(\mathbf{0}, \Sigma^{-1})$. Here we have assumed that the observations are centered without loss of generality, so that their mean is the zero vector. In this case the probability density for the Gaussian distribution simplifies to:

$$p(\mathbf{x}) = (2\pi)^{-p/2} \det(\Sigma)^{-1/2} \exp\left(-\frac{1}{2}\mathbf{x}^T \Sigma^{-1} \mathbf{x}\right).$$

The likelihood function that describes the chance to observe a given data set $\mathcal{D} = \{\mathbf{x}^1, \mathbf{x}^2, \ldots, \mathbf{x}^n\}$ from this distribution is,

$$L(\Sigma^{-1}, \mathcal{D}) = \prod_{i=1}^{n} p(\mathbf{x}^i)$$

$$\sim \prod_{i=1}^{n} \det(\Sigma)^{-1/2} \exp\left(-\frac{1}{2}(\mathbf{x}^i)^T \Sigma^{-1} \mathbf{x}^i\right).$$

Constants can be ignored since they do not affect estimation. Taking logarithm in both sides and scaling by $2/n$ leads to a so-called log likelihood function,

$$LL(\Sigma^{-1}, \mathcal{D}) = \log \det(\Sigma^{-1}) - \mathrm{tr}(S\Sigma^{-1}), \tag{2}$$

where $S := \frac{1}{n}\sum_{i=1}^{n} \mathbf{x}^i(\mathbf{x}^i)^T$ is the sample covariance matrix and $\mathrm{tr}(A)$ is the trace (the sum of diagonal elements) of a square matrix $A$. Note that we have used a property of determinant that $\det(\Sigma^{-1}) = \det(\Sigma)^{-1}$.

## 3.3   Promoting Sparsity in $\Sigma^{-1}$

While searching for $\Sigma^{-1}$ that maximizes the (log) likelihood function, it is preferable to consider such a $\Sigma^{-1}$ that contains as many zero entries as possible. In other words, a *sparse* $\Sigma^{-1}$ is preferred as a solution since otherwise the resulting GMRF will have densely connected graph, which is very hard to understand and visualize.

A sparse $\Sigma^{-1}$ can be obtained by minimizing the $\ell_1$ norm of the matrix while maximizing the log likelihood (or equivalently minimizing the negative log likelihood.) These goals can be described as a convex optimization problem,

$$\min_{\Theta \in \Re^{p \times p}} \quad -LL(\Theta, \mathcal{D}) + \lambda \|\Theta\|_1$$

$$\text{subject to} \quad \Theta \succ 0, \ \Theta^T = \Theta. \tag{3}$$

Here we have replaced $\Theta := \Sigma^{-1}$ to simplify notations, and $LL(\Theta, \mathcal{D})$ is the log likelihood function from Eq. (2). The $\ell_1$ norm of $\Theta$ is defined by

$$\|\Theta\|_1 := \sum_{i=1}^{p} \sum_{j=1}^{p} |\Theta_{ij}|, \tag{4}$$

whose value becomes smaller if $\Theta$ is sparser (note that this definition is different from vector-induced matrix norms.) In effect, the parameter $\lambda > 0$ controls sparsity in $\Theta$: the larger $\lambda$ is, the sparser the outcome becomes. The constraints $\Theta = \Theta^T$ and $\Theta \succ 0$ specifies that the matrix $\Theta$ should be symmetric and positive definite, i.e. all of its eigenvalues are strictly positive. These constraints originate from the fact that $\Sigma$ is a covariance matrix (which is symmetric positive semidefinite) and that $\Sigma^{-1}$ must be nonsingular so that $(\Sigma^{-1})^{-1} = \Sigma$ exists.

The term $\lambda \|\Theta\|_1$ added to the original objective function is often called a *regularizer*, and this particular type tends to induce sparsity in solutions. The use of regularizers goes back to the work of Tikhonov [39], however, $\ell_1$ regularizers have been popularized only recently, for example, in lasso regression [40], elastic net [41], online manifold identification [42], spatio-temporal Markov random fields [43], and compressed sensing [44, 45], just to name a few.

### 3.4    Graph Representation of Feature Structure

Structure learning with GMRFs can be summarized by collecting Eq. (2) and (3) as follows:

$$\min_{\Theta \in \Re^{p \times p}} \quad -\log \det \Theta + \text{tr}(S\Theta) + \lambda \|\Theta\|_1$$

$$\text{subject to} \quad \Theta \succ 0, \ \Theta^T = \Theta. \tag{5}$$

As we can see, the only input required for structure learning is the sample covariance matrix $S := \frac{1}{n} \sum_{i=1}^{n} \mathbf{x}^i (\mathbf{x}^i)^T$. Such a matrix can be easily computed from data in feature vector representation.

To demonstrate structure learning with GMRFs, we use a gene expression data set from the Gene Expression Omnibus (GEO, http://www.ncbi.nlm.nih.gov/geo/) with the accession ID GSE31210 [46, 47], which contains 226 lung cancer (adenocarcinoma) patient profiles measured by the Affymetrix Human Genome U133 Plus 2.0 Array platform (GPL570). The data were preprocessed with the frozen RMA (robust multiarray analysis) algorithm [48], and 22 microarrays with the GNUSE (global normalized unscaled standard error) scores [49] > 1.0 were discarded for quality control. Figure 1 shows the structure of features in the data

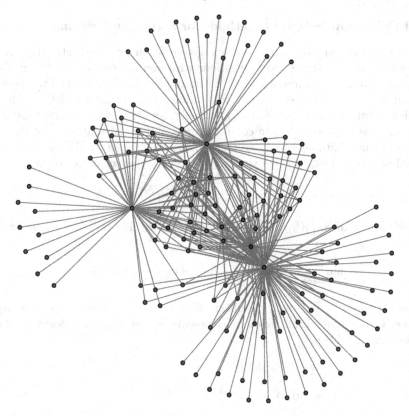

**Fig. 1.** Graph representation of gene features in lung adenocarcinoma data set from the Gene Expression Omnibus (GSE31210), obtained by the sparse inverse covariance estimation (structure learning with the Gaussian Markov random field.) Nodes represent genes and edges represent nonzero conditional dependency between genes.

set, constructed by sparse inverse covariance estimation. Each node corresponds to a gene (more specifically, a transcript) and the existence of a connection between two nodes implies that the correlation between the two corresponding genes is still informative even after having seen all the other genes.

# 4   Open Problems

There are two major open challenges for solving the sparse inverse covariance estimation problem in high-dimensions: development of efficient optimization algorithms and consideration of statistical stability of solutions.

## 4.1    Efficient Optimization Methods for Structure Learning

Structure learning in Eq. (5) is a convex optimization problem, estimating parameters and finding the support (positions with nonzero entries) of the inverse covariance matrix $\Sigma^{-1}$ simultaneously. Yuan and Lin [14] approached the problem as an instance of the determinant-maximization (so-called maxdet) problem for which an interior point method was available [50]. However, the complexity of these solvers is $\mathcal{O}(p^6 \log(1/\epsilon))$ to compute an $\epsilon$-suboptimal solution, and therefore they are not suitable for large dimensions $p$. Banerjee et al. [15] constructed the dual problem of Eq. (5) by expressing the $\ell_1$ regularizer in Eq. (4) as

$$\|\Theta\|_1 = \max_{\|U\|_\infty \leq 1, U^T = U} \operatorname{tr}(U\Theta),$$

where $\|U\|_\infty := \max_{i,j} |U_{ij}|$. Then the structure learning problem Eq. (5) can be rewritten as

$$\min_{\Theta \succ 0, \Theta^T = \Theta} \max_{\|U\|_\infty \leq 1, U^T = U} -\log \det \Theta + \operatorname{tr}((S + U)\Theta).$$

Exchanging the min and max, we obtain $\Theta = (S + U)^{-1}$ from the optimality condition of the inner minimization. Replacing $W := S + U$, it leads to the following dual problem,

$$\max_{W \in \Re^{p \times p}} \log \det W \tag{6}$$
$$\text{subject to } W \succ 0, \ W^T = W, \ \|W - S\|_\infty \leq \lambda.$$

Compared to the primal problem Eq. (5), the dual formulation above has a smooth objective function (the nondifferentiable $\ell_1$ term is removed), which is typically easier to optimize. A coordinate descent algorithm [15] has been proposed to solve the dual, and the equivalence of its subproblems to the lasso regression has led to another coordinate descent algorithm based on lasso [17]. However, their subproblems are quadratic programs involving quite large $(p-1) \times (p-1)$ matrices, resulting in $\mathcal{O}(Kp^4)$ complexity for $K$ sweeps of all variables.

A new algorithm was proposed by Duchi et al. [16] based on the projected gradient method [51] to solve the dual formulation, improving the complexity to $\mathcal{O}(p^3)$ but without showing iteration complexity bound. Nesterov's optimal first order method [52] and smoothing techniques [53] have been adapted to sparse inverse covariance learning, e.g. [54,55], but their practical performance was not appealing. Alternating direction methods [19,56] have been proposed equipped with interior point subproblem solvers, resulting in $\mathcal{O}(p^3/\epsilon)$ total complexity. Dinh et al. [21] reduced iteration complexity from $\mathcal{O}(p^3)$ to $\mathcal{O}(p^2)$ by means of a carefully designed proximal Newton framework, eliminating the need for matrix inversion in the previous methods. Other types of methods using the second order information of the objective have shown faster convergence [57,58], notably being able to handle up to a million variables [59].

Although optimization methods have been improved over the past few years, challenges still remain: in particular, the memory requirement $\mathcal{O}(p^2)$ is rather prohibitive when the dimensionality $p$ is large. Also, more efficiency in computation is still in demand, since the structure learning problem Eq. (5) or Eq. (6) typically has to be solved for several values of the parameter $\lambda$ for a given data set.

## 4.2  Statistical Stability of Estimation

Another important challenge in structure learning with GMRFs is how to obtain statistically stable solutions. This is a different issue to solving optimization problems discussed above: here we ask how close a solution of Eq. (5) or Eq. (6) is, if obtained with $n$ examples, to the "true" solution we would have obtained if we had an access to infinite examples.

Stability of estimation algorithms is often investigated in different perspectives. A classical type is called the *consistency in terms of parameter estimation.* For a solution matrix obtained with $n$ examples, denoted by $\widetilde{\Theta}_n$, and the true solution (so-called the population parameter which could be obtained with infinite examples) denoted by $\Theta^*$, it asks if the following property holds:

$$P(\widetilde{\Theta}_n = \Theta^*) \to 1 \ \text{ as } \ n \to \infty.$$

Another type of stability is called the *consistency in terms of variable selection,* which fits better for our interest. Here we ask if the following is true:

$$P\left(\{(i,j): [\widetilde{\Theta}_n]_{ij} \neq 0\} = \{(i,j): [\Theta^*]_{ij} \neq 0\}\right) \to 1 \ \text{ as } \ n \to \infty.$$

In other words, if the nonzero pattern of the estimate $\widetilde{\Theta}_n$ approaches the true nonzero pattern, then the estimation algorithm is considered to be stable. Since the nonzero patterns determine the structure of GMRFs, this guarantees that the algorithm will eventually discover the true graphical structure as $n$ increases. The two types of consistency are not necessarily the same [60], and often the variable selection consistency is easier to satisfy than the other [42].

When the dimensionality $p$ is much larger than the number of examples $n$ in data, there could exist multiple solutions (with different graphical structures) from an estimation procedure, and therefore stability plays an important role for discovering the truthful structure. The stability in the sense of variable selection has been shown for the neighborhood selection method [13] and the graph lasso algorithm [18] for structure learning with GMRFs. Therefore the optimization methods discussed in the previous section that solve the graph lasso problem (Eq. (5)) exactly share the same stability property. However, the stability of inexact solvers is unknown, although they may handle much larger number of variables. Also, when the ratio $p/n$ is too large, it becomes very hard to extract any meaningful graph structure from data using the graph lasso [18]. Therefore it still remains as an open challenge how to properly handle a very large number of features.

# 5    Future Work

Despite recent developments, structure learning of GMRFs via sparse inverse covariance estimation has not been well accepted in practical applications. One reason is that efficient solution methods for high dimensional problems have not been available until recently, whereas modern high-throughput biomedical studies involve few hundred thousands of features. The other reason is that the required number of examples (patients) for stable selection is often too large for biomedical applications, given a very large number of features. Finally, visual inspection tools customized for the structure of GMRFs showing associated clinical information (age, gender, tumor type, reactions to treatments, etc.) have not been well developed, preventing practitioners from accessing the technology.

Optimization methods for structure learning still require improvements with respect to their computation and memory requirements. Especially, if the memory footprint can be reduced from $\mathcal{O}(p^2)$ to $\mathcal{O}(pn)$ for the cases where the sample size $n$ is much smaller than the dimensionality $p$, then more efficient implementations will be possible. For instance, small memory footprint is preferable for using modern graphical processing units (GPUs), which have been applied successfully for accelerating various applications (e.g. compressed sensing and image recovery [45]), leveraging massive parallelism.

Stability of sparse inverse covariance estimation for high-dimensional cases is likely to be improved by using ensemble approaches. In particular, several different graphical structures can be estimated from different subsamples of patient data. If the estimation were for a parameter vector, bootstrapping [61, 62] and bagging [63, 64] would allow for using a simple average of estimates obtained with subsamples, leading to better stability. However, for structure learning it is not very clear if such simple "averaging" over graphs will lead to the best answer. Rather, data mining approaches on the patterns identified by small connected components over bootstrap estimates may give us more information, such as the set of common or rare patterns that would be relevant for prediction or for the discovery of personalized medicine.

Data mining of subgraphs will require not only statistically well-thought algorithms (which include, for example, a proper handling of multiple hypotheses testing), but also computationally efficient ways to compare subgraphs. In particular, comparison of subgraphs involves (sub)graph isomorphism problems [65–67], which have gained focus recently in computational theory [68, 69], machine learning [70], and data mining [71].

The basis architecture discussed above would not be successful without the support from interactive visualization systems to present outcomes in informative ways and allow users to explore complex systems for better understanding. Such tools will be required to provide clustering, grouping and coloring of nodes/edges in terms of clinical information, multiple graph embedding algorithms for different layouts, and graph theoretic measures for deeper investigation. A successful implementation of such systems will be only possible with tight integration of optimization, data mining, and visualization, which is the key element in the HCI-KDD approach [72].

**Acknowledgments.** This research was supported by Deutsche Forschungsgemeinschaft (DFG) within the Collaborative Research Center SFB 876 "Providing Information by Resource-Constrained Analysis", project C1.

# References

1. Grunenwald, H., Baas, B., Caruccio, N., Syed, F.: Rapid, high-throughput library preparation for next-generation sequencing. Nature Methods 7(8) (2010)
2. Soon, W.W., Hariharan, M., Snyder, M.P.: High-throughput sequencing for biology and medicine. Molecular Systems Biology 9, 640 (2013)
3. Guyon, I., Elisseeff, A.: An introduction to variable and feature selection. Journal of Machine Learning Research 3, 1157–1182 (2003)
4. Khatri, P., Draghici, S.: Ontological analysis of gene expression data: Current tools, limitations, and open problems. Bioinformatics 21(18), 3587–3595 (2005)
5. Altman, T., Travers, M., Kothari, A., Caspi, R., Karp, P.D.: A systematic comparison of the MetaCyc and KEGG pathway databases. BMC Bioinformatics 14(1), 112 (2013)
6. Koller, D., Friedman, N.: Probabilistic Graphical Models: Principles and Techniques. MIT Press (2009)
7. Pearl, J.: Probabilistic Reasoning in Intelligent Systems: Networks of Plausible Inference. Morgan Kaufmann Publishers Inc. (1988)
8. Friedman, N., Linial, M., Nachman, I., Pe'er, D.: Using Bayesian networks to analyze expression data. Journal of Computational Biology: A Journal of Computational Molecular Cell Biology 7(3-4), 601–620 (2000)
9. Sachs, K., Perez, O., Pe'er, D., Lauffenburger, D.A., Nolan, G.P.: Causal protein-signaling networks derived from multiparameter single-cell data. Science 308(5721), 523–529 (2005)
10. Jiang, X., Cooper, G.F.: A Bayesian spatio-temporal method for disease outbreak detection. Journal of the American Medical Informatics Association 17(4), 462–471 (2010)
11. Chickering, D.: Learning equivalence classes of Bayesian-network structures. Journal of Machine Learning Research, 445–498 (2002)
12. Chickering, D., Heckerman, D., Meek, C.: Large- sample learning of Bayesian networks is NP-hard. Journal of Machine Learning Research 5, 1287–1330 (2004)
13. Meinshausen, N., Bühlmann, P.: High-dimensional graphs and variable selection with the lasso. Annals of Statistics 34, 1436–1462 (2006)
14. Yuan, M., Lin, Y.: Model selection and estimation in the gaussian graphical model. Biometrika 94(1), 19–35 (2007)
15. Banerjee, O., Ghaoui, L.E., d'Aspremont, A.: Model selection through sparse maximum likelihood estimation for multivariate gaussian or binary data. Journal of Machine Learning Research 9, 485–516 (2008)
16. Duchi, J., Gould, S., Koller, D.: Projected subgradient methods for learning sparse gaussians. In: Conference on Uncertainty in Artificial Intelligence (2008)
17. Friedman, J., Hastie, T., Tibshirani, R.: Sparse inverse covariance estimation with the graphical lasso. Biostatistics 9(3), 432–441 (2008)
18. Meinshausen, N., Bühlmann, P.: Stability selection. Journal of the Royal Statistical Society (Series B) 72(4), 417–473 (2010)
19. Scheinberg, K., Ma, S., Goldfarb, D.: Sparse inverse covariance selection via alternating linearization methods. In: Advances in Neural Information Processing Systems 23, pp. 2101–2109. MIT Press (2010)

20. Johnson, C., Jalali, A., Ravikumar, P.: High-dimensional sparse inverse covariance estimation using greedy methods. In: Proceedings of the 15th International Conference on Artificial Intelligence and Statistics (2012)
21. Dinh, Q.T., Kyrillidis, A., Cevher, V.: A proximal newton framework for composite minimization: Graph learning without cholesky decompositions and matrix inversions. In: International Conference on Machine Learning (2013)
22. Dempster, A.P.: Covariance selection. Biometrika 32, 95–108 (1972)
23. Whittaker, J.: Graphical Models in Applied Multivariate Statistics. Wiley (1990)
24. Giudici, P., Green, P.J.: Decomposable graphical Gaussian model determination. Biometrika 86(4), 785–801 (1999)
25. Dobra, A., Hans, C., Jones, B., Nevins, J.R., Yao, G., West, M.: Sparse graphical models for exploring gene expression data. Journal of Multivariate Analysis 90(1), 196–212 (2004)
26. Verzelen, N., Villers, F.: Tests for gaussian graphical models. Computational Statistics and Data Analysis 53(5), 1894–1905 (2009)
27. Hunt, B.R.: The application of constrained least squares estimation to image restoration by digital computer. IEEE Transactions on Computers C-22(9), 805–812 (1973)
28. Chellappa, R., Chatterjee, S.: Classification of textures using Gaussian Markov random fields. IEEE Transactions on Acoustics, Speech and Signal Processing 33(4), 959–963 (1985)
29. Cross, G.R., Jain, A.K.: Markov random field texture models. IEEE Transactions on Pattern Analysis and Machine Intelligence 5(1), 25–39 (1983)
30. Manjunath, B.S., Chellappa, R.: Unsupervised texture segmentation using Markov random field models. IEEE Transactions on Pattern Analysis and Machine Intelligence 13(5), 478–482 (1991)
31. Dryden, I., Ippoliti, L., Romagnoli, L.: Adjusted maximum likelihood and pseudo-likelihood estimation for noisy Gaussian Markov random fields. Journal of Computational and Graphical Statistics 11(2), 370–388 (2002)
32. Cox, D.R., Wermuth, N.: Multivariate Dependencies: Models, Analysis and Interpretation. Chapman and Hall (1996)
33. Edwards, D.M.: Introduction to Graphical Modelling. Springer (2000)
34. Rue, H., Held, L.: Gaussian Markov Random Fields: Theory and Applications. Monographs on Statistics and Applied Probability, vol. 104. Chapman & Hall (2005)
35. Wasserman, L.: All of statistics: A concise course in statistical inference. Springer (2010)
36. Lauritzen, S.L.: Graphical Models. Oxford University Press (1996)
37. Nocedal, J., Wright, S.J.: Numerical Optimization. 2nd edn. Springer (2006)
38. Aldrich, J.: R.A. Fisher and the making of maximum likelihood 1912–1922. Statistical Science 12(3), 162–176 (1997)
39. Tikhonov, A.N.: On the stability of inverse problems. Doklady Akademii Nauk SSSR 5, 195–198 (1943)
40. Tibshirani, R.: Regression shrinkage and selection via the lasso. Journal of the Royal Statistical Society (Series B) 58, 267–288 (1996)
41. Zou, H., Hastie, T.: Regularization and variable selection via the elastic net. Journal of the Royal Statistical Society (Series B) 67, 301–320 (2005)
42. Lee, S., Wright, S.J.: Manifold identification in dual averaging methods for regularized stochastic online learning. Journal of Machine Learning Research 13, 1705–1744 (2012)
43. Piatkowski, N., Lee, S., Morik, K.: Spatio-temporal random fields: compressible representation and distributed estimation. Machine Learning 93(1), 115–139 (2013)

44. Candés, E.J., Romberg, J., Tao, T.: Stable signal recovery from incomplete and inaccurate measurements. Comm. Pure Appl. Math. 59, 1207–1223 (2005)

45. Lee, S., Wright, S.J.: Implementing algorithms for signal and image reconstruction on graphical processing units. Technical report, University of Wisconsin-Madison (2008)

46. Okayama, H., Kohno, T., Ishii, Y., Shimada, Y., Shiraishi, K., Iwakawa, R., Furuta, K., Tsuta, K., Shibata, T., Yamamoto, S., Watanabe, S.I., Sakamoto, H., Kumamoto, K., Takenoshita, S., Gotoh, N., Mizuno, H., Sarai, A., Kawano, S., Yamaguchi, R., Miyano, S., Yokota, J.: Identification of genes upregulated in ALK-positive and EGFR/KRAS/ALK-negative lung adenocarcinomas. Cancer Res. 72(1), 100–111 (2012)

47. Yamauchi, M., Yamaguchi, R., Nakata, A., Kohno, T., Nagasaki, M., Shimamura, T., Imoto, S., Saito, A., Ueno, K., Hatanaka, Y., Yoshida, R., Higuchi, T., Nomura, M., Beer, D.G., Yokota, J., Miyano, S., Gotoh, N.: Epidermal growth factor receptor tyrosine kinase defines critical prognostic genes of stage I lung adenocarcinoma. PLoS ONE 7(9), e43923 (2012)

48. McCall, M.N., Bolstad, B.M., Irizarry, R.A.: Frozen robust multiarray analysis (fRMA). Biostatistics 11(2), 242–253 (2010)

49. McCall, M., Murakami, P., Lukk, M., Huber, W., Irizarry, R.: Assessing affymetrix genechip microarray quality. BMC Bioinformatics 12(1), 137 (2011)

50. Vandenberghe, L., Boyd, S., Wu, S.P.: Determinant maximization with linear matrix inequality constraints. SIAM Journal on Matrix Analysis and Applications 19(2), 499–533 (1998)

51. Levitin, E., Polyak, B.: Constrained minimization methods. USSR Computational Mathematics and Mathematical Physics 6(5), 1–50 (1966)

52. Nesterov, Y.: Introductory Lectures on Convex Optimization: A Basic Course. Kluwer Academic Publishers (2004)

53. Nesterov, Y.: Smooth minimization of non-smooth functions. Mathematical Programming 103, 127–152 (2005)

54. d'Aspremont, A., Banerjee, O., El Ghaoui, L.: First-order methods for sparse covariance selection. SIAM Journal on Matrix Analysis and Applications 30(1), 56–66 (2008)

55. Lu, Z.: Smooth optimization approach for sparse covariance selection. SIAM Journal on Optimization 19(4), 1807–1827 (2009)

56. Yuan, X.: Alternating direction method for covariance selection models. Journal of Scientific Computing 51(2), 261–273 (2012)

57. Hsieh, C.J., Dhillon, I.S., Ravikumar, P.K., Sustik, M.A.: Sparse inverse covariance matrix estimation using quadratic approximation. In: Advances in Neural Information Processing Systems 24, pp. 2330–2338. MIT Press (2011)

58. Oztoprak, F., Nocedal, J., Rennie, S., Olsen, P.A.: Newton-like methods for sparse inverse covariance estimation. In: Advances in Neural Information Processing Systems 25, pp. 764–772. MIT Press (2012)

59. Hsieh, C.J., Sustik, M.A., Dhillon, I., Ravikumar, P., Poldrack, R.: BIG & QUIC: Sparse inverse covariance estimation for a million variables. In: Advances in Neural Information Processing Systems 26, pp. 3165–3173. MIT Press (2013)

60. Zhao, P., Yu, B.: On model selection consistency of lasso. Journal of Machine Learning Research 7, 2541–2563 (2006)

61. Efron, B.: Bootstrap methods: Another look at the jackknife. Annals of Statistics 7(1), 1–26 (1979)

62. Efron, B., Tibshirani, R.: Cross-validation and the bootstrap: Estimating the error rate of a prediction rule. Technical report. Department of Statistics, Stanford University (May 1995)
63. Breiman, L.: Bagging predictors. Machine Learning 24, 123–140 (1996)
64. Emmert-Streib, F., Simoes, R.D.M., Glazko, G., Mcdade, S., Holzinger, A., Dehmer, M., Campbell, F.C.: Functional and genetic analysis of the colon cancer network. BMC Bioinformatics, 1–24 (to appear 2014)
65. Whitney, H.: Congruent graphs and the connectivity of graphs. American Journal of Mathematics 54(1), 150–168 (1932)
66. Ullmann, J.R.: An algorithm for subgraph isomorphism. Journal of the ACM 23(1), 31–42 (1976)
67. Spielman, D.A.: Faster isomorphism testing of strongly regular graphs. In: Proceedings of the Twenty-eighth Annual ACM Symposium on Theory of Computing, pp. 576–584 (1996)
68. Arvind, V., Kurur, P.P.: Graph isomorphism is in SPP. Information and Computation 204(5), 835–852 (2006)
69. Datta, S., Limaye, N., Nimbhorkar, P., Thierauf, T., Wagner, F.: Planar graph isomorphism is in log-space. In: 24th Annual IEEE Conference on Computational Complexity, pp. 203–214 (2009)
70. Narayanamurthy, S.M., Ravindran, B.: On the hardness of finding symmetries in Markov decision processes. In: Proceedings of the 25th International Conference on Machine Learning, pp. 688–696 (2008)
71. Cook, D.J., Holder, L.B.: Mining Graph Data. John Wiley & Sons (2006)
72. Holzinger, A.: Human–computer interaction & knowledge discovery (HCI-KDD): What is the benefit of bringing those two fields to work together? In: Cuzzocrea, A., Kittl, C., Simos, D.E., Weippl, E., Xu, L. (eds.) CD-ARES 2013. LNCS, vol. 8127, pp. 319–328. Springer, Heidelberg (2013)

# Multi-touch Graph-Based Interaction for Knowledge Discovery on Mobile Devices: State-of-the-Art and Future Challenges

Andreas Holzinger[1], Bernhard Ofner[1], and Matthias Dehmer[2]

[1] Research Unit Human-Computer Interaction, Institute for Medical Informatics, Statistics & Documentation, Medical University Graz, Austria
{a.holzinger,b.ofner}@hci4all.at

[2] Department of Computer Science, Universität der Bundeswehr München Neubiberg, Germany
matthias.dehmer@unibw.de

**Abstract** Graph-based knowledge representation is a hot topic for some years and still has a lot of research potential, particularly in the advancement in the application of graph-theory for creating benefits in the biomedical domain. Graphs are most powerful tools to map structures within a given data set and to recognize relationships between specific data objects. Many advantages of graph-based data structures can be found in the applicability of methods from network analysis, topology and data mining (e.g. small-world phenomenon, cluster analysis). In this paper we present the state-of-the-art in graph-based approaches for multi-touch interaction on mobile devices and we highlight some open problems to stimulate further research and future developments. This is particularly important in the medical domain, as a conceptual graph analysis may provide novel insights on hidden patterns in data, hence support interactive knowledge discovery.

**Keywords:** Graph Based Interaction, Graph Theory, Graph-based Data Mining, Multi-Touch, Interactive Node-Link Graph Visualization.

## 1 Introduction and Motivation

Graphs and Graph-Theory [1] are powerful tools to map data structures and to find novel connections between single data objects [2,3]. The inferred graphs can be further analyzed by using graph-theoretical and statistical techniques [4]. A mapping of already existing and in medical practice approved *knowledge spaces* as a conceptual graph and the subsequent visual and graph-theoretical analysis may bring novel insights on hidden patterns in the data, which exactly is the goal of knowledge discovery [5]. Another benefit of the graph-based data structure is in the applicability of methods from network topology and network analysis and data mining, e.g. small-world phenomenon [6,7], and cluster analysis [8,9]. The main contribution of this paper is a blend of graph-theory and multi-touch

A. Holzinger, I. Jurisica (Eds.): Knowledge Discovery and Data Mining, LNCS 8401, pp. 241–254, 2014.
© Springer-Verlag Berlin Heidelberg 2014

interaction to stimulate further research; these ideas follows exactly the HCI-KDD approach of bringing together "the best of two worlds" [10]; both concepts applied together can offer enormous benefits for practical applications.

This paper is organized as follows: In section 2 we provide a short glossary to ensure a common understanding; in section 3 we discuss the state-of-the-art in multi-touch interaction, multi-touch gesture primitives, and multi-touch graph interaction. In section 4 we present the state-of-the-art in node-link graphs and interactive node-link graph visualization. In section 5 we provide an example of an empirically proved biomedical knowledge space and in section 6 we discuss some open problems in order to stimulate further research; we conclude the paper with a short future outlook.

## 2   Glossary and Key Terms

*Network:* Synonym for a graph, which can be defined as an ordered or unordered pair $(N, E)$ of a set $N$ of nodes and a set $E$ of edges [3]. Engineers often mention: Data + Graph = Network, or call at least directed graphs as networks; however, in theory, there is no difference between a graph and a network.

*Undirected Graph:* each edge is an unordered pair of nodes, i.e., $E \subseteq \{(x, y) | x, y \in N\}$ [1].

*Directed Graph:* each edge is an ordered pair, i.e., $E \subseteq \{(x, y) | x, y \in N\}$, and the edge $(x, y)$ is distinct from the edge $(y, x)$ [1].

*Relative Neighbourhood Graphs (RNG):* introduced by Toussaint (1980) [11], they capture the proximity between points by connecting nearby points with a graph edge; the various possible notions of "nearby" lead to a variety of related graphs.

*Sphere-of-Influence Graph (SIG(V)):* Let $C_p$ be the circle centered on $p$ with radius equal to the distance to a nearest neighbour of $p$. SIG(V) has node set $V$ and an edge $(p, q)$ iff $C_p$ and $C_q$ intersect in at least two points.

*Multi-touch:* refers to the abilities of a touch-screen [12], to recognize the presence of two or more points of contact. This plural-point awareness is often used to implement advanced functionalities such as pinch to zoom or activating certain subroutines attached to predefined multi-touch gestures [13].

*Graph Mining:* is the application of graph-based methods to structural data sets [14], a survey on graph mining can be found here [15].

*Pattern Discovery:* subsumes a plethora of data mining and machine learning methods to detect complex patterns in data sets [16]; applications thereof are, for instance, subgraph graph mining [14] and string matching [17].

*Frequent Subgraph Mining:* is a major challenge of graph mining and relates to determine all frequent subgraphs of a given class of graphs. Their occurrence should be according to a specified threshold [14].

*Small World Networks:* are generated based on certain rules with high clustering coefficient [3, 18] but the distances among the vertices are rather short in average, hence they are somewhat similar to random networks and they have been found in several classes of biological networks, see [19].

*Cluster Analysis Problem:* refers to partitioning a collection of $n$ points in some fixed-dimensional space into $m < n$ groups that are "natural" in some sense ($m \ll n$) [8, 9].

*Cyclicity:* Graph property measuring structural complexity, introduced by Bonchev et al. [20].

*Branching:* a precise definition of the concept of branching still remains a challenge [21, 22], but several indices have been suggested to measure branching in trees, including the Bonchev-Trinajstić index [23] and the Wiener index [24].

# 3    State-of-the-Art I: From Multi-touch Interaction to Multi-touch Graph Interaction

## 3.1    Multi-touch Interaction

Multi-touch input is a classic topic in Human–Computer Interaction and an active area of research with a history of several decades [13], [25].

Touch screens put the fingers in touch with the content in computer screens, consequently are considered as the most natural of all input devices [12]. The most obvious advantage of touch screens is that the input device is also the output device. Enhancing the advantages of the touch paradigm even more, multi-touch input can sense the degree of contact in a continuous manner along with the amount and location of a number of simultaneous points of contact [13]. A good introduction into multi-touch technologies can be found at the Natural User Interface Group, an open source HCI community [26].

Inspired by studies on human-short term memory requirements during keyboard operation by Alden et al. (1972) [27], Mehta et al. (1982) [28] laid the foundations for the triumph of multi-touch technologies, which today dominate the input technology of smartphones and tablets, and their success is also related to the renaissance in stylus-based input technologies [29].

Several studies have shown that multi-touch can be beneficial for interaction [30], [31], [32], and can particularly be useful for applications in the biomedical domain [33], [34], [35], [36].

However, this area is still a not well covered research area, e.g. a search for title= "multi-touch interaction" on the Web of Science (WoS) resulted in only 13 hits, topic = "multi-touch interaction" brought still only 47 results (as of April, 19, 2014). The most recent work is "A Fast and Robust Fingertips Tracking Algorithm for Vision-Based Multi-touch Interaction" by [37]. The oldest paper is on "Flowfield and beyond: Applying pressure-sensitive multi-point touchpad interaction" by [38], and the most cited (17 references as of April, 19, 2014) is "ThinSight: Versatile Multi-touch Sensing for Thin Form-factor Displays" by [39].

Most relevant for our paper are the recent advances in the development of multi-touch *gesture sets*. There is a lot of research available on sketch recognition and free-hand gesture recognition, see e.g. [40], [41], [42], [43], [44], but there are only few works on the construction of gesture sets for multi-touch applications: Wu et al. (2006) [45] identify the creation of multi-touch gesture sets as a relevant problem, and provide guidelines to build effective sets, and a more recent work is [46], a very recent work is [47].

### 3.2   Multi-touch Gesture Primitives

Kammer et al. [48] defined the basic information supplied for gesture recognition as coordinates on a two-dimensional surface, and proposed strategies for formalization of gestural interaction on multi-touch surfaces. The resulting Gesture Formalization For Multi-Touch language (GeForMT) attempts to describe continued contacts by introducing five language elements:

1. the Pose Function, which describes the shape of the recognized contact on the touch device,
2. Atomic Gestures, such as `MOVE`, `POINT`, `DEPOINT`, `LINE`, `CIRCLE`
3. Composition Operators,
4. the Focus of the gesture,
5. and Area Constraints, which describe the relative movement of atomic gestures.

The basic multi-touch gestures, common across all different devices, are shown in Fig. 1, ranging form simple tapping to the more complex rotation gesture [49].

1. *Tap*: A single tap is recognized by quickly touching the device (`POINT`) and immediately releasing the finger (`DEPOINT`); typically used to press an input control or select an item.
2. *Double/Multi Tap*: Repeated taps and releases with a single finger (`1F`).
3. *Tap and Hold*: Defined as touching and holding (`HOLD`) the multi-touch surface. Also referred to as "Press and Hold" or "Long Press".
4. *Two/Multi Finger Tap*: A single touch down with two (`2F`) or more fingers.
5. *Drag*: The drag gesture is defined as touching down and moving the finger in an arbitrary direction, whilst keeping contact with the touch device. Stopping the movement and releasing the dragged object ends the gesture. Dragging is typically used for scrolling and panning.

6. *Two/Multi Finger Drag*: Drag gesture executed with multiple fingers.
7. *Flick*: A drag gesture which adds momentum by releasing the moved object before stopping the finger movement; generally used for faster scrolling and panning.
8. *Pinch*: The pinch gesture is recognized by touching down with two fingers, usually thumb and index finger, and either close (JOIN) or open (SPREAD) both fingers without releasing the touch device. The gesture ends once both fingers are stopped and released. "Pinch open" and "Pinch close" gestures are usually paired with the zoom function.
9. *Rotate*: Defined as touching down with two fingers and performing a clockwise or counter-clockwise rotation with both fingers, stopping the movement and releasing both fingers.

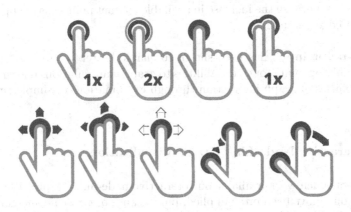

**Fig. 1.** Multi-touch Interaction Primitives: Tap – Double Tap – Tap and Hold – Two Finger Tap; Drag – Double Finger Drag – Flick – Pinch – Rotate

### 3.3    Multi-touch Graph Interaction

A search for TI="multi-touch graph interaction" as well as TS="multi-touch graph interaction" on the WoS resulted in 0 hits. Even TI="touch graph interaction" (and TS as well) did not return any results. The Google search allintitle: "Multi-touch Graph Interaction" resulted in exactly one hit – a paper by [50] presented at the 2010 ACM International Conference on Interactive Tabletops and Surfaces, which received so far 18 citations as of April, 2, 2014.

Schmidt et al. [50] focus in their paper on redesigning node-link graph exploration interfaces for use with multi-touch input.

# 4  State-of-the-Art II: From Node-Link Graphs to Interactive Node-Link Graph Visualization

## 4.1  Node-Link Graphs

**Node-link graphs** are critical in many domains and raise specific interaction challenges; for example:

1. congestion of nodes and links [51],
2. crossing of links [52], and
3. overview and detail [53].

The use of multi-touch input to address these challenges is a hot and promising research issue, because the increase in available contact points may support more significant edge detangling.

**Multi-point input** has been shown to enable better collaborative analysis [54]. By applying multi-touch capabilities to graph manipulations one can extend the possibilities of graph interaction through combinations of simple actions.

## 4.2  Interactive Node-Link Graph Visualization

There is not much work available on Interactive node-link Graph Visualization: Graph layouts have been often applied, but because of the scale and complexity of real world data, these layouts tend to be dense and often contain difficult to read edge configurations [55].

Much previous work on graph layouts has focused on algorithmic approaches for the creation of readable layouts and on issues such as edge crossings and bends in layout aesthetics [56, 57].

There are only a few interactive approaches which try to mitigate problems such as edge congestion include zoom and local magnification techniques [55, 58–60]. These approaches **tend to work on the graph as a whole or focus on the nodes**, despite the fact that edges had been identified as one of the central aesthetic issues.

Recent interaction advances that deal directly with edges in connected diagrams include Wong et al.'s EdgeLens [51] and EdgePlucking [61], Holten's edge bundling [62] and Moscovich et al.'s link-based navigation techniques [63]. EdgeLens and EdgePlucking aim to reduce edge congestion by interactively moving and bending edges while preserving the location of nodes; in edge bundling, adjacent edges are bent and grouped into bundles, in order to reduce visual clutter in node-link diagrams. While the former approaches provide techniques to clarify the graph structure, Moscovich et al. focus on content-aware navigation in large networks.

# 5  Example of an Empirically Proved Biomedical Knowledge Space

Our experiences with a large data set clearly showed the advantages of graph-based data structures for the representation of medical information content. The graph is derived from a standard quick reference guide for emergency doctors and paramedics in the German speaking area; tested in the field, and constantly improved for 20 years: The handbook "Medikamente und Richtwerte in der Notfallmedizin" [64] (German for Drugs and Guideline Values in Emergency Medicine, currently available in the 11th edition accompanies every German-speaking emergency doctor as well as many paramedics and nurses. It has been sold 58,000 times in the German-speaking area. The 92-pages handbook (size: 8 x 13 cm) contains a comprehensive list of emergency drugs and proper dosage information. Additionally, important information for many emergency situations is included. The data includes more than 100 essential drugs for emergency medicine, together with instructions on application and dosage depending on the patient condition, complemented by additional guidelines, algorithms, calculations of medical scores, and unit conversion tables of common values. However, due to the traditional list-based interaction style, the interaction is limited to a certain extent. Collecting all relevant information may require multiple switches between pages and chapters, and knowledge about the entire content of the booklet. In consequence to the alphabetical listing of drugs by active agents, certain tasks, like finding all drugs with common indications, proved to be inefficient and time consuming.

Modeling relationships between drugs, patient conditions, guidelines, scores and medical algorithms as a graph (cf. Fig. 2) gives valuable insight into the structure of the data set.

Each drug is associated with details about its active agent and pharmacological group; brand name, strengths, doses and routes of administration of different products; indications and contraindication, as well as additional remarks on application. Consequently, a single drug itself can be represented as connected concepts. Shared concepts create links between multiple drugs with medical relevance, and provide a basis for content-aware navigation.

The interconnection of two drugs, namely adrenaline and dobutamine, is shown in Fig. 3. The left-hand side illustrates the main three types of relations inducing medical relevance; shared indications, shared contra-indications and shared pharmacological groups. Different node colors are used to distinguish between types of nodes such as active agents, pharmacological groups, applications, dosages, indications and contra-indications. The right-hand side highlights the connection of adrenaline and dobutamine by a shared indication.

Links to and between clinical guidelines, tables and calculations of medical scores, algorithms and other medical documents, follow the same principle. On the contrast to a list-based interaction style, these connections can be used for identification and visualization of relevant medical documents, to reorganize the presentation of the medical content and to provide a fast and reliable contextual navigation.

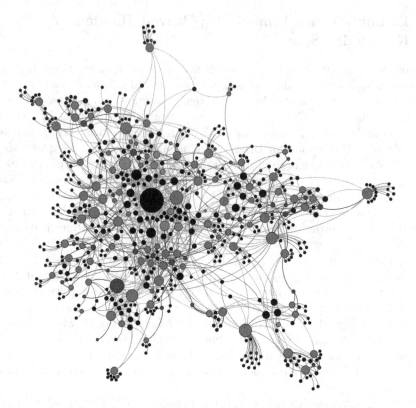

**Fig. 2.** Graph of the medical data set showing the relationship between drugs, guidelines, medical scores and algorithms

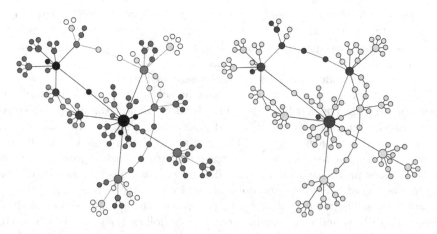

**Fig. 3.** Interconnection between two drugs, "Adrenaline" and "Dobutamine"; connections to and between clinical guidelines, tables and calculations of medical scores, algorithms and other medical documents, follow the same principle

# 6   Open Problems

Still unsolved problems include:

*Problem 1.* What is the maximum number of edges of an RNG in $\mathbb{R}^3$? It is known that it has at most $O(n^{\frac{4}{3}})$ edges, but no supra-linear lower bound is known.

*Problem 2.* That the SIG has at most $15n$ edges in the plane follows from a theorem of Erdös & Panwitz [65], but the best lower bound is $9n$. It is also known that the SIG has a linear number of edges in any fixed dimension [66], and bounds on the expected number of edges are known [67], but again tight results are not available.

*Problem 3.* What is the structural interpretation of graph measures [19, 68]? Graph measures are mappings which maps graphs to the reals. Thus, they can be understood as graph complexity measures [19, 68–70]. Investigating their structural interpretation relates to understand what kind of structural complexity they detect. Cyclicity, branching and linearity (path-like) are examples theoreof.

*Problem 4.* Multi-touch graph-based interaction requires to visualize large networks meaningfully. So far, there has been a lack of interest to develop efficient software beyond the available commercial software.

*Problem 5.* Can we generate unique fingerprints of multi-touch interaction graphs? Similar work but in the context of structural chemistry has already been performed by Dehmer et al. [71, 72].

*Problem 6.* Which structural properties possess the multi-touch interaction graphs? This calls for investigating graph classes beyond small world and random networks.

*Problem 7.* Which known graph classes are appropriate to model multi-touch interaction graphs properly? For instance, small world networks or special hypergraphs seem to be applicable. What kind of structural properties do the multi-touch interaction graphs have?

*Problem 8.* Are multi-touch interaction graphs structurally similar to other graphs (from known graph classes)? This calls for a comparison of graph classes and their structural characteristics.

*Problem 9.* Which graph measures are suitable to determine the complexity of multi-touch interaction graphs? Does this lead to any meaningful classification based on their topology?

*Problem 10.* What is interesting? Where to start the interaction with the graph?

# 7 Conclusion and Future Outlook

The explosive growth of complexity of networks have overwhelmed conventional visualization methods and future research should focus on developing more robust and efficient temporally aware clustering algorithms for dynamic graphs, i.e. good clustering will produce layouts that meet general criteria, such as cluster colocation and short average edge length, as well as minimize node motion between time steps [73].

Attacking aforementioned open problems, introduces several exciting and unique challenges. As an example, extensive investigation of structural properties of multi-touch interaction graphs, using large sets of generated graphs, seems to be an ideal starting point in addressing multiple unsolved problems. A comparison of these graph measures might give insightful conclusions, and might lead to a distinct characterization of multi-touch interaction graphs (problems 5 and 6). By further investigation of these structural characteristics, one could identify existing graph classes which are suitable to model multi-touch interaction, or reveal the need for a distinct graph class (problems 7 and 8). This requires an exhaustive comparison of known graph classes and their structural properties, as well as their limitations.

As mentioned above, the complexity of multi-touch interaction graphs should be investigated by using numerical graph invariants [19]. By using some distinct graph invariants such as graph entropy, distance measures and degree-based measures, one could determine their characteristic distributions and compare them with other graphs. This leads us to the question whether the structure of multi-touch interaction graphs is really different, i.e., whether these graphs have a different characteristic compared to others.

**Acknowledgments.** The authors are grateful for many fruitful, lively and enjoyable discussions with the hci4all.at Team at the Institutes meetings.

# References

1. Harary, F.: Structural models, An introduction to the theory of directed graphs. Wiley (1965)
2. Strogatz, S.H.: Exploring complex networks. Nature 410(6825), 268–276 (2001)
3. Dorogovtsev, S., Mendes, J.: Evolution of networks: From biological nets to the Internet and WWW. Oxford University Press (2003)
4. Dehmer, M., Emmert-Streib, F., Mehler, A.: Towards an Information Theory of Complex Networks: Statistical Methods and Applications. Birkhaeuser Boston (2011)
5. Holzinger, A., Dehmer, M., Jurisica, I.: Knowledge discovery and interactive data mining in bioinformatics - state-of-the-art, future challenges and research directions. BMC Bioinformatics 15(suppl. 6), 11 (2014)
6. Barabasi, A.L., Albert, R.: Emergence of scaling in random networks. Science 286(5439), 509–512 (1999)
7. Kleinberg, J.: Navigation in a small world. Nature 406(6798), 845–845 (2000)

8. Koontz, W., Narendra, P., Fukunaga, K.: A graph-theoretic approach to nonparametric cluster analysis. IEEE Transactions on Computers 100(9), 936–944 (1976)
9. Wittkop, T., Emig, D., Truss, A., Albrecht, M., Boecker, S., Baumbach, J.: Comprehensive cluster analysis with transitivity clustering. Nature Protocols 6(3), 285–295 (2011)
10. Holzinger, A.: Human computer interaction & knowledge discovery (hci-kdd): What is the benefit of bringing those two fields to work together? In: Cuzzocrea, A., Kittl, C., Simos, D.E., Weippl, E., Xu, L. (eds.) CD-ARES 2013. LNCS, vol. 8127, pp. 319–328. Springer, Heidelberg (2013)
11. Toussaint, G.T.: The relative neighbourhood graph of a finite planar set. Pattern Recognition 12(4), 261–268 (1980)
12. Holzinger, A.: Finger instead of mouse: Touch screens as a means of enhancing universal access. In: Carbonell, N., Stephanidis, C. (eds.) UI4ALL 2002. LNCS, vol. 2615, pp. 387–397. Springer, Heidelberg (2003)
13. Lee, S., Buxton, W., Smith, K.: A multi-touch three dimensional touch-sensitive tablet. In: ACM SIGCHI Bulletin, vol. 16, pp. 21–25. ACM (1985)
14. Cook, D., Holder, L.B.: Mining Graph Data. Wiley Interscience (2007)
15. Chakrabarti, D., Faloutsos, C.: Graph mining: Laws, generators, and algorithms. ACM Computing Surveys (CSUR) 38(1), 2 (2006)
16. Duda, R.O., Hart, P.E., Stork, D.G.: Pattern Classification. Wiley, New York (2001)
17. Gusfield, D.: Algorithms on Strings, Trees, and Sequences: Computer Science and Computational Biology. Cambridge University Press (1997)
18. Watts, D.J., Strogatz, S.H.: Collective dynamics of 'small-world' networks. Nature 393, 440–442 (1998)
19. Emmert-Streib, F., Dehmer, M.: Networks for systems biology: Conceptual connection of data and function. IET Systems Biology 5, 185–207 (2011)
20. Bonchev, D., Mekenyan, O., Trinajstić, N.: Topological characterization of cyclic structures. International Journal of Quantum Chemistry 17(5), 845–893 (1980)
21. Schutte, M., Dehmer, M.: Large-scale analysis of structural branching measures. Journal of Mathematical Chemistry 52(3), 805–819 (2014)
22. Kirby, E.C.: Sensitivity of topological indexes to methyl group branching in octanes and azulenes, or what does a topological index index? Journal of Chemical Information and Computer Sciences 34(5), 1030–1035 (1994)
23. Bonchev, D., Trinajstić, N.: Information theory, distance matrix, and molecular branching. The Journal of Chemical Physics 67(10), 4517–4533 (1977)
24. Wiener, H.: Structural determination of paraffin boiling points. J. Am. Chem. Soc. 69(1), 17–20 (1947)
25. Buxton, B.: A touching story: A personal perspective on the history of touch interfaces past and future. In: SID Symposium, vol. 41, pp. 444–448. Wiley (2010)
26. Cetin, G., Bedi, R.: Multi-touch Technologies. NUIgroup.com (2009)
27. Alden, D.G., Daniels, R.W., Kanarick, A.F.: Keyboard design and operation: A review of the major issues. Human Factors: The Journal of the Human Factors and Ergonomics Society 14(4), 275–293 (1972)
28. Mehta, N., Smith, K., Holmes, F.: Feature extraction as a tool for computer input. In: IEEE International Conference on Acoustics, Speech, and Signal Processing (ICASSP 1982), vol. 7, pp. 818–820. IEEE (1982)
29. Holzinger, A., Searle, G., Peischl, B., Debevc, M.: An answer to "Who needs a stylus?" on handwriting recognition on mobile devices. In: Obaidat, M.S., Sevillano, J.L., Filipe, J. (eds.) ICETE 2011. CCIS, vol. 314, pp. 156–167. Springer, Heidelberg (2012)

30. Moscovich, T.: Multi-touch interaction. In: Conference on Human Factors in Computing Systems: CHI 2006 Extended Abstracts on Human Factors in Computing Systems, vol. 22, pp. 1775–1778 (2006)

31. Wang, F., Ren, X.S.: Empirical evaluation for finger input properties in multi-touch interaction. In: Greenberg, S., Hudson, S.E., Hinkley, K., RingelMorris, M., Olsen, D.R. (eds.) Proceedings of the 27th Annual Chi Conference on Human Factors in Computing Systems, pp. 1063–1072. Assoc Computing Machinery (2009)

32. Park, W., Han, S.H.: Intuitive multi-touch gestures for mobile web browsers. Interacting With Computers 25(5), 335–350 (2013)

33. Holzinger, A., Höller, M., Schedlbauer, M., Urlesberger, B.: An investigation of finger versus stylus input in medical scenarios. In: Luzar-Stiffler, V., Dobric, V.H., Bekic, Z. (eds.) ITI 2008: 30th International Conference on Information Technology Interfaces, pp. 433–438. IEEE (2008)

34. Crisan, S., Tarnovan, I.G., Tebrean, B., Crisan, T.E.: Optical multi-touch system for patient monitoring and medical data analysis. In: Vlad, S., Ciupa, R., Nicu, A.I. (eds.) MEDITECH 2009. IFMBE Proceedings, vol. 26, pp. 279–282. Springer, Heidelberg (2009)

35. Lundstrom, C., Rydell, T., Forsell, C., Persson, A., Ynnerman, A.: Multi-touch table system for medical visualization: Application to orthopedic surgery planning. IEEE Transactions on Visualization and Computer Graphics 17(12), 1775–1784 (2011)

36. Crisan, S., Tarnovan, I.G.: Optimization of a multi-touch sensing device for biomedical applications. In: Vlaicu, A., Brad, S. (eds.) Interdisciplinary Research in Engineering: Steps Towards Breakthrough Innovation for Sustainable Development. Advanced Engineering Forum, vol. 8-9, pp. 545–552. Trans Tech Publications Ltd, Stafa-Zurich (2013)

37. Xie, Q.Q., Liang, G.Y., Tang, C., Wu, X.Y.: A fast and robust fingertips tracking algorithm for vision-based multi-touch interaction. In: 10th IEEE International Conference on Control and Automation (ICCA), pp. 1346–1351 (2013)

38. Chen, T.T.H., Fels, S., Min, S.S.: Flowfield and beyond: applying pressure-sensitive multi-point touchpad interaction. In: Proceedings of 2003 International Conference on Multimedia and Expo., ICME 2003, vol. 1, pp. 49–52 (July 2003)

39. Hodges, S., Izadi, S., Butler, A., Rrustemi, A., Buxton, B.: Thinsight: Versatile multi-touch sensing for thin form-factor displays. In: Proceedings of the 20th Annual ACM Symposium on User Interface Software and Technology, UIST 2007, pp. 259–268. ACM (2007)

40. Baudel, T., Beaudouinlafon, M.: Charade - remote control of objects using free-hand gestures. Communications of the ACM 36(7), 28–35 (1993)

41. Long Jr., A.C., Landay, J.A., Rowe, L.A.: Implications for a gesture design tool. In: Proceedings of the SIGCHI Conference on Human Factors in Computing Systems, pp. 40–47. ACM (1999)

42. Alvarado, C., Davis, R.: Sketchread: A multi-domain sketch recognition engine. In: Proceedings of the 17th Annual ACM Symposium on User Interface Software and Technology, pp. 23–32. ACM (2004)

43. Paulson, B., Hammond, T.: Paleosketch: Accurate primitive sketch recognition and beautification. In: Proceedings of the 13th International Conference on Intelligent user Interfaces, pp. 1–10. ACM (2008)

44. Fernández-Pacheco, D., Albert, F., Aleixos, N., Conesa, J.: A new paradigm based on agents applied to free-hand sketch recognition. Expert Systems with Applications 39(8), 7181–7195 (2012)

45. Wu, M., Shen, C., Ryall, K., Forlines, C., Balakrishnan, R.: Gesture registration, relaxation, and reuse for multi-point direct-touch surfaces. In: First IEEE International Workshop on Horizontal Interactive Human-Computer Systems, TableTop 2006. IEEE (2006)
46. Wobbrock, J.O., Morris, M.R., Wilson, A.D.: User-defined gestures for surface computing. In: Greenberg, S., Hudson, S.E., Hinkley, K., RingelMorris, M., Olsen, D.R. (eds.) CHI2009: Proceedings of the 27th Annual Conference on Human Factors in Computing Systems, pp. 1083–1092. Assoc Computing Machinery (2009)
47. Park, W., Han, S.H.: An analytical approach to creating multitouch gesture vocabularies in mobile devices: A case study for mobile web browsing gestures. International Journal of Human-Computer Interaction 30(2), 126–141
48. Kammer, D., Wojdziak, J., Keck, M., Groh, R., Taranko, S.: Towards a formalization of multi-touch gestures. In: ACM International Conference on Interactive Tabletops and Surfaces, ITS 2010, pp. 49–58. ACM (2010)
49. Hoggan, E., Williamson, J., Oulasvirta, A., Nacenta, M., Kristensson, P.O., Lehtiö, A.: Multi-touch rotation gestures: Performance and ergonomics. In: Proceedings of the SIGCHI Conference on Human Factors in Computing Systems, CHI 2013, pp. 3047–3050. ACM, New York (2013)
50. Schmidt, S., Nacenta, M., Dachselt, R., Carpendale, S.: A set of multi-touch graph interaction techniques. In: ACM International Conference on Interactive Tabletops and Surfaces, pp. 113–116. ACM (2010)
51. Wong, N., Carpendale, S., Greenberg, S.: Edgelens: An interactive method for managing edge congestion in graphs. In: IEEE Symposium on Information Visualization, INFOVIS 2003, pp. 51–58. IEEE (October 2003)
52. Purchase, H.C., Carrington, D., Allder, J.: Evaluating graph drawing aesthetics: Defining and exploring a new empirical research area. Computer Graphics and Multimedia, 145–178 (2004)
53. Cockburn, A., Karlson, A., Bederson, B.B.: A review of overview plus detail, zooming, and focus plus context interfaces. ACM Computing Surveys, 41–1 (2008)
54. Isenberg, P., Carpendale, S., Bezerianos, A., Henry, N., Fekete, J.D.: Coconuttrix: Collaborative retrofitting for information visualization. IEEE Computer Graphics and Applications 29(5), 44–57 (2009)
55. Herman, I., Melanon, G., Marshall, M.: Graph visualization and navigation in information visualization: A survey. IEEE Transactions on Visualization and Computer Graphics 6(1), 24–43 (2000)
56. Tollis, I., Eades, P., Di Battista, G., Tollis, L.: Graph drawing: Algorithms for the visualization of graphs, vol. 1. Prentice-Hall, New York (1998)
57. Purchase, H.C.: Which aesthetic has the greatest effect on human understanding? In: DiBattista, G. (ed.) GD 1997. LNCS, vol. 1353, pp. 248–261. Springer, Heidelberg (1997)
58. Bederson, B.B., Hollan, J.D.: Pad++: A zooming graphical interface for exploring alternate interface physics. In: Proceedings of the 7th Annual ACM Symposium on User Interface Software and Technology, pp. 17–26. ACM (1994)
59. Sarkar, M., Brown, M.H.: Graphical fisheye views of graphs. In: Proceedings of the SIGCHI Conference on Human Factors in Computing Systems, pp. 83–91. ACM (1992)
60. Purchase, H.C.: Metrics for graph drawing aesthetics. Journal of Visual Languages & Computing 13(5), 501–516 (2002)
61. Wong, N., Carpendale, S.: Supporting interactive graph exploration with edge plucking. In: Proceedings of SPIE, vol. 6495, pp. 235–246 (2007)

62. Holten, D.: Hierarchical edge bundles: Visualization of adjacency relations in hierarchical data. IEEE Transactions on Visualization and Computer Graphics 12(5), 741–748 (2006)
63. Moscovich, T., Chevalier, F., Henry, N., Pietriga, E., Fekete, J.: Topology-aware navigation in large networks. In: Proceedings of the 27th International Conference on Human Factors in Computing Systems, pp. 2319–2328. ACM (2009)
64. Müller, R.: Medikamente und Richtwerte in der Notfallmedizin, 11th edn. Ralf Müller Verlag, Graz (2012)
65. Soss, M.A.: On the size of the euclidean sphere of influence graph. In: Proceedings Eleventh Canadian Conference on Computational Geometry, pp. 43–46 (1999)
66. Guibas, L., Pach, J., Sharir, M.: Sphere-of-influence graphs in higher dimensions. Intuitive Geometry 63, 131–137 (1994)
67. Dwyer, R.A.: The expected size of the sphere-of-influence graph. Computational Geometry 5(3), 155–164 (1995)
68. Dehmer, M.: Information theory of networks. Symmetry 3, 767–779 (2012)
69. Mowshowitz, A.: Entropy and the complexity of the graphs I: An index of the relative complexity of a graph. Bull. Math. Biophys. 30, 175–204 (1968)
70. Holzinger, A., Ofner, B., Stocker, C., Calero Valdez, A., Schaar, A.K., Ziefle, M., Dehmer, M.: On graph entropy measures for knowledge discovery from publication network data. In: Cuzzocrea, A., Kittl, C., Simos, D.E., Weippl, E., Xu, L. (eds.) CD-ARES 2013. LNCS, vol. 8127, pp. 354–362. Springer, Heidelberg (2013)
71. Dehmer, M., Grabner, M., Varmuza, K.: Information indices with high discriminative power for graphs. PLoS ONE 7, e31214 (2012)
72. Dehmer, M., Grabner, M., Mowshowitz, A., Emmert-Streib, F.: An efficient heuristic approach to detecting graph isomorphism based on combinations of highly discriminating invariants. Advances in Computational Mathematics (2012)
73. Ma, K.L., Muelder, C.W.: Large-scale graph visualization and analytics. Computer 46(7), 39–46 (2013)

# Intelligent Integrative Knowledge Bases: Bridging Genomics, Integrative Biology and Translational Medicine

Hoan Nguyen[1,3,*], Julie D. Thompson[1,2], Patrick Schutz[3], and Olivier Poch[1,2]

[1] Laboratoire de Bioinformatique et Génomique Intégratives (LBGI), ICube UMR 7357- Laboratoire des sciences de l'ingénieur, de l'informatique et de l'imagerie, Strasbourg, France
[2] Faculté de Médecine, Strasbourg, France
[3] Département Biologie structurale intégrative, Institut de Génétique et de Biologie Moléculaire et Cellulaire (IGBMC), Illkirch-Graffenstaden, France
nguyen@igbmc.fr

**Abstract.** Successful application of translational medicine will require understanding the complex nature of disease, fueled by effective analysis of multidimensional 'omics' measurements and systems-level studies. In this paper, we present a perspective — the intelligent integrative knowledge base (I2KB) — for data management, statistical analysis and knowledge discovery related to human disease. By building a bridge between patient associations, clinicians, experimentalists and modelers, I2KB will facilitate the emergence and propagation of systems medicine studies, which are a prerequisite for large-scaled clinical trial studies, efficient diagnosis, disease screening, drug target evaluation and development of new therapeutic strategies.

**Keywords:** Knowledge discovery, Knowledge Base, Translational bioinformatics, Biological database, I2KB, SM2PH, DIKW, HCI-KDD.

## 1 Introduction

Personalized health monitoring and treatment, the so-called P4 (predictive, preventive, personalized and participatory) medicine[1] or 'precision medicine', aims to treat patients based on their individual characteristics, including patient-specific molecular and genomic data, environmental factors and clinical history[2, 3]. This ambitious goal can only be achieved by the effective application of large-scale biomedical data analysis and systems biology approaches, in order to link the genome and other 'omics' data to individual physiology and physiopathology[4, 5]. Indeed, modern biomedical studies are often performed by large consortia that produce large amounts of data to describe the status of individual genomes, transcriptomes, proteomes or metabolites in diverse situations. To derive meaning from this vast catalogue will require original bioinformatics systems for managing and sharing data, information, and knowledge

---

* Correspondence author.

A. Holzinger, I. Jurisica (Eds.): Knowledge Discovery and Data Mining, LNCS 8401, pp. 255–270, 2014.

across the translational medicine continuum, with the ultimate goal of obtaining predictive biological models and system-level analyses applicable to biomedical studies and predictive medicine (Fig. 1).

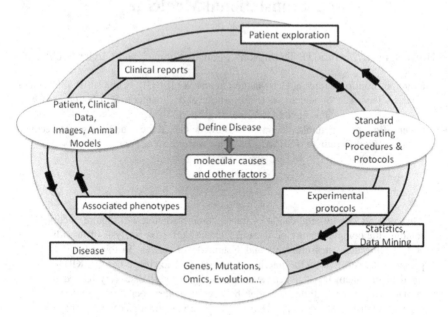

**Fig. 1.** Modern medicine aims to define diseases more precisely, based on their underlying molecular causes and other factors. This requires integrative analysis of gene-related data, patient data and non gene-related data, and operating protocols with computational and analytical tools to extract useful information and knowledge.

In the information science and artificial intelligence fields, models for data, information, knowledge and ultimately wisdom (DIKW)[6] have been developed to extract meaning from large data sets using specialized techniques, such as Data Mining[7], Integrative Data Mining [8], Knowledge Discovery from Databases[9] or Intelligent Data Analysis[10]. The application of these models will be essential for transforming raw biomedical data into information and knowledge about the nature of complex biological systems[11, 12] and their behavior in the development of genetically complex diseases[13]. Efforts in biomedical DIKW studies have traditionally focused on the transformation of the large-scale raw data into standardized information[14]. This involves identifying different objects, naming and categorizing them, via shared data formats or ontologies (e.g. HUPO Proteomics Standards Initiative[15], Protein Structure Initiative[16]), as well as structuring and organizing the data to give them meaning (Human Gene Mutation Database[17]).

A critical need is now to address the problem of extracting useful knowledge, and ultimately wisdom, from this organized information [18]. While information can be defined as 'organized or structured data', the concept of knowledge is more difficult to describe formally. Some proposed definitions include 'relevant information, that an individual or actor uses to interpret situations', 'organization and processing to convey understanding', or 'a mix of contextual information, values, experience and rules'[19]. All these definitions include notions of semantic interoperability between data and information from very diverse origins, as well as some form of processing to make the information useful[20]. Systems that exploit information in a relational database architecture, together with computational data analysis, data mining and knowledge discovery techniques are known as Intelligent Knowledge Bases (I2KB). An I2KB is not merely a space for data storage, but promotes the collection, organization and retrieval of knowledge. It includes real-time querying and reasoning services for intelligent inference and decision support. The output is not a list of data, but a proposed answer to a question, in the form of information (statistics, graphs, rules, etc.).

The field of P4 medicine is vast, and designing a single I2KB system that covers all the existing knowledge in the domain is clearly not feasible. As a result, current systems are generally designed for specific fields, tasks or applications. As an example, the public pharmacogenomics knowledge base[21] provides a central repository for clinical and genetic information that could help researchers understand how genetic variation among individuals contributes to differences in reactions to drugs. Another example is the G2P Knowledge Centre[22], which oversees the collection and use of data from community research investigating the links between genetic variation and health. The G2P I2KB is based on a hybrid centralized/federated network strategy, providing the data standards, database components, tools for data analysis and data access protocols to ensure that all relevant research results can be properly integrated and made available for the scientific community. A similar initiative has been launched recently by the US Department of Energy Systems Biology Knowledge base (KBase) to share and integrate data and analytical tools for predictive biology applied to microbes, microbial communities, and plants (genomicscience.energy.gov/compbio).

In spite of these recent developments, efficient system-level analyses of human disease and translational medicine studies are still hindered by a number of important issues. First, formalized and computerized descriptions of phenotypic and clinical data are still limited. While genomic and other 'omics' data have been the subject of intense efforts towards standardized formalisms and automated management, most phenotypic and clinical data are still defined by individual human experts. Second, there is a lack of integrative computer platforms that are capable of coupling advanced analysis tools and methods with the diverse data related to human disease and associated animal models. In the remainder of this section, we present an overview and describe the basic requirements of I2KB for precision medicine studies. We then illustrate how these principles were used to design and implement our I2KB solution and finally, we describe its application in a use case scenario.

## 2    Glossary and Key Terms

**Translational Medicine:** 'Often described as an effort to carry scientific knowledge 'from bench to bedside,' translational medicine builds on basic research advances - studies of biological processes using cell cultures, for example, or animal models - and uses them to develop new therapies or medical procedures'. (sciencemag.org/site/marketing/stm/definition.xhtml)

**Genomics:** refers to the study of the entire genome of an organism whereas genetics refers to the study of a particular gene.

**Transcriptomics:** 'allows for the examination of whole transcriptome changes across a variety of biological conditions'.

**Omics:** 'is a general term for a broad discipline of science and engineering for analyzing the interactions of biological information objects in various 'omes'(genome, transcriptome..). The main focus is on: 1) mapping information objects such as genes, proteins, and ligands; 2) finding interaction relationships among the objects; 3) engineering the networks and objects to understand and manipulate the regulatory mechanisms; and 4) integrating various omes and 'omics' subfields' (nature.com/omics/)

**Integrative biology:** 'is both an approach to and an attitude about the practice of science. Integrative approaches seek both diversity and incorporation. They deal with integration across all levels of biological organization, from molecules to the biosphere, and with diversity across taxa, from viruses to plants and animals' [23].

**Pharmacogenomics:**'is the study of how genes affect a person's response to drugs. This relatively new field combines pharmacology (the science of drugs) and genomics (the study of genes and their functions) to develop effective, safe medications and doses that will be tailored to a person's genetic makeup' (ghr.nlm.nih.gov/handbook).

**KNODWAT**: KNOwledge Discovery With Advanced Techniques
**HCI-KDD**: Human–Computer Interaction and Knowledge Discovery
**KD4v**: Comprehensible Knowledge Discovery System for Missense Variant
**LVOD**: Leiden Open (source) Variation Database
**UMD**: Universal Mutation Database
**MSV3d**: Database of human MisSense Variants mapped to 3D protein structure
**OBO**: Open Biomedical Ontologies
**BIRD**: Biological Integration and Retrieval of Data
**SM2PH**: from Structural Mutation to Pathology Phenotypes in Human
**GxDB**:Gene eXpression DataBase
**HUPO**: Human Proteome Organization
**MIAME**: Minimum Information About a Microarray Experiment
**SOA**:Service-Oriented Architecture

## 3    Requirements for I2KB in Translational Medicine

An I2KB can be used to transform raw data into useful knowledge that can be applied to answer specific questions, to solve a specific problem or to give advice about actions to be taken in a specific situation. A useful I2KB for translationnal medicine studies should combine two major functionalities (Fig. 2).

First, state-of-the-art data integration technologies are needed to collect and organize the heterogeneous data required to decipher the complex relationships between a patient's genetic background, environment and clinical history. A good data management strategy should ensure the integrity, consistency and currentness of this huge volume of continuously updated data[24]. The I2KB should also include standardization protocols (biomedical taxonomies, ontologies) to facilitate data sharing and evaluation, as well as knowledge representations (in the form of rules or other fact representations) to formalize expert knowledge in the domain. The knowledge should be usable, on the one hand, by a computer for automated deductive reasoning, and on the other hand, by human experts via an intuitive query language and user-friendly visualization tools[25].

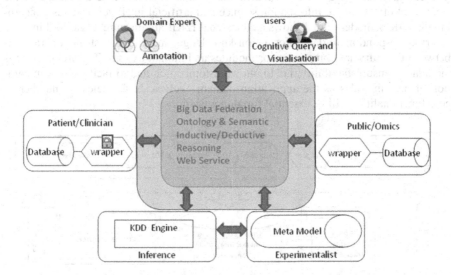

**Fig. 2.** Requirements for I2KB in modern medicine. The I2KB combines the data integration and organization capabilities of knowledge bases, with the analytical power of intelligent computational tools for knowledge discovery.

Second, efficient computational analyses based on DIKW models will be crucial to allow rapid processing of complex queries, efficient extraction of relevant information and effective inference of new knowledge in the form of predictions, models and decision support tools. In the long term, such analyses should help to provide answers to important healthcare questions: what are the genetic/environmental factors underlying the disease? which patients are at risk? what is the most effective treatment? This will clearly involve an iterative process, including many stages of data collection, validation, analysis and interpretation, where each iteration leads to a new understanding that is likely to restart the whole process.

The development of I2KB in precision medicine will clearly require collaborations between specialists with complementary expertise in clinics, genetics and 'omics' analysis, as well as in knowledgebase management and computer sciences to promote modeling and systems biology approaches. The major challenge will be to develop an integrative architecture that will allow efficient data capture, information representation and prior knowledge creation[26], providing an appropriate software platform to facilitate the interplay between 'omics' and large-scaled phenotype and clinical data related to human diseases. The I2KB should thus represent an innovative system integrating the definition of phenotypes in human diseases and model animals, similarities and differences in disease structures and phenotypic alterations, cellular and tissular contexts, gene and gene-product regulations and interactions.

## 4     Design Strategies

The design of an I2KB for precision medicine studies should take advantage of the significant efforts in the information science and artificial intelligence fields concerning the DIKW model. Fig. 3 shows a conceptual I2KB architecture, organized in three layers corresponding to data-information-knowledge, and allowing strong interactions between the software components or modules and human experts. The architecture is modular to ensure flexibility, i.e. to allow customization and to facilitate the integration of new modules as the application domain evolves. Nevertheless, a number of core functionalities will be essential for all applications:

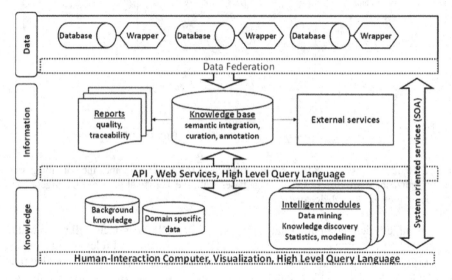

**Fig. 3.** Conceptual architecture of I2KB for the precision medicine community. The three layer model facilitates independent management of data, information and knowledge. Input data resources are interfaced via database-specific wrappers to ensure modularity and flexibility. Data federation should use a hybrid architecture approach, combining relational databases and flat file repositories. The knowledge base represents a central repository, facilitating semantic integration, curation and annotation of data to create useful information. This is an essential step in the knowledge discovery process, which implies the use of computational tools to extract hidden patterns or rules.

**Data Federation:** The deployment of standardized data, such as gene, mutation, polymorphism, pathology, tissue and cellular expression as well as animal models and literature, in a centralized, federated database means that links or relations can be created between them. The scale of biomedical data is a major challenge, calling for the use of an effective information federation system, such as IBM's WebSphere, which acts as a virtual database across connected databases and allows queries to be made as if they were on a single database. This IBM technology could be exploited under an academic license by The IBM Academic Initiative which is a program for university professors and researchers. In the case of external databases, such as LOVD[27] or UMD[28] and other private databases, including clinical databases, it is not always possible to duplicate or to transfer the data over the network for obvious ethical reasons and confidentiality[29]. Private or sensitive information should therefore remain under the control of the provider, with restricted access for other users. This can be achieved by the configuration of data resources as virtual nodes with node-specific wrappers, which essentially define specific access rights to different data and ensure that adequate privileges are defined.

**Semantic Integration, Curation and Annotation:** Biomedical data are stored in a large number of diverse, independent databases and significant efforts are now being made to achieve interoperability between them[30]. This is generally achieved by the definition of domain ontologies[31], which formally represent the data as a set of concepts and the relationships between concepts. This conceptualization is fundamental to resolve semantic ambiguities and to facilitate data sharing, data management and automated knowledge discovery systems and will rely on specific ontologies for biomedical semantics, such as the Variation Ontology (variationontology.org), the Disease Ontology (disease-ontology.org) or the Medline Unified Medical Language System (nlm.nih.gov/research/umls). Furthermore, the links between raw data, e.g. sequence variants or gene expression measurements, and an individual's phenotypic characteristics are not easily deducible without extensive description, validation and interpretation of the data, either by automatic annotation systems or by expert curation. To ensure quality and traceability, all experimental procedures from biochemistry to clinical practices need to be stored and standardized, for example by following Minimum Information specifications[32]. The I2KB should thus provide a central repository for metadata, standard procedures and operating protocols and offer user-friendly tools for their upload and retrieval.

**Knowledge Discovery from Data (KDD), Statistics and Modeling:** KDD approaches are now being applied in some biomedical domains to extract information from large-scale, heterogeneous data[33]. KDD is commonly defined as the 'non trivial process of identifying valid, novel, potentially useful and ultimately understandable patterns in data'[9]. The KDD process involves three main operations: selection and preparation of the data, data mining, and finally interpretation of the extracted units. Some common KDD algorithms include Bayesian networks, neural networks and rule based systems, such as Inductive Logic Programming (ILP)[34]. ILP combines Machine Learning and Logic Programming [35]. ILP has several advantages. Firstly, using logic programming allows encoding more general forms of background knowledge such as recursions, functions or quantifiers. Secondly, the learned rules, which are based on first-order logic, are comprehensible by humans and computers and can be interpreted without the need for visualization [36]. ILP has been applied successfully to various bioinformatics problems including breast cancer studies[37], gene function prediction[38], protein-protein interaction prediction[39], protein-ligand interaction prediction[40] and microarray data classification[41]. Recently, we implemented the ILP method in the KD4v system[42] for the interpretation and prediction of the phenotypic effects of missense variants.

The interpretation of large-scale, high-dimensional data sets also requires the development of original algorithms in the fields of biostatistics, mathematical modeling and systems biology, e.g.[43]. The integration and exploitation of these techniques will pave the way to deciphering and understanding the functional mechanisms implicated in complex systems and diseases.

**Human-Computer Interaction with Knowledge Discovery (HCI-KDD):**
The integration of domain-specific knowledge from human experts in the I2KB should facilitate researcher communication and will provide a solid basis for an atmosphere of trust and a continuous flow of information that will in turn simplify the collection of data and medical information from clinicians and patient associations. This will require efficient access to DIKW via human-computer interaction (HCI) which 'deals with aspects of human perception, cognition, intelligence, sense-making and most of all the interaction between human and machine' [44]. Recently, a new approach, called HCI-KDD [45], was developed by combining HCI and KDD solutions in the unified framework in order to enhance human intelligence by computational intelligence. The goal of HCI-KDD is to enable end users to find and recognize previously unknown and potentially useful and usable DIKW. HCI-KDD is a process of identifying novel, valid and potentially useful DIKW patterns, with the goal of understanding these DIKW patterns. In this context, the new KDD framework such as KNODWAT [8] should be coupled to biomedical workflows such as Taverna[46] or Galaxy[47], provide useful integrative solutions for I2KB.

**System Oriented Services:** A Service-Oriented Architecture (SOA)[48] facilitates the interconnection and maintenance of local and remote databases, as well as computational tools and complex workflows, by providing standardized methods and services. The SOA is essential for simultaneous analysis of multilevel data/information, in order to enhance existing knowledge or to infer new associative patterns, behavior or knowledge. It also allows to dynamically integrate incoming data with the existing data set, the validated hypotheses and models (along with metadata) and the software used for creating and manipulating them.

**High Level Biological Query Language:** The heterogeneous data included in the I2KB system are stored in relational tables and XML/flat files. The exploitation of these data by standard query languages (e.g. SQL- Structured Query Language) is not obvious, requiring expert developers or users. For this reason, the I2KB should be equipped with a declarative query language which allows users to easily express complex queries across heterogeneous datasets and retrieve information, without requiring detailed knowledge of the underlying structure of the tables in the database system.

# 5    Knowledge Identification and Acquisition

An essential aspect of any I2KB is the formalization of existing knowledge and human expertise. This is achieved by knowledge engineering, a discipline concerned with the process of formalizing an expert's knowledge in a form that can be exploited by a computer system to solve complex problems. Knowledge engineering activities include assessment of the problem, acquisition and structuring of pertinent information and knowledge, and their integration in the knowledge base, under the supervision of database curators and biological experts. To facilitate knowledge identification and acquisition in the context of modern medicine, specific axes need to be addressed:

**Phenotypic Descriptions:** Phenotypes are not well defined or standardized in most biological databases and are generally described by individual clinicians using natural language. For example, in the case of retinal pathologies, phenotypic definitions could include descriptions of retinal images or patterns, in combination with medical data from techniques such as optical coherence, tomography, psychophysics or electrophysiology. Clearly, as of now, phenotyping relies strongly on clinical experience, educated pattern recognition and an evolving assessment of genotype-phenotype correlations. Biological data models and tools are needed to ensure automated integration, traceability of data sources (organization, treatment protocol, etc.) and subsequent automated analysis of these rich, but complex, knowledge resources. Efforts are now underway to develop formalisms, such as the specifications in the UMD and LOVD databases, or the Human Variome Project[49].

**Genotype/Phenotype Associations:** Comprehensive information about mutations and associated phenotypes are available from the literature or from patient cohorts implicated in the molecular diagnosis of the specific diseases. Traditional database systems dedicated to the analysis of the relationships between genotypes and phenotypes generally include a regularly updated collection of sequence variants and allow rapid identification of previous pathogenicity reports for diagnostic purposes. The advantage of the I2KB architecture is that it can be used to infer new relationships by integrating computational tools, e.g. Polyphen[50], Sift[51] or KD4v[52], for the analysis of existing mutation data and novel sequence variants.

**Relevance of Model Animal Knowledge to Human Disease:** For many pathologies and diseases, model animal systems represent an important source of information, including gene-related data (genome location, mutation, omics), phenotypic description of mutation effects, experimental protocols and images. Functional annotation, curation and formalization of data from animal models is needed[53, 54], as well as the definition of complex use-cases (e.g. comparison/propagation of 'omics' data from animal to human pathologies) in order to train and validate the knowledge base. This will require the design of ontology network and knowledge extraction tools to facilitate the efficient association and subsequent querying, automated analysis and pertinent inference of knowledge related to the human pathology analysis.

**Ontology Network for DIKW:** This work involves (1) the identification and curation of currently available DIKW (for each phenotype or disease) sets from diverse types ['omics', phenotypics (textual description, images...), clinical...] and about the choice of the gene-related and non-gene related DIKW required in the framework of the three synergistic axes (see above) (2) the design of the ontology network for DIKW using the open-source Protégé platform to capture knowledge and populate I2KB with instances in a tractable and accessible format compatible with the OBO consortium standards., (3) the design of data models and tools suitable for automated integration, traceability of data sources and subsequent automated analysis, (4) the definition of complex test-cases (e.g. propagating 'omics' data from animal or simulation to human pathologies, design of clinical trials...) in order to train and validate the knowledge base. All DIKW will be integrated under the supervision of database curators and biological experts by dedicated knowledge management experts that will participate in the development of novel bioinformatics features to respond to specific questions related to knowledge acquisition and formalization in diagnostics.

## 6    A Use Case Scenario: Discovering Phenotype-Genotype

In this section, we present an use case scenario, designed to improve our understanding of the complex relationships between genetic mutations and disease phenotypes, an ambitious endeavor central to many disease descriptions and a domain that has attracted significant efforts recently, e.g.[55-57]. Our I2KB (Fig. 4) is the SM2PH-Central knowledge base[58], which is part of an overall strategy aimed at the development of a transversal system to better understand and describe the networks of causality linking a particular phenotype, and one or various genes or networks.

The I2KB incorporates tools and data related to all human genes, including their evolution, tissue expressions, genomic features and associated phenotypes, in a single infrastructure. Data federation of private and public databases is achieved by the IBM WebSphere and BIRD systems [59]. The generalist data is integrated, indexed and structured in SM2PH-Central, which represents the central repository for the DIKW considered to be universal by a panel of experts. SM2PH-Central also provides access to systematic annotation tools, including sequence database searches, multiple alignment and 3D model exploitation, physico-chemical, functional, structural and evolutionary characterizations of missense variants. All information is accessible via standardized reports (gene profiles, error reports, etc.), as well as automated services for specific applications, such as gene prioritization.

The structuration of the data and information in the I2KB facilitates the application of intelligent modules to search for hidden patterns and extract pertinent knowledge. For instance, we can cite MSV3d[60], devoted to the characterization of all missense variants, and the KD4v system[52], which uses the available or modeled 3D structures and information provided by the MSV3d pipeline to characterize and predict the phenotypic effect of a mutation. The modular architecture of the I2KB is designed to allow the integration of other data resources or analytical tools, thus ensuring the future evolution of the system in response to new technological developments in the computer science and health fields.

A crucial feature of this architecture is the ability to create specialized I2KB, called SM2PH-Instances, which can be managed independently and allow the integration, management and distribution of domain-specific data and knowledge. In the context of a specific pathology, a SM2PH-Instance facilitates the creation of detailed ontologies, as well as the construction of test sets to develop, and optimize methods to identify the genes and processes involved in the disease[61]. The potential of the I2KB has been demonstrated in a number of recent studies devoted to specific human diseases, including complete congenital stationary night blindness[62, 63]).

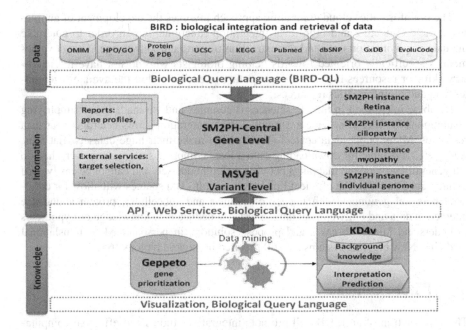

**Fig. 4.** I2KB infrastructure based on the SM2PH Central knowledge base. Data from public (in blue) and inhouse (gene expression in GxDB: gx.igbmc.fr, or evolutionary barcodes [64] in green) biomedical databases are federated using the BIRD system. The SM2PH-Central can automatically generate any SM2PH database instance (i.e. a specialized database centered on a thematic use case, for example genes involved in a specific human disease or an individual genome). Intelligent modules have been incorporated (MSV3d, KD4v) to characterize and predict the phenotypic effects of genetic variants.

# 7    Open Problems

Precision medicine relies on efficient genome annotation, 'omics' data integration and system level analyses to develop new approaches for personalized health care in which patients are treated based on their individual characteristics. In this perspective, we proposed a conception for a deployable environment for I2KB, providing an open solution that has the ability to evolve to embrace future developments in biomedical informatics and translational medicine.

The I2KB allows to share and to manage clinical and scientific DIKW. Due to the multiple data resources, the heterogeneous formats and the access restrictions of each user, the content and organization of the DIKW cannot be fixed in advance. Furthermore, at each stage of the I2KB project, the extent and pertinence of data exchanges between the different researchers groups must be well defined. For this reason, the establishment of common standards and procedures for the consortium are essential. The I2KB should therefore be designed to provide different levels of integration, starting with low correlated information, and progressively constructing more extensive relations between data throughout the duration of the project.

The bioinformatics cloud computing approach involves the development of an interoperable architecture and high-level integration functionalities in order to automate the data acquisition process and the extraction of pertinent knowledge. This development is specifically oriented towards helping biologists who do not have the necessary skills or resources in scientific computing to easily exploit the available genomics data and bioinformatics resources.

Database integration in the life sciences is complex and we made many simplifying assumptions in order to provide a certain level of integration across heterogeneous data resources. Many public data centers (NCBI, EBI) make their huge datasets (flat files, XML, etc.) available for downloading onto a local computer system. However, they do not generally provide the mappings between different datasets and cannot be easily used to integrate data types. An efficient link between multi-data sources will allow for correlated personal genomics with images of cellular and subcellular, protein abundance interaction data and other clinical data in order to deduce new knowledge or hypotheses to understand human diseases and propose solutions in personalized or translational medicine. New big-data systems are still required in modern biology [65].

# 8    Future Outlook

The construction of an I2KB will promote integrative studies and effective computational biology approaches to decipher the underlying molecular networks and processes in the context of complex diseases. This I2KB approach has been applied in SM2PH-Central knowledge base providing complex data integration for the comprehensive analysis of genetic mutations in human diseases. Such integrative studies are a prerequisite for the large-scaled clinical trial studies, efficient diagnosis, disease screening, drug target evaluation and development of new therapeutic strategies that will bring us within touching distance of achieving the goal of precision medicine. This would have a huge impact on the training of health professionals, the development of predictive and personalized medicine and the shaping of a growing body of validated accurate models for complex disease processes.

In the future, the integration of knowledge discovery functionalities within the biological query language will provide a powerful declarative workflow for I2KB development. In this model, large data centers share their datasets and their computational services via the declarative query language. The development of data update protocol to ensure the synchronization with the public data sources and computation service is a challenge in the context of big data.

**Acknowledgements.** The work was performed within the framework of the Décrypthon program, co-funded by Association Française contre les Myopathies (AFM, 14390-15392), IBM and Centre National de la Recherche Scientifique (CNRS). We acknowledge financial support from the ANR (Puzzle-Fit: ANR-09-PIRI-0018-02, BIPBIP: ANR-10-BINF-03-02, FRISBI: ANR-10-INSB-05-01), Labex INRT, and Institute funds from the CNRS, INSERM, Université de Strasbourg and Faculté de Médecine de Strasbourg. The IGBMC common services and platforms are acknowledged for their assistance.

# References

1. Hood, L., Balling, R., Auffray, C.: Revolutionizing medicine in the 21st century through systems approaches. Biotechnol. J. 7, 992–1001 (2012)
2. Council, N.R.: Toward Precision Medicine: Building a Knowledge Network for Biomedical Research and a New Taxonomy of Disease, Washington, DC (2011)
3. Robinson, P.N.: Deep phenotyping for precision medicine. Hum. Mutat. 33, 777–780 (2012)
4. Auffray, C., Caulfield, T., Khoury, M.J., Lupski, J.R., Schwab, M., Veenstra, T.: Genome Medicine: Past, present and future. Genome. Med. 3, 6 (2011)
5. Chen, R., Snyder, M.: Systems biology: Personalized medicine for the future? Curr. Opin. Pharmacol. 12, 623–628 (2012)
6. Zins, C.: Conceptual Approaches for Defining Data, Information, and Knowledge. J. Am. Soc. Inf. Sci. 58, 479–493 (2007)
7. Han, J., Kamber, M.: Data Mining, Concepts and Techniques. Morgan Kaufmann Publishers, San Francisco (2006)
8. Holzinger, A., Zupan, M.: KNODWAT: A scientific framework application for testing knowledge discovery methods for the biomedical domain. BMC Bioinformatics 14, 191 (2013)
9. Fayyad, U.M., Piatetsky-Shapiro, G., Smyth, P., Uthurusamy, R.: Advances in Knowledge Discovery and Data Mining. AAAI Press (Year)
10. Berthold, M., Hand, D.J.: Intelligent Data Analysis: An Introduction. Springer, New York (2003)
11. Kitano, H.: Systems biology: A brief overview. Science 295, 1662–1664 (2002)
12. Smolke, C.D., Silver, P.A.: Informing biological design by integration of systems and synthetic biology. Cell 144, 855–859 (2011)
13. Clermont, G., Auffray, C., Moreau, Y., Rocke, D.M., Dalevi, D., Dubhashi, D., Marshall, D.R., Raasch, P., Dehne, F., Provero, P., Tegner, J., Aronow, B.J., Langston, M.A., Benson, M.: Bridging the gap between systems biology and medicine. Genome. Med. 1, 88 (2009)
14. Trelles, O., Prins, P., Snir, M., Jansen, R.C.: Big data, but are we ready? Nat. Rev. Genet. 12, 224 (2011)
15. Orchard, S., Hermjakob, H., Taylor, C., Aebersold, R., Apweiler, R.: Human Proteome Organisation Proteomics Standards Initiative. In: Pre-Congress Initiative. Proteomics, vol. 5, pp. 4651–4652. Proteomics (2005)
16. Gifford, L.K., Carter, L.G., Gabanyi, M.J., Berman, H.M., Adams, P.D.: The Protein Structure Initiative Structural Biology Knowledgebase Technology Portal: a structural biology web resource. J. Struct. Funct. Genomics 13, 57–62 (2012)
17. Stenson, P.D., Ball, E.V., Mort, M., Phillips, A.D., Shaw, K., Cooper, D.N.: The Human Gene Mutation Database (HGMD) and its exploitation in the fields of personalized genomics and molecular evolution. Curr. Protoc. Bioinformatic, ch. 1, Unit1 13 (2012)
18. Schadt, E.E., Bjorkegren, J.L.: NEW: network-enabled wisdom in biology, medicine, and health care. Sci. Transl. Med. 4, 115rv111 (2012)
19. Wallace, D.P.: Knowledge Management: Historical and Cross-Disciplinary Themes. Libraries Unlimited (2007)
20. Stein, L.D.: Towards a cyberinfrastructure for the biological sciences: progress, visions and challenges. Nat. Rev. Genet. 9, 678–688 (2008)

21. Hernandez-Boussard, T., Whirl-Carrillo, M., Hebert, J.M., Gong, L., Owen, R., Gong, M., Gor, W., Liu, F., Truong, C., Whaley, R., Woon, M., Zhou, T., Altman, R.B., Klein, T.E.: The pharmacogenetics and pharmacogenomics knowledge base: accentuating the knowledge. Nucleic Acids Res. 36, D913-D918 (2008)

22. Webb, A.J., Thorisson, G.A., Brookes, A.J.: An informatics project and online Knowledge Centre supporting modern genotype-to-phenotype research. Human Mutation 32, 543–550 (2011)

23. Wake, M.H.: What is "Integrative Biology"? Integr. Comp. Biol. 43, 239–241 (2003)

24. Harel, A., Dalah, I., Pietrokovski, S., Safran, M., Lancet, D.: Omics data management and annotation. Methods Mol. Biol. 719, 71–96 (2011)

25. Jeanquartier, F., Holzinger, A.: On Visual Analytics And Evaluation In Cell Physiology: A Case Study. In: Cuzzocrea, A., Kittl, C., Simos, D.E., Weippl, E., Xu, L. (eds.) CD-ARES 2013. LNCS, vol. 8127, pp. 495–502. Springer, Heidelberg (2013)

26. AlAama, J., Smith, T.D., Lo, A., Howard, H., Kline, A.A., Lange, M., Kaput, J., Cotton, R.G.: Initiating a Human Variome Project Country Node. Hum. Mutat. 32, 501–506 (2011)

27. Fokkema, I.F., den Dunnen, J.T., Taschner, P.E.: LOVD: Easy creation of a locus-specific sequence variation database using an LSDB-in-a-box approach. Human Mutation 26, 63–68 (2005)

28. Beroud, C., Collod-Beroud, G., Boileau, C., Soussi, T., Junien, C.: UMD (Universal mutation database): A generic software to build and analyze locus-specific databases. Human Mutation 15, 86–94 (2000)

29. Lunshof, J.E., Chadwick, R., Vorhaus, D.B., Church, G.M.: From genetic privacy to open consent. Nat. Rev. Genet. 9, 406–411 (2008)

30. Mons, B., van Haagen, H., Chichester, C., Hoen, P.B., den Dunnen, J.T., van Ommen, G., van Mulligen, E., Singh, B., Hooft, R., Roos, M., Hammond, J., Kiesel, B., Giardine, B., Velterop, J., Groth, P., Schultes, E.: The value of data. Nat. Genet. 43, 281–283 (2011)

31. Whetzel, P.L., Noy, N.F., Shah, N.H., Alexander, P.R., Nyulas, C., Tudorache, T., Musen, M.A.: BioPortal: Enhanced functionality via new Web services from the National Center for Biomedical Ontology to access and use ontologies in software applications. Nucleic Acids Res. 39, W541-W545 (2011)

32. Taylor, C.F., Field, D., Sansone, S.A., Aerts, J., Apweiler, R., Ashburner, M., Ball, C.A., Binz, P.A., Bogue, M., Booth, T., Brazma, A., Brinkman, R.R., Michael Clark, A., Deutsch, E.W., Fiehn, O., Fostel, J., Ghazal, P., Gibson, F., Gray, T., Grimes, G., Hancock, J.M., Hardy, N.W., Hermjakob, H., Julian Jr., R.K., Kane, M., Kettner, C., Kinsinger, C., Kolker, E., Kuiper, M., Le Novere, N., Leebens-Mack, J., Lewis, S.E., Lord, P., Mallon, A.M., Marthandan, N., Masuya, H., McNally, R., Mehrle, A., Morrison, N., Orchard, S., Quackenbush, J., Reecy, J.M., Robertson, D.G., Rocca-Serra, P., Rodriguez, H., Rosenfelder, H., Santoyo-Lopez, J., Scheuermann, R.H., Schober, D., Smith, B., Snape, J., Stoeckert Jr., C.J., Tipton, K., Sterk, P., Untergasser, A., Vandesompele, J., Wiemann, S.: Promoting coherent minimum reporting guidelines for biological and biomedical investigations: the MIBBI project. Nat. Biotechnol 26, 889–896 (2008)

33. Jensen, P.B., Jensen, L.J., Brunak, S.: Mining electronic health records: Towards better research applications and clinical care. Nat. Rev. Genet. 13, 395–405 (2012)

34. Muggleton, S.: Inductive logic programming: issues, results and the challenge of learning language in logic. Artif. Intell. 114, 283–296 (1999)

35. Lloyd, J.W.: Foundations of logic programming, 2nd edn. Springer, New York (1987)

36. Nguyen, H., Luu, T.D., Poch, O., Thompson, J.D.: Knowledge discovery in variant databases using inductive logic programming. Bioinform Biol. Insights 7, 119–131 (2013)

37. Woods, R.W., Oliphant, L., Shinki, K., Page, D., Shavlik, J., Burnside, E.: Validation of Results from Knowledge Discovery: Mass Density as a Predictor of Breast Cancer. J. Digit Imaging (2009)

38. King, R.D.: Applying inductive logic programming to predicting gene function. AI. Mag. 25, 57–68 (2004)

39. Nguyen, T.P., Ho, T.B.: An integrative domain-based approach to predicting protein-protein interactions. J. Bioinform. Comput. Biol. 6, 1115–1132 (2008)

40. Kelley, L.A., Shrimpton, P.J., Muggleton, S.H., Sternberg, M.J.: Discovering rules for protein-ligand specificity using support vector inductive logic programming. Protein Eng. Des. Sel. 22, 561–567 (2009)

41. Ryeng, E., Alsberg, B.K.: Microarray data classification using inductive logic programming and gene ontology background information. Journal of Chemometrics 24, 231–240 (2010)

42. Luu, T.D., Rusu, A., Walter, V., Linard, B., Poidevin, L., Ripp, R., Moulinier, L., Muller, J., Raffelsberger, W., Wicker, N., Lecompte, O., Thompson, J.D., Poch, O., Nguyen, H.: KD4v: Comprehensible knowledge discovery system for missense variant. Nucleic Acids Res. (2012)

43. Wilkinson, D.J.: Bayesian methods in bioinformatics and computational systems biology. Brief Bioinform. 8, 109–116 (2007)

44. Holzinger, A., Pasi, G. (eds.): HCI-KDD 2013. LNCS, vol. 7947. Springer, Heidelberg (2013)

45. Holzinger, A.: Human–Computer Interaction & Knowledge Discovery (HCI-KDD): What is the benefit of bringing those two fields to work together? In: Cuzzocrea, A., Kittl, C., Simos, D.E., Weippl, E., Xu, L. (eds.) CD-ARES 2013. LNCS, vol. 8127, pp. 319–328. Springer, Heidelberg (2013)

46. Oinn, T., Addis, M., Ferris, J., Marvin, D., Senger, M., Greenwood, M., Carver, T., Glover, K., Pocock, M.R., Wipat, A., Li, P.: Taverna: A tool for the composition and enactment of bioinformatics workflows. Bioinformatics 20, 3045–3054 (2004)

47. Giardine, B., Riemer, C., Hardison, R.C., Burhans, R., Elnitski, L., Shah, P., Zhang, Y., Blankenberg, D., Albert, I., Taylor, J., Miller, W., Kent, W.J., Nekrutenko, A.: Galaxy: A platform for interactive large-scale genome analysis. Genome Res. 15, 1451–1455 (2005)

48. Nadkarni, P.M., Miller, R.A.: Service-oriented architecture in medical software: promises and perils. J. Am. Med. Inform. Assoc. 14, 244–246 (2007)

49. Vihinen, M., den Dunnen, J.T., Dalgleish, R., Cotton, R.G.: Guidelines for establishing locus specific databases. Human Mutation 33, 298–305 (2012)

50. Adzhubei, I.A., Schmidt, S., Peshkin, L., Ramensky, V.E., Gerasimova, A., Bork, P., Kondrashov, A.S., Sunyaev, S.R.: A method and server for predicting damaging missense mutations. Nat. Methods. 7, 248–249 (2010)

51. Kumar, P., Henikoff, S., Ng, P.C.: Predicting the effects of coding non-synonymous variants on protein function using the SIFT algorithm. Nat. Protoc. 4, 1073–1081 (2009)

52. Luu, T.D., Rusu, A., Walter, V., Linard, B., Poidevin, L., Ripp, R., Moulinier, L., Muller, J., Raffelsberger, W., Wicker, N., Lecompte, O., Thompson, J.D., Poch, O., Nguyen, H.: KD4v: Comprehensible knowledge discovery system for missense variant. Nucleic. Acids. Res. 40, W71–W75 (2012)

53. Oellrich, A., Gkoutos, G.V., Hoehndorf, R., Rebholz-Schuhmann, D.: Quantitative comparison of mapping methods between Human and Mammalian Phenotype Ontology. J. Biomed. Semantics 3(suppl. 2), S1 (2012)

54. Washington, N.L., Haendel, M.A., Mungall, C.J., Ashburner, M., Westerfield, M., Lewis, S.E.: Linking human diseases to animal models using ontology-based phenotype annotation. PLoS Biol. 7, e1000247 (2009)

55. Lyon, G.J., Wang, K.: Identifying disease mutations in genomic medicine settings: Current challenges and how to accelerate progress. Genome Med. 4, 58 (2012)

56. Gilissen, C., Hoischen, A., Brunner, H.G., Veltman, J.A.: Disease gene identification strategies for exome sequencing. Eur. J. Hum. Genet. 20, 490–497 (2012)

57. Sifrim, A., Van Houdt, J.K., Tranchevent, L.C., Nowakowska, B., Sakai, R., Pavlopoulos, G.A., Devriendt, K., Vermeesch, J.R., Moreau, Y., Aerts, J.: Annotate-it: A Swiss-knife approach to annotation, analysis and interpretation of single nucleotide variation in human disease. Genome Med. 4, 73 (2012)

58. Friedrich, A., Garnier, N., Gagniere, N., Nguyen, H., Albou, L.P., Biancalana, V., Bettler, E., Deleage, G., Lecompte, O., Muller, J., Moras, D., Mandel, J.L., Toursel, T., Moulinier, L., Poch, O.: SM2PH-db: An interactive system for the integrated analysis of phenotypic consequences of missense mutations in proteins involved in human genetic diseases. Hum. Mutat. 31, 127–135 (2010)

59. Nguyen, H., Michel, L., Thompson, J.D., Poch, O.: Heterogeneous Biological Data Integration with High Level Query Language. IBM Journal of Research and Development 58 (2014)

60. Luu, T.D., Rusu, A.M., Walter, V., Ripp, R., Moulinier, L., Muller, J., Toursel, T., Thompson, J.D., Poch, O., Nguyen, H.: MSV3d: Database of human MisSense variants mapped to 3D protein structure. Database (Oxford) 2012, bas018 (2012)

61. Moreau, Y., Tranchevent, L.C.: Computational tools for prioritizing candidate genes: boosting disease gene discovery. Nat. Rev. Genet. 13, 523–536 (2012)

62. Audo, I., Bujakowska, K., Orhan, E., Poloschek, C.M., Defoort-Dhellemmes, S., Drumare, I., Kohl, S., Luu, T.D., Lecompte, O., Zrenner, E., Lancelot, M.E., Antonio, A., Germain, A., Michiels, C., Audier, C., Letexier, M., Saraiva, J.P., Leroy, B.P., Munier, F.L., Mohand-Said, S., Lorenz, B., Friedburg, C., Preising, M., Kellner, U., Renner, A.B., Moskova-Doumanova, V., Berger, W., Wissinger, B., Hamel, C.P., Schorderet, D.F., De Baere, E., Sharon, D., Banin, E., Jacobson, S.G., Bonneau, D., Zanlonghi, X., Le Meur, G., Casteels, I., Koenekoop, R., Long, V.W., Meire, F., Prescott, K., de Ravel, T., Simmons, I., Nguyen, H., Dollfus, H., Poch, O., Leveillard, T., Nguyen-Ba-Charvet, K., Sahel, J.A., Bhattacharya, S.S., Zeitz, C.: Whole-exome sequencing identifies mutations in GPR179 leading to autosomal-recessive complete congenital stationary night blindness. American Journal of Human Genetics 90, 321–330 (2012)

63. Zeitz, C., Jacobson, S.G., Hamel, C., Bujakowska, K., Orhan, E., Zanlonghi, X., Lancelot, M.E., Michiels, C., Schwartz, S.B., Bocquet, B., Consortium, C.N.S.B., Antonio, A., Audier, C., Letexier, M., Saraiva, J.P., Luu, T.D., Sennlaub, F., Nguyen, H.O.P., Dollfus, H., Lecompte, O., Kohl, S., Sahel, J.A., Bhattacharya, S.S.I.A.: Whole exome sequencing identifies mutations in LRIT3 as a cause for autosomal recessive complete congenital stationary night blindness. Am. J. Hum. Genet. (2012)

64. Linard, B., Nguyen, N.H., Prosdocimi, F., Poch, O., Thompson, J.D.: EvoluCode: Evolutionary Barcodes as a Unifying Framework for Multilevel Evolutionary Data. Evol. Bioinform Online. 8, 61–77 (2011)

65. Boyle, J.: Biology must develop its own big-data systems. Nature 499, 7 (2013)

# Biomedical Text Mining: State-of-the-Art, Open Problems and Future Challenges

Andreas Holzinger[1], Johannes Schantl[1], Miriam Schroettner[1],
Christin Seifert[2], and Karin Verspoor[3,4]

[1] Research Unit Human-Computer Interaction, Institute for Medical Informatics,
Statistics and Documentation Medical University Graz, Austria
{a.holzinger,j.schantl,m.schroettner}@hci4all.at
[2] Chair of Media Informatics, University of Passau, Germany
christin.seifert@uni-passau.de
[3] Department of Computing & Information Systems, University of Melbourne,
Australia
[4] Health and Biomedical Informatics Centre, University of Melbourne, Australia
karin.verspoor@unimelb.edu.au

**Abstract.** Text is a very important type of data within the biomedical domain. For example, patient records contain large amounts of text which has been entered in a non-standardized format, consequently posing a lot of challenges to processing of such data. For the clinical doctor the written text in the medical findings is still the basis for decision making – neither images nor multimedia data. However, the steadily increasing volumes of unstructured information need machine learning approaches for data mining, i.e. text mining. This paper provides a short, concise overview of some selected text mining methods, focusing on statistical methods, i.e. Latent Semantic Analysis, Probabilistic Latent Semantic Analysis, Latent Dirichlet Allocation, Hierarchical Latent Dirichlet Allocation, Principal Component Analysis, and Support Vector Machines, along with some examples from the biomedical domain. Finally, we provide some open problems and future challenges, particularly from the clinical domain, that we expect to stimulate future research.

**Keywords:** Text Mining, Natural Language Processing, Unstructured Information, Big Data, Knowledge Discovery, Statistical Models, Text Classification, LSA, PLSA, LDA, hLDA, PCA, SVM.

## 1 Introduction and Motivation

Medical doctors and biomedical researchers of today are confronted with increasingly large volumes of high-dimensional, heterogeneous and complex data from various sources, which pose substantial challenges to the computational sciences [1], [2]. The majority of this data, particularly in classical business enterprise hospital information systems, is unstructured information. It is often imprecisely called unstructured data, which is used in industry as a similar buzz word as "big data". In the clinical domain it is colloquially called *"free-text"*,

A. Holzinger, I. Jurisica (Eds.): Knowledge Discovery and Data Mining, LNCS 8401, pp. 271–300, 2014.
© Springer-Verlag Berlin Heidelberg 2014

which should be more correctly defined as *non-standardized data* [3], [?]. However, this unstructured information is particularly important for decision making in clinical medicine, as it captures details, elaborations, and nuances that cannot be captured in discrete fields and predefined nomenclature [5]. All essential documents of the patient records contain large portions of complex text, which makes manual analysis very time-consuming and frequently practically impossible, hence computational approaches are indispensable [6]. Here it is essential to emphasize that for the clinical doctor the written text in the medical findings is still the basis for decision making – neither images nor multimedia data [7].

## 2   Glossary and Key Terms

*Bag-of-Words:* A representation of the content of a text in which individual words (or terms) and word (or term) counts are captured, but the linear (sequential) structure of the text is not maintained. Processing of linguistic structure is not possible in this representation.

*Classification:* Identification to which set of categories (sub-populations) a new observation belongs, on the basis of a training set of data containing observations (or instances) whose category membership is known. Supervised machine learning technique.

*Clustering:* Grouping a set of objects in such a way that objects in the same group (cluster) are more similar to each other than to those in other groups (clusters). Unsupervised machine learning technique.

*Corpus:* A collection of (text) documents. In a vector space model, each document can be mapped into a point (vector) in $\mathbb{R}^n$. For specific applications, documents or portions of documents may be associated with labels that can be used to train a model via machine learning.

*Knowledge Discovery:* Exploratory analysis and modelling of data and the organized process of identifying valid, novel, useful and understandable patterns from these data sets.

*Machine Learning:* Study of systems that can learn from data. A sub-field of computational learning theory, where agents learn when they change their behaviour in a way that makes them perform better in the future.

*Metric space:* A space is where a notion of distance between two elements (a metric) is defined. The distance function is required to satisfy several conditions, including positive definiteness and the triangle inequality.

*Optimization:* The selection of a best element (with regard to some criteria) from some set of available alternatives.

*Text:* Text is a general term for sequences of words. Text may be further structured into chapters, paragraphs and sentences as in books. Texts may contain some structure easily identifiable for humans, including linguistic structure. However, from the computer science point of view, text is unstructured information because the structure is not directly accessible for automatic processing.

*Term:* Units of text, often representing entities. Terms may be words, but also may be compound words or phrases in some application scenarios (e.g., "IG-9", "Rio de Janeiro", "Hodgkin's Lymphoma"). Relevant terms may be defined by a dictionary; the dictionary subsequently defines the dimension of the vector space for representation of documents.

*Text Mining (TM):* or Text Data Mining. The application of techniques from machine learning and computational statistics to find useful patterns in text data [8].

*Vector Space Model (VSM):* Representation of a set of documents $D$ as vectors in a common vector space. Approach whose goal is to make objects comparable by establishing a similarity measure between pairs of documents by using vector algebra (Euclidean distance, cosine similarity etc.). Most common vector space is the n-dimensional vector space of real numbers $\mathbb{R}^n$.

## 2.1   Notation

Document set or corpus $D$, $d \in D$
Vocabulary/Dictionary: $V$ vocabulary, $t \in V$ term, $|V|$ size of the vocabulary
$\mathbb{R}^n$ n-dimensional space of real numbers
$N$ - number of documents
$\overrightarrow{d}$ - vector representation of document d

# 3   Computational Representation of Text

In this chapter, we will introduce a selection of text mining methods, with an emphasis on statistical methods that utilise a matrix-like representation of the input data. In the case of text this representation is called the Vector Space Model (VSM). The general processing steps from textual data to the vector-space representation is described in section 3, the VSM itself is introduced in section 3.2. Specific algorithms applied to this representation of text will be presented in section 4.

There are a large number of linguistic approaches to processing of biomedical text, known as *biomedical natural language processing* (BioNLP) methods. Such approaches make extensive use of linguistic information such as grammatical relations and word order, as well as semantic resources such as ontologies and controlled vocabularies. These methods have been demonstrated to be particularly effective for extraction of biomedical concepts, events and relations, where the linguistic structure of the text can be particularly important. There are a number of resources that explore BioNLP methods, including a short encyclopedia chapter [9] and two recently published books [10, 12]. We therefore point the reader to those resources for more detail on such methods.

### 3.1   The Text Processing Pipeline

Text processing in the biomedical domain applies the same pipeline as for general text processing, an overview of which can be found in [13]. A detailed analysis of the steps in the context of information retrieval is available in [14]. Figure 1 shows and overview of a typical text processing pipeline assumed for statistical modeling of text. In the following we present each step in detail focusing on the content of the documents (and not the meta data).

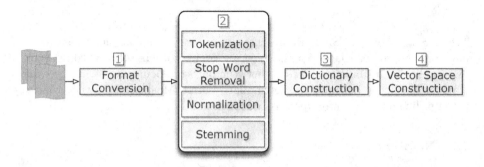

**Fig. 1.** Text processing pipeline. After converting documents of various source formats [1], the terms for the dictionary are defined [2], the dictionary is constructed [3], which leads to the vector space representation for the documents [4].

**Format Conversion:** Text comes in various formats, some of which can be accessed only by humans, such as paper books or lecture notes on a notepad. But even where text is digitally available, the formats vary and need to be normalized to apply text analysis methods. For instance, web pages contain not only the actual text content but also layout information (e.g., HTML tags, JavaScript code) and in HTML 5 the format has been defined with focus on layout and semantic structure [15]. On the other hand, Adobe's PDF format is optimized for layout and optimized printing [16]. In both HTML and PDF files, additional content, such as images or tables may be embedded. Source documents also come with various character encodings, like plain-text in Latin-1 encoding.

All such variants of texts have to be unified to make them accessible and the content available to text analysis methods. Plain text can be extracted from PDFs or Word documents, layout information is typically removed or ignored, and character encodings must be carefully handled, in particular to ensure correct treatment of special characters such as Greek letters or mathematical symbols. Depending on the source format this step may take considerable effort when the documents are in non-standard format. The output of the format conversion step are documents in a plain-text format with a standardized encoding suitable for further processing.

**Tokenization:** Vector space models typically use words as their basic representational element. Words must be identified from a text document, or a sequence of characters. This requires splitting those sequences into word-like pieces, a process called tokenization. In the simplest case tokenization involves splitting on non-alphanumeric characters (e.g., white spaces, punctuation marks, quotation marks). However, the process may be difficult in detail, e.g., using such simple splitting rules would split the words `O'Connor` and `isn't` in the same way with very different meaning. Further, specific tokenization rules may be necessary for some domains, e.g. by not splitting email addresses. The outcome of this step is a sequence of tokens for each document.

**Stop Word Removal:** Words that are thought not to carry any meaning for the purpose of text analysis are called "stop words". They are considered to be unnecessary and are typically removed before constructing a dictionary of relevant tokens. Removing those words serves two purposes: first, the reduced number of terms decreases the size of the vector space (reduced storage space) and second, the subsequent processes operating on the smaller space are more efficient. Stop words can be either removed by using predefined lists or applying a threshold to the frequency of words in the corpus and removing high-frequent words. Stop word removal is an optional step in text preprocessing. The outcome of this step is a sequence of tokens for each document (which may be smaller than the sequence obtained after tokenization).

**Normalization:** The process of normalization aims at finding a canonical form for words with the same semantic meaning but different character sequences. For instance, the character sequences `Visualization` and `visualisation`, and `IBM` and `I.B.M.` contain different characters but carry the same semantic meaning. Normalization methods include case-folding (convert all letters to lower case letters), and removing accents and diacritics, but their applicability depends of the language of the texts.

**Stemming and Lemmatization:** The underlying assumption for stemming and lemmatization is that for the purpose of machine text analysis the meaning of the words is not influenced by their grammatical form in the text. Stemming is the process of heuristically removing suffices from words to reduce the word to a common form (the word stem), while lemmatization refers to more sophisticated methods using vocabularies and morphological analysis. The BioLemmatizer [17] is a tool for lemmatization that is tailored to biomedical texts. The most common used stemming algorithm for the English language is the Porter stemmer [18]. The outcome of this step is the representation of documents as a sequence of (normalized, base) terms.

**Building the Dictionary:** Having obtained a sequence of terms for each document, a dictionary can be constructed from the document texts themselves. It is simply the set of all terms in all documents. Generally in machine learning one would refer to the dictionary terms as features. Details on how to obtain the vector space model of the document corpus given a dictionary and the documents are presented in section 3.2.

Note that in more linguistic approaches to text analysis, the dictionary may be an externally-specified collection of terms, potentially including multi-word terms, that reflect standard vocabulary terms for a given domain. For biomedicine, dictionaries of terms may include disease or drug names, or lists of known proteins. This dictionary may be used as a basis for identifying meaningful terms in the texts, rather than the more data-driven methodology we have introduced here. We will not consider this complementary approach further but again refer the reader to other resources [10, 12].

## 3.2 The Vector Space Model

The Vector space model aka term vector model is an algebraic model for representing any data objects in general, and text documents specifically, as vectors of so-called identifiers, e.g. index terms. The VSM is state-of-the-art in information retrieval, text classification and clustering for a long time [14, 19, 20]. In practice VSM's usually have the following properties, (1) a high dimensional features space, (2) few irrelevant features and (3) sparse instance vectors [21]. The VSM has been often combined with theoretical, structural and computational properties of connectionist networks in order to provide a natural environment for representing and retrieving information [22].

**Functionality:** Documents $d$ in a corpus $D$ are represented as vectors in a vector-space. The dimensionality of the vector space equals the number of terms in the dictionary $V$. The two most common vector space models used are the Boolean model and the real-valued vector-space. Figure 2 shows two example documents $d_1$ and $d_2$ in a three-dimensional vector space spanned by terms $t_1$, $t_2$ and $t_3$. In a metric vector space, similarities or distances between documents can be calculated, a necessary ingredient for most algorithms in information retrieval, text clustering and classification.

In a Boolean vector space, documents are representing as binary vectors, i.e. $d \in \{0,1\}^{|V|}$. This model can only capture whether a certain term occurs in a document or not. On the contrary for documents in a real-valued vector space $d \in \mathbb{R}^{|V|}$ more information about the term-document relation can be captured by weighting the term occurrences. Several different ways of computing the term weights, have been developed. The most prominent weighting schemes are tf-idf weighting [19] and the BM-25 family of weighting schemes [23].

The intuition behind *tf-idf weighting* is that (i) terms that occur multiple times in a document should have a higher influence on the document (tf) and (i) terms that occur in many documents should have lower influence because they

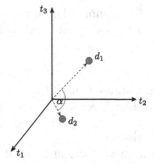

**Fig. 2.** A simple three-dimensional vector space with two documents. The angle between two documents can be used a similarity measure (cf. cosine similarity).

are less discriminating between documents (idf). More precisely, the $tf - idf$ weight of term $t$ for document $d$ is determined by

$$\text{tf-idf}_{t,d} = \text{tf}_{t,d} \cdot \text{idf}_t \qquad (1)$$

$$\text{idf}_t = \log \frac{N}{\text{df}_t} \qquad (2)$$

where tf-idf$_{t,d}$ is the number of occurrences of term $t$ in document $d$, $N$ is the number of documents and df$_t$ the number of documents that contain term $t$.

In *BM-25 weighting* additional statistics of the text corpus, i.e. a document length-normalization, is incorporated in the weighting formula. For more details about BM-25 weighting variants see [23].

*Cosine similarity* The cosine similarity between document $d_i$ and $d_j$ corresponds to the angle between the documents (see figure 2 and is defined as

$$sim(d_i, d_j) = \frac{\vec{d_i} \cdot \vec{d_j}}{|\vec{d_i}||\vec{d_j}|} \qquad (3)$$

where $\vec{d_i}, \vec{d_j}$ is the vector space representation and $|\vec{d_i}|, |\vec{d_j}|$ the Euclidean length of document $d_i$ and $d_j$ respectively. For normalized vectors the cosine similarity is equal to the dot product of those vectors, because the denominator in formula 3 becomes 1. Other similarity measure include Euclidean distance, which works similar well to cosine similarity for normalized document vectors and the dot product [14].

**Examples in the Biomedical Domain:** In Hlioautakis et al. (2006) [24] a good application example of the vector space model is explained. A medical knowledge finder which is based on the vector space model was evaluated in a clinical setting and compared with a gold standard by Hersh et al. [25]. In Müller et al. [26] content based image retrieval systems in the medical domain are compared with each other where some are based on vector space models.

According to Cunha et al. [27] a combination of vector space model, statistical physics and linguistics lead to a good hybrid approach for text summarization of medical articles.

**Discussion:** The VSM is the state-of-the art representation for text in information retrieval and text mining. *Advantages* of the model include:

- The model is simple and clear.
- The representation is a matrix that can be easily used by many machine learning algorithms.
- A continuous ranking of documents can be achieved according to their similarity to a query vector.
- A general representation of a document as a real-valued vector allows for different weighting schemes, which are used for instance to incorporate users' relevance feedback.

The *limitations* of the VSM are the following:

- The method is calculation intensive and needs a lot of processing time compared to a binary text representation. E.g., two passes over the document-term matrix are necessary for tf-idf weighting.
- The vector space for text has a high dimensionality (for natural language texts in the order of $10^4$), and the matrix is a sparse matrix, since only a very small number of terms occur in each document. Thus, a sparse representation of the matrix is usually required to keep the memory consumption low.
- Adding new documents to the search space, means to recalculate/re-dimension the global term document matrix.
- Each document is seen as a bag of words, words are considered to be statistically independent. The meaning of the word sequence is not reflected in the model.
- Assumption a single term represents exactly one word sense, which is not true for natural language texts, which contain synonymous and polysemous words. Methods like word sense disambiguation have to applied in the pre-processing step.

**Similar Spaces:** The Semantic Vector Space Model (SVSM) is a text representation and searching technique based on the combination of Vector Space Model (VSM) with heuristic syntax parsing and distributed representation of semantic case structures. In this model, both documents and queries are represented as semantic matrices. A search mechanism is designed to compute the similarity between two semantic matrices to predict relevancy [28].

Latent semantic mapping (LSM) is a data-driven framework to model globally meaningful relationships implicit in large volumes of (often textual) data [29]. It is a generalization of latent semantic analysis.

# 4  Text Mining Methods

There are many different methods to deal with text, e.g. Latent Semantic Analysis (LSA), Probabilistic latent semantic analysis (PLSA), Latent Dirichlet allocation (LDA), Hierarchical Latent Dirichlet Allocation (hLDA), Semantic Vector Space Model (SVSM), Latent semantic mapping (LSM) and Principal component analysis (PCA) to name only a few.

## 4.1  Latent Semantic Analysis (LSA)

Latent Semantic Analysis (LSA) is both: a theory and a method for both extracting and representing the meaning of words in their contextual environment by application of statistical analysis to a large amount of text LSA is basically a general theory of acquired similarities and knowledge representations, originally developed to explain learning of words and psycholinguistic problems [30,31]. The general idea was to induce global knowledge indirectly from local co-occurrences in the representative text. Originally, LSA was used for explanation of textual learning of the English language at a comparable rate amongst schoolchildren. The most interesting issue is that LSA does not use any prior linguistic or perceptual similarity knowledge; i.e., it is based exclusively on a general mathematical learning method that achieves powerful inductive effects by extracting the right number of dimensions to represent both objects and contexts. The fundamental suggestion is that the aggregate of all words in contexts in which a given word does and does not appear provides a set of mutual constraints that largely determines the similarity of meaning of words and sets of words to each other. For the combination of Informatics and Psychology it is interesting to note that the adequacy of LSA's reflection of human knowledge has been established in a variety of ways [32]. For example, the scores overlap closely to those of humans on standard vocabulary and subject matter tests and interestingly it emulates human word sorting behaviour and category judgements [30]. Consequently, as a practical outcome, it can estimate passage coherence and the learnability of passages, and both the quality and quantity of knowledge contained in an textual passage (originally this were student essays).

**Functionality:** Latent Semantic Analysis (LSA) is primarily used as a technique for measuring the coherence of texts. By comparing the vectors for 2 adjoining segments of text in a high-dimensional semantic space, the method provides a characterization of the degree of semantic relatedness between the segments. LSA can be applied as an automated method that produces coherence predictions similar to propositional modelling, thus having potential as a psychological model of coherence effects in text comprehension [32].

Having $t$ terms and $d$ documents one can build a $t \times d$ matrix $X$. Often the terms within this matrix are weighted according to term frequency - inverse document frequency (fd-idf) [x]. The main method now is to apply the singular value decomposition (SVD) on $X$ [y]. Therefore $X$ can be disjointed into tree components $X = TSD^T$. $T$ and $D^T$ are orthonormal matrices with the eigenvectors of $XX^T$ and $X^TX$ respectively. $S$ contains the roots of the eigenvalues of $XX^T$ and $X^TX$.

Reducing the dimensionality can now be achieved by step-by-step eliminating the lowest eigenvalue with the corresponding eigenvectors to a certain value $k$. See relatedness to PCA (section 4.5).

A given Query $q$ can now be projected into this space by applying the equation:

$$\frac{Q = q^T U_k}{diag(S_k)} \quad (4)$$

Having $Q$ and the documents in the same semantic space a similarity measure can now be applied. Often used for example is the so called cosine similarity between a document in the semantic space and a query $Q$. Having two vectors $A$ and $B$ in the $n$ dimensional space the cosine similarity is defined as:

$$cos(\phi) = \frac{A \cdot B}{\|A\| \|B\|} \quad (5)$$

**Examples in the Biomedical Domain:** Latent semantic analysis can be used to automatically grade clinical case summaries written by medical students and therefore proves to be very useful [33]. In [34] latent semantic analysis is used to extract clinical concepts from psychiatric narrative. According to [35] LSA was used to extract semantic word and semantic concepts for developing a ontology-based speech act identification in a bilingual dialogue system. Furthermore, latent semantic analysis combined with hidden Markov models lead to good results in topic segmentation and labelling in the clinical field [36]. In [37] the characteristics and usefulness of distributional semantics models (like LSA, PLSA, LDA) for clinical concept extraction are discussed and evaluated.

**Discussion:** The *advantages* of LSA are:

- LSA tends to solve the synonym problem [38].
- LSA reflects the semantic of the texts, so similar concepts are found.
- Finds latent classes.
- Reduction of dimensionality of Vector Space Model.

LSA has the following *limitations*:

- High mathematical complexity (SVD).
- Recalculation of the singular value decomposition when adding new documents or terms.
- Offers only a partial solution to the polsemy problem [38].
- The estimation of $k$, that means how many eigenvalues to keep to get good information retrieval results.
- It has a bad statistical foundation [39].

## 4.2   Probabilistic Latent Semantic Analysis (PLSA)

The probabilistic latent semantic analysis (PLSA) is a statistical method for factor analysis of binary and count data which is closely related to LSA, however, in contrast to LSA which stems from linear algebra and performs a Singular Value Decomposition of co-occurrence tables, the PLSA technique uses a generative latent class model to perform a probabilistic mixture decomposition [40, 41]. This results in a more principled approach with a solid foundation in statistical inference. PLSA has many applications, most prominently in information retrieval, natural language processing, machine learning from text, see e.g, [42–45]).

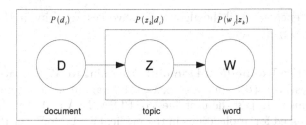

**Fig. 3.** Two level generative model

**Functionality:** The PLSA is a unsupervised technique that forms a two level generative model (see picture 3). In contrast to the LSA model, it builds up a clear probability model of the underlying documents, concepts (topics) and words and therefore is more easy to interpret. Abstractly spoken every document can talk about different concepts to a different extend as well as words form different topics. So having a document collection $D = \{d_1, d_2, d_i..., d_M\}$ we can define a co-occurrence table using a vocabulary $W = \{w_1, w_2, w_j..., w_N\}$. Furthermore each observation, where an observation is defined as occurrence of a word in a document is associated with an unobservable class variable $Z = \{z_1, z_2, z_k..., z_K\}$. We can now define a joint probability $P(d_i, z_k, w_j)$ as:

$$P(d_i, z_k, w_j) = P(w_j|z_k)P(z_k|d_i)P(d_i) \tag{6}$$

Getting rid of the unobservable variable $z_k$ we can rewrite the equation as:

$$P(d_i, w_j) = \sum_{k=1}^{K} P(w_j|z_k)P(z_k|d_i)P(d_i) \tag{7}$$

The probability of the entire text corpus can now be rewritten as:

$$P(d, w) = \prod_{i=1}^{M} \prod_{j=1}^{N} P(d_i) \sum_{k=1}^{K} P(w_j|z_k)P(z_k|d_i) \tag{8}$$

Rewriting the probability of the text corpus in terms of a log likelihood yields:

$$L = log \prod_{i=1}^{M} \prod_{j=1}^{N} P(d_i, w_j)^{n(d_i, wj)} \tag{9}$$

Maximizing L is done by using the expectation maximization algorithm [46]. The algorithm basically consists of two steps:

**Expectation-Step:** Expectation for the latent variables are calculated given the observations by using the current estimates of the parameters.

**Maximization-Step:** Update the parameters such that L increases using the posterior probabilities in the E-Step.

The steps are repeated until the algorithm converges, resulting in the quantities $P(w_j|z_k)$ and $P(z_k|d_i)$.

**Examples in the Biomedical Domain:** According to [47] probabilistic latent semantic analysis is used to find and extract data about human genetic diseases and polymorphism. In [48] the usefulness of PLSA, LSA and other data mining method is discussed for applications in the medical field. Moreover PLSA counts to one of the well-known topic models that are used to explore health-related topics in online health communities [49]. According to Masseroli et al. [50] PLSA is also used for prediction of gene ontology annotations and provides good results.

**Discussion:** The *advantages* of PLSA include:

- Can deal with the synonym and polysemy problem [39].
- PLSA performs better than LSA [39].
- PLSA is based on a sound statistical foundation [39].
- Finds latent topics.
- Topics are easily interpretable.

PLSA has the following *limitations*:

- The underlying iterative algorithm of PlSA converges only logically [51].

### 4.3   Latent Dirichlet Allocation (LDA)

Latent Dirichlet allocation (LDA) is a generative probabilistic model for collections of discrete data such as text corpora, based on a three-level hierarchical Bayesian model, in which each item of a collection is modelled as a finite mixture over an underlying set of topics [52]. Each topic is, in turn, modelled as an infinite mixture over an underlying set of topic probabilities. In the context of text modelling, the topic probabilities provide an explicit representation of a document, consequently LDA can be seen as a 'bag-of-words' type of language modelling and dimension reduction method [53] (TODO: get pdf). One interesting application of LDA was fraud detection in the telecommunications industry in order to build user profile signatures and assumes that any significant unexplainable deviations from the normal activity of an individual end user is strongly correlated with fraudulent activity; thereby, the end user activity is represented as a probability distribution over call features which surmises the end user calling behaviour [54] (TODO: get pdf). LDA is often assumed to be better performing than e.g. LSA or PLSA [55].

**Functionality:** The basic idea behind LDA is that documents can be represented as a mixture of latent topics, which are represented by a distribution across words [52]. Similar to LSA and PLSA, the number of latent topics used in the model has to be fixed a-priori. But in contrast, for instance, to LSA which uses methods of linear algebra, LDA uses probabilistic methods for inferring the mixture of topics and words. According to Blei et al. [52], the assumed generative process for each word $w$ in a document within a corpus $D$ contains the following steps: (1) Choose $N$, the number of words for a document, estimated by a Poisson distribution. (2) Choose a topic mixture $\theta$ according to a Dirichlet distribution over $\alpha$, a Dirichlet prior over all documents. (3) Each of the $N$ words $w_n$ are selected by first choosing a topic which is represented as multinomial random variable $z$, and second by choosing a word from $p(w_n|z_n, \beta)$, a multinomial probability conditioned on the topic $z_n$.

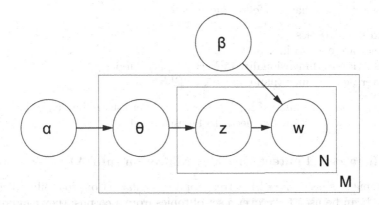

**Fig. 4.** LDA graphical model. The outer box represents documents, while the inner box represents the iterative choice of topics and words in a document. [52]

Figure 4, shows the probabilistic graphical model of LDA. The LDA representation contains three levels. The corpus level parameters $\alpha$ and $\beta$ are sampled once within the process of generating a corpus. The document level variable $\theta$ is sampled once per document, and the word level parameters $z_n$ and $w_n$ are sampled once for each word within a document.

The goal of inference in the LDA model is to find the values of $\phi$, the probability of word $w$ occurring in topic $z$ and $\theta$, the distribution of topics over a document. There are several algorithms proposed for solving the inference problem for LDA, including a variational Expectation-Maximization algorithm [52], an Expectation-Propagation algorithm [56] or an collapsed Gibbs sampling algorithm of Griffiths and Steyvers [57].

**Examples in the Biomedical Domain:** In [58], Wu et al. apply LDA to predict protein-protein relationships from literature. One of their features to rank candidate gene-drug pairs was the topic distance derived from LDA. Case-based information retrieval from clinical documents due to LDA can be used to discover relevant clinical concepts and structuring in patient's health record [59]. In [60] [get pdf and check if LDA is used for topic model], Arnold and Speier present a topic model tailored to the clinical reporting environment which allows for individual patient timelines. In [61] unsupervised relation discovery with sense disambiguation is processed with the help of LDA which can be used in different areas of application. Moreover with LDA a genomic analysis of time-to-event outcomes can be processed [62]. According to [63] big data is available for research purposes due to data mining of electronic health records, but it has to pre-processed to be useful with the help of different mining techniques including LDA.

**Discussion:** LDA has the following *advantages*:

- Find latent topics.
- Topics are easy to interpret.
- Reduction of dimensionality of Vector Space Model.
- Better performance than e.g. LSA or PLSA [55].

The main *disadvantage* of LDA is the parameter estimation, e.g., the number of topics has to be known or needs to be estimated.

### 4.4   Hierarchical Latent Dirichlet Allocation (hLDA)

While topic models such as LDA treat topics as a flat set of probability distributions and can be used to recover a set of topics from a corpus, they can not give insight about the abstraction of a topic or how the topics are related. The hierarchical LDA (hLDA) model is a non-parametric generative probabilistic model and can be seen as an extension of LDA. One advantage of non-parametric models is, that these models do not assume a fixed set of parameters such as the number of topics, instead the number of parameters can grow as the corpus grows [64]. HLDA is build on the nested Chinese restaurant process (nCRP) to additionally organize topics as a hierarchy. HLDA arranges topics into a tree, in which more general topics should appear near the root and more specialized ones closer to the leaves. This model can be useful e.g. for text categorization, comparison, summarization, and language modelling for speech-recognition [64].

**Functionality:** HLDA uses the nCRP, a distribution on hierarchical partitions, as a non-parametric prior for the hierarchical extension to the LDA model [64]. A nested Chinese restaurant process can be illustrated by an infinite tree where each node denotes to a restaurant with an infinite number of tables. One restaurant is identified as the root restaurant, and on each of its tables lies a card with the name of another restaurant. Further, on each table of these restaurants are again cards to other restaurants and this structure repeats infinite times, with the restriction that each restaurant is referred only one time. In this way all restaurants are structured into an infinity deep and infinitely branched tree. Every tourist starts by selecting a table in the root restaurant according to the CRP distribution defined as:

$$p(\text{occupied table } i | \text{previous customer}) = \frac{m_i}{\gamma + m - 1}$$
$$p(\text{next occupied table} | \text{previous customer}) = \frac{\gamma}{\gamma + m - 1} \tag{10}$$

where $m_i$ denotes to the number of previous customers at table $i$, and $\gamma$ is a parameter [64]. Next, the tourist chooses in the same way a table in the referred restaurant from the last restaurants table. This process repeats infinity many times. After M tourists go through this process the collection of paths describes a random sub-tree of the infinite tree [64].

According to [64], the nCRP is augmented in two ways to obtain a generative model for documents. (1) Each node in the tree is associated with a topic, which is a probability distribution across words. A path in the tree samples an infinite collection of topics. (2) The GEM distribution [65] is used to define a probability distribution on the topics along the path. A document is then generated by repeatedly sampling topics according to the probabilities defined by one draw of the GEM distribution, and further sampling each word from the probability distribution from the selected topic.

For detailed information about the inference in hLDA, it is referred to the original description of HLDA from Blei et.al [64].

**Examples in the Biomedical Domain:** Due to hLDA individual and population level traits are extracted from clinical temporal data and used to track physiological signals of premature infants and therefore gain clinical relevant insights [66]. According to [67] clinical document labelling and retail product categorization tasks on large-scale data can be performed by hLDA .

**Discussion:** Hierarchical LDA has the same advantages and limitations as LDA (see section 4.3), additionally *advantages* are:

- Organics topics in a hierarchy depending on their abstraction level.
- Number of topics does not need be fixed a-priori.

## 4.5   Principal Components Analysis

Principal component analysis (PCA) is a technique used to reduce multidimensional data sets to lower dimensions for analysis. Depending on the field of application, it is also named the discrete Karhunen-Loève transform, the Hotelling transform [68] or proper orthogonal decomposition (POD).

PCA was introduced in 1901 by Karl Pearson [69]. Now it is mostly used as a tool in exploratory data analysis and for making predictive models. PCA involves the calculation of the eigenvalue decomposition of a data covariance matrix or singular value decomposition of a data matrix, usually after mean centering the data for each attribute. The results of a PCA are usually discussed in terms of component scores and loadings.

**Functionality:** In this section we give a brief mathematical introduction into PCA, presuming mathematical knowledge about: standard deviation, covariance, eigenvectors and eigenvalues. Lets assume to have M observations of an object gathering at each observation N features. So at any observation point we can collect a N-dimensional feature vector $\Gamma$. All feature Vectors together form the $N \times M$ observation matrix $\Theta(\Gamma_1, \Gamma_2, ..., \Gamma_M)$. Furthermore the average feature vector is given by:

$$\Psi = \frac{1}{M} \sum_{n=1}^{M} \Gamma_n \tag{11}$$

So by mean-adjusting every feature vector $\Gamma_i$ by $\Phi_i = \Gamma_i - \Psi$ one can form the covariance matrix of the mean adjusted data by:

$$C = \frac{1}{M} \sum_{n=1}^{M} \Phi_n \Phi_n^T \tag{12}$$

Basically the PCA is done by following steps:

- Calculate the eigenvalues and the corresponding eigenvectors of C, resulting in $\lambda_1, \lambda_2, ..., \lambda_M$ eigenvalues with the corresponding eigenvectors $u_1, u_2, ..., u_M$
- Keep the the highest eigenvalues $M' < M$ forming a matrix $P = [u_1, u_2, ..., u_{M'}]^T$ with the corresponding eigenvectors where $\lambda_1 > \lambda_2 > ...\lambda_{M'}$.
- Transform the data into the reduced space applying $Y = PC$

An important thing to mention is that $cov(Y) = \frac{1}{M'} YY^T$ is a Diagonalmatrix. That means we found a representation of the data with minimum redundancy and noise (off diagonal elements of the covariance matrix are zero). Remember that one diagonal element of the covariance matrix represent the variance of one typical feature measured. Another thing to mention for a better understanding is that the eigenvectors try to point toward the direction of greatest variance of the data and that all eigenvectors are orthonormal. See figure 5 for an illustrative example. PCA is closely related to SVD, so LSA is one of the typical examples in the field of information retrieval where PCA is used.

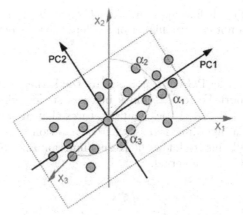

**Fig. 5.** Eigenvectors pointing to direction of maximum variance

**Examples in the Biomedical Domain:** Examples in medicine span a lot of different areas, due to the case that PCA is a base statistical mathematical tool. Especially used as space dimension reduction method, high dimensional parameter space can be reduced to a lower one. Nevertheless we want to give some recent research papers in various fields of medicine to show that even though the mathematical principles are know more than 100 years old [69], its appliance in modern medical informatics is still essential. According to [70] the principal components analysis is used to explicitly model ancestry differences between cases and controls to enable detection and correction of population stratification on a genome-wide scale. Moreover PCA is used in [71] to investigate a large cohort with the Tourette syndrome and evaluate the results. In [72] lay requests to gain medical information or advice from sick or healthy persons are automatically classified due to different text-mining methods including PCA. Furthermore, with the help of PCA and other text mining methods drug re-purposing can be identified trough analysing drugs, targets and clinical outcomes [73].

**Discussion:** PCA is widely used for dimensionality reduction and generally has the following *advantages*:

- Finds the mathematically optimal methods in the sense of minimizing the squared error.
- The measurement of the variance along each principle component provides a means for comparing the relative importance of each dimension.
- PCA is completely non-parametric.
- PCA provides the optimal reduced representation of the data.

However, the following *limitations* have to be considered when considering to apply PCA:

- Sensitive to outliers.
- Removing the outliers before applying the PCA can be a difficult task.
- Standard PCA can not capture higher order dependencies between the variables.

**Similar Methods:** Kernel PCA [74] is based on the kernel trick which comes from the field of Support Vector Machines but has successfully been applied to the PCA. Basically the kernel trick maps features that are not separable in the current space into a high dimensional where separation is possible. For this purpose one has basically just to know the Kernel function $K(x, y)$. A often used kernel function is the Gaussian kernel,

$$K(x, y) = e^{\frac{-||x-y||^2}{2\sigma^2}} \tag{13}$$

but other Kernels can also be used that at least that they have to fulfil the condition that the dot product between two components in feature space has the same results applying the kernel function between two components in the original space. The main advantage of kernel PCA is the fact that it is able to separate components, where normal PCA failures.

### 4.6  Classification of Text Using Support Vector Machines

Support Vector Machines are first introduced in the year 1995 by Vapnik and Cortes [75], and are one of the most commonly used classification methods. They are based on well founded computational learning theory and are analysed in research in very detail. SVMs can easily deal with sparse and high dimensional data sets, therefore, they fit very well for text mining applications [21].

**Functionality:** The task of a SVM is to find an hyperplane which separates the positive and negative instances (in case of a two class input data set) with the maximum margin. Therefore SVMs are also called maximum margin classifiers. The margin is defined as the distance between the hyperplane and the closest point to the hyperplane among both classes denoted by $x_+$ and $x_-$. Assuming that $x_+$ and $x_-$ are equidistant to the hyperplane with a distance of 1, the margin is defined as:

$$m_D(f) = 1/2\hat{w}^T(x_+ - x_-) = \frac{1}{||w||} \tag{14}$$

where $\hat{w}$ is a unit vector in the direction of $w$ which is known as the weight vector [76]. Maximizing the margin $\frac{1}{||w||}$, which is equivalent to minimizing $||w||^2$, will maximize the separability between the classes. In this context, one can distinguish between the hard margin SVM, which can be applied for linearly separably data sets, and the soft margin SVM which works also for not linearly separably data by allowing also misclassifications. The optimization task of a hard margin SVM is to minimize $1/2||w||^2$ subject to

$$y_i(w^T x_i + b) \geq 1, i = 1, ...., n \tag{15}$$

where $y_i$ denotes the label of an example [76]. In case of the soft margin SVM the objective of minimizing $1/2||w||^2$. is augmented with the term $C\sum_{i=1}^{n} \xi_i$ to penalize misclassification and margin errors, where $\xi_i$ are slack variables that allow an example to be in the margin ($0 \leq \xi_i \leq 1$) or to be misclassified ($\xi_i > 1$) and the parameter $C$ sets the relative importance of minimizing the amount of slack and maximizing the margin [76]. The optimization task of a soft margin SVM is then to minimize $1/2||w||^2 + C\sum_{i=1}^{n} \xi_i$ subject to

$$y_i(w^T x_i + b) \geq 1 - \xi_i, x_i \geq 0 \tag{16}$$

The SVM algorithm as presented above is inherently a binary classifier. SVM has been successfully applied to multi-class classification problems by using the multiple one-vs-all or one-vs-one classifiers, a true multi-class SVM approach has been proposed by Crammer & Singer [77]. In many applications a non-linear classifier provides better accuracy than a linear one. SVMs use also the kernel trick, to transfer the input space into a higher dimensional space in which the data is linearly separable by a hyperplane. In this way SVMs fit also very well as a non-linear classifier.

**Examples in the Biomedical Domain:** According to Guyon et al. [78] a new method of gene selection based on support vector machines was proposed and evaluated. In a text classification task, Ghanem et al. [79], used SVMs in combination with regular expressions to evaluate whether papers from the Fly-Base data set should be curated based on the presence of evidence of Dosophila gene products. Support vector machine is also used for mining biomedical literature for protein-protein interactions Donaldson et al. [80]. To discover protein functional regions, Eskin and Agichtein [81] combined text and sequence analysis by using an SVM classifier. In Joshi et al. [82] support vector machines are explored for the use in the domain of medical text and compared with other machine learning algorithm. Further, SVMs are also used in the most effective approaches for the assertion checking and and relation extraction subtask in the i2b2 2011 challenge which are tasks of biomedical NLP [83]. Also in the i2b2 co-reference challenge 2012, SVM was used among the leading approaches [83].

**Discussion:** The SVM is considered state-of-the-art in text classification due to the following *advantages*:

- Can deal with many features (more than 10000).
- Can deal with sparse document vectors.
- Not restricted to linear models due to the kernel functions.

The only *disadvantage* of SVM classification is the interpretable of the classification model compared to easily interpretable models like Naive Bayes [84] or Decision trees [85].

# 5  Open Problems

## 5.1  Deployment and Evaluation of Text Mining in Clinical Context

Evaluation of text mining systems is substantially more mature in the context of analysis of the published biomedical literature than in the clinical context. A number of community evaluations, with shared tasks and shared data sets, have been performed to assess the performance of information extraction and information retrieval from the biomedical literature (e.g. the BioNLP shared tasks [86], BioCreative [87], and TREC Genomics [88]). Especially when dealing with supervised machine learning methods, one needs substantial quantities of labelled training data and again there are growing large-scale richly annotated training data resources (e.g. the GENIA [89] and CRAFT [90, 91] corpora, as well as a increasing number of more specific resources such as the SCAI chemical compounds corpus [92] and the Variome genetic variants corpus [93]).

Such tasks and resources have been far more limited on the clinical side. The 2012 TREC Medical Records track [94], i2b2 natural language processing shared tasks addressing clinical discharge summaries [95, 96], and the ShARE/CLEF eHealth evaluation lab 2013 [97] provide examples of the importance of such evaluations in spurring research into new methods development on real-world problems. The availability of de-identified clinical records that can be shared publicly is critical to this work, but has posed a stumbling block to open assessment of systems on the same data. Copyright restrictions and especially data privacy also interfere with the research progress [98]. Indeed, much more work is needed into evaluation measures to determine how valuable a text mining tool is for the actual user [98]. Some examples exist (e.g., for biocuration [99] and systematic reviews [100]) but limited work addresses deployment in a clinical context, which poses significant challenges. To find the right trade-off between the processing speed and the accuracy of a text mining algorithm is a challenging task, especially for online applications which must be responsive [101]. Furthermore, text mining tools should not only focus on English text documents, but should be able to process other languages too [102]. Recently, there have been some efforts to explore adaptation of predominantly English vocabulary resources and tools to other languages [103] and to address multilingual text processing in the health context [104] but there is significantly more to be done in this area, in particular to support integration of clinical information across language-specific data sets.

## 5.2  Specific Characteristics of Biomedical Texts

Clinical texts, in contrast to edited published articles, are in often not grammatically correct, use locally used abbreviations and have misspellings [11]. This poses huge challenges for transferring tools that have been developed for text analysis in the literature mining context to the clinical context. At a minimum, it requires appropriate normalization and spelling correction methods for text [105]. Even well-formed medical texts have different characteristics from general domain texts, and require tailored solutions. The BioLemmatizer [17] was developed specifically for handling inflectional morphology in biomedical texts; general English solutions do not have adequate coverage of the domain-specific vocabulary. Within clinical texts, there can be substantial variation in how 'regular' they are from a text processing perspective; emergency department triage notes written during a two-minute assessment of a patient will be substantially noisier than radiology reports or discharge summaries. More work is required to address adaptation of text processing tools to less well-formed texts. The biomedical literature also has certain characteristics which require specialised text processing strategies [106]. Enrichment and analysis of specific document parts such as tables gives access to a wealth of information, but cannot be handled using standard vector space or natural language processing strategies [107–110]. Similarly, it has recently been shown that substantial information in the biomedical literature actually resides in the *supplementary files* associated with publications rather than the main narrative text [111]; due to the varied and unpredictable nature of such files accessing this information will pose challenges to existing methods for information extraction.

## 5.3   Linguistic Issues and Semantic Enrichment

When extracting information from text documents one has to deal with several challenges arising from the complexities of natural language communication. One issue, which is particularly problematic for instance when trying to find relations among entities, is that language is very rich and one can express the same underlying concepts in many different ways. In addition, such relations expressed over multiple sentences which makes it even more difficult to find them and typically requires co-reference resolution. Ambiguity of words, phrases and entire sentences is one of the leading challenges in text mining that emerges because of the complexity of natural language itself. Some progress on ambiguity, especially term ambiguity, has been made; there exists a disambiguation module in the UMLS MetaMap concept recognition tool as well as other proposed approaches [112,113]. On the other hand, substantial challenges remain. For instance, although disambiguation of gene names in the biomedical literature (also known as gene normalization, in which mentions of genes are linked to a reference entity in a gene database) has been addressed in a recent challenge [114], the performance of the state-of-the-art systems has left room for improvement. Gene names are heavily overloaded, re-used across organisms and often confused with the function of the gene (e.g. "transcription growth factor"). An approach for entity disambiguation in the biomedical domain has been presented in [115]. Higher-level ambiguity such as processing of coordination structures and attachment of modifiers will require more linguistic methods and has been addressed in few systems [116,117] but remains a stumbling block. Co-reference resolution has been addressed in limited contexts [118–120] and also continues to pose a substantial challenge to integration of information from across a text.

# 6 Conclusion and Future Outlook

Biomedical text mining has benefited from substantial interest from the research community and from practical needs of the clinical domain, particularly in the last ten years. However, there remain substantial opportunities to progress the field further. One important direction is in the continued improvement of existing methods, supported through new creation of *gold standards* as benchmark sets [6]. Such resources are urgently needed to enable further improvement of methods, particularly in the clinical context where only a limited range of text types and tasks have been rigorously explored. Of particular importance are open data sets that can internationally be used [121], [106].

Another area of great opportunity is in methodological hot topics such as the graph-theoretical and topological text mining methods which are very promising approaches, yet not much studied [122]. Much potential for further research has the application of evolutionary algorithms [123], for text mining [124].

There are in addition a large number of opportunities to apply text mining to new problems and new text types. Text analysis of Web 2.0 and social media [125] is an emerging focus in biomedicine, for instance for detecting influenza-likes illnesses [126] or adverse drug events [127, 128], [129].

In practice we need *integrated solutions* [130] of content analytics tools [131] into the clinical workplace. Integration of text mining with more general data mining is also a fruitful direction. In the clinical context drawing signals from both text, structured patient data (e.g. biometrics or laboratory results), and even biomedical images, will likely enable a more complete picture of a patient and his or her disease status for clinical decision support or outcome modeling. Such applications will require new strategies for multi-modal data integration and processing that incorporate text mining as a fundamental component. These tasks will result in solutions that will have substantial real-world impact and will highlight the importance of text mining for biomedicine.

**Acknowledgments.** We thank the Austrian IBM Watson Think Group for fruitful discussions and for the support of Gottfried Prohaska, Alberto Brabenetz and Michael Grosinger. We are grateful for comments from Michael Granitzer from the University of Passau, Germany. Part of the presented work was developed within the EEXCESS project funded by the European Union Seventh Framework Programme FP7/2007-2013 under grant agreement number 600601.

# References

1. Holzinger, A., Dehmer, M., Jurisica, I.: Knowledge discovery and interactive data mining in bioinformatics: State-of-the-art, future challenges and research directions. BMC Bioinformatics 15(suppl. 6), I1 (2014)
2. Holzinger, A.: Biomedical Informatics: Discovering Knowledge in Big Data. Springer, New York (2014)
3. Holzinger, A.: On Knowledge Discovery and Interactive Intelligent Visualization of Biomedical Data - Challenges in Human Computer Interaction and Biomedical Informatics, pp. 9–20. INSTICC, Rome (2012)

4. Holzinger, A., Stocker, C., Dehmer, M.: Big complex biomedical data: Towards a taxonomy of data. In: Springer Communications in Computer and Information Science. Springer, Heidelberg (in print, 2014)
5. Resnik, P., Niv, M., Nossal, M., Kapit, A., Toren, R.: Communication of clinically relevant information in electronic health records: a comparison between structured data and unrestricted physician language. In: CAC Proceedings of the Perspectives in Health Information Management (2008)
6. Kreuzthaler, M., Bloice, M., Faulstich, L., Simonic, K., Holzinger, A.: A comparison of different retrieval strategies working on medical free texts. Journal of Universal Computer Science 17(7), 1109–1133 (2011)
7. Holzinger, A., Geierhofer, R., Modritscher, F., Tatzl, R.: Semantic information in medical information systems: Utilization of text mining techniques to analyze medical diagnoses. Journal of Universal Computer Science 14(22), 3781–3795 (2008)
8. Witten, I., Frank, E., Hall, M.: Data Mining: Practical machine learning tools and techniques. Morgan Kaufmann, San Francisco (2011)
9. Verspoor, K., Cohen, K.: Natural language processing. In: Dubitzky, W., Wolkenhauer, O., Cho, K.H., Yokota, H. (eds.) Encyclopedia of Systems Biology, pp. 1495–1498. Springer, Heidelberg (2013)
10. Cohen, K.B., Demner-Fushman, D.: Biomedical Natural Language Processing. John Benjamins (2014)
11. Holzinger, A., Geierhofer, R., Errath, M.: Semantische Informationsextraktion in medizinischen Informationssystemen. Informatik Spektrum 30(2), 69–78 (2007)
12. Kumar, V., Tipney, H. (eds.): Biomedical Literature Mining. Methods in Molecular Biology, vol. 1159. Springer (2014)
13. Seifert, C., Sabol, V., Kienreich, W., Lex, E., Granitzer, M.: Visual analysis and knowledge discovery for text. In: Gkoulalas-Divanis, A., Labbi, A. (eds.) Large Scale Data Analytics, pp. 189–218. Springer (2014)
14. Manning, C.D., Raghavan, P., Schütze, H.: Introduction to Information Retrieval. Cambridge University Press, New York (2008)
15. W3C: HTML5 : a vocabulary and associated APIs for HTML and XHTML (2012)
16. Adobe Systems, I.: Pdf reference, 6th edn., version 1.23. (2006)
17. Liu, H., Christiansen, T., Baumgartner Jr., W.A., Verspoor, K.: BioLemmatizer: a lemmatization tool for morphological processing of biomedical text. Journal of Biomedical Semantics 3(3) (2012)
18. Porter, M.: An algorithm for suffix stripping. Program 14(3), 130–137 (1980)
19. Salton, G., Wong, A., Yang, C.: A vector space model for automatic indexing. Communications of the ACM 18(11), 620 (1975)
20. Boerjesson, E., Hofsten, C.: A vector model for perceived object rotation and translation in space. Psychological Research 38(2), 209–230 (1975)
21. Joachims, T.: Text categorization with suport vector machines: Learning with many relevant features. In: Nédellec, C., Rouveirol, C. (eds.) ECML 1998. LNCS, vol. 1398, pp. 137–142. Springer, Heidelberg (1998)
22. Crouch, C., Crouch, D., Nareddy, K.: Connectionist model for information retrieval based on the vector space model. International Journal of Expert Systems 7(2), 139–163 (1994)
23. Spärk Jones, K., Walker, S., Robertson, S.E.: A probabilistic model of information retrieval: development and comparative experiments. Inf. Process. Manage. 36(6) (2000)

24. Hliaoutakis, A., Varelas, G., Voutsakis, E., Petrakis, E., Milios, E.: Information Retrieval by Semantic Similarity. Intern. Journal on Semantic Web and Information Systems (IJSWIS) 3(3), 55–73 (2006); Special Issue of Multimedia Semantics
25. Hersh, W., Buckley, C., Leone, T.J., Hickam, D.: Ohsumed: An interactive retrieval evaluation and new large test collection for research. In: Proceedings of the 17th Annual International ACM SIGIR Conference on Research and Development in Information Retrieval, SIGIR 1994, pp. 192–201. Springer-Verlag New York, Inc., New York (1994)
26. Müller, H., Michoux, N., Bandon, D., Geissbuhler, A.: A review of content-based image retrieval systems in medical applications - clinical benefits and future directions. International Journal of Medical Informatics 73(1), 1–23 (2003)
27. da Cunha, I., Fernández, S., Velázquez Morales, P., Vivaldi, J., SanJuan, E., Torres-Moreno, J.-M.: A new hybrid summarizer based on vector space model, statistical physics and linguistics. In: Gelbukh, A., Kuri Morales, Á.F. (eds.) MICAI 2007. LNCS (LNAI), vol. 4827, pp. 872–882. Springer, Heidelberg (2007)
28. Liu, G.: Semantic Vector Space Model: Implementation and Evaluation. Journal of the American Society for Information Science 48(5), 395–417 (1997)
29. Bellegarda, J.: Latent semantic mapping (information retrieval). IEEE Signal Processing Magazine 22(5), 70–80 (2005)
30. Landauer, T., Dumais, S.: A solution to Plato's problem: The latent semantic analysis theory of acquisition, induction, and representation of knowledge. Psychological Review 104(2), 211–240 (1997)
31. Landauer, T., Foltz, P., Laham, D.: An introduction to latent semantic analysis. Discourse Processes 25, 259–284 (1998)
32. Foltz, P., Kintsch, W., Landauer, T.: The measurement of textual coherence with latent semantic analysis. Discourse Processes 25, 285–308 (1998)
33. Kintsch, W.: The potential of latent semantic analysis for machine grading of clinical case summaries. Journal of Biomedical Informatics 35(1), 3–7 (2002)
34. Cohen, T., Blatter, B., Patel, V.: Simulating expert clinical comprehension: adapting latent semantic analysis to accurately extract clinical concepts from psychiatric narrative. Journal of Biomedical Informatics 41(6), 1070–1087 (2008)
35. Yeh, J.F., Wu, C.H., Chen, M.J.: Ontology-based speech act identification in a bilingual dialog system using partial pattern trees. J. Am. Soc. Inf. Sci. Technol. 59(5), 684–694 (2008)
36. Ginter, F., Suominen, H., Pyysalo, S., Salakoski, T.: Combining hidden markov models and latent semantic analysis for topic segmentation and labeling: Method and clinical application. I. J. Medical Informatics 78(12), 1–6 (2009)
37. Jonnalagadda, S., Cohen, T., Wu, S., Gonzalez, G.: Enhancing clinical concept extraction with distributional semantics. Journal of biomedical informatics 45(1), 129–140 (2012)
38. Deerwester, S., Dumais, S.T., Furnas, G.W., Landauer, T.K., Harshman, R.: Indexing by latent semantic analysis. Journal of the American Society for Information Science 41(6), 391–407 (1990)
39. Hofmann, T.: Probabilistic latent semantic indexing. In: Proceedings of the 22Nd Annual International ACM SIGIR Conference on Research and Development in Information Retrieval, SIGIR 1999, pp. 50–57. ACM, New York (1999)
40. Papadimitriou, C., Raghavan, P., Tamaki, H., Vempala, S.: Latent semantic indexing: A probabilistic analysis. Journal of Computer and System Sciences 61(2), 217–235 (2000)
41. Hofmann, T.: Unsupervised Learning by Probabilistic Latent Semantic Analysis. Machine Learning 42, 177–196 (2001)

42. Xu, G., Zhang, Y., Zhou, X.: A web recommendation technique based on prob-abilistic latent semantic analysis. In: Ngu, A.H.H., Kitsuregawa, M., Neuhold, E.J., Chung, J.-Y., Sheng, Q.Z. (eds.) WISE 2005. LNCS, vol. 3806, pp. 15–28. Springer, Heidelberg (2005)

43. Si, L., Jin, R.: Adjusting mixture weights of gaussian mixture model via regu-larized probabilistic latent semantic analysis. In: Ho, T.-B., Cheung, D., Liu, H. (eds.) PAKDD 2005. LNCS (LNAI), vol. 3518, pp. 622–631. Springer, Heidelberg (2005)

44. Lin, C., Xue, G., Zeng, H., Yu, Y.: Using Probabilistic Latent Semantic Analysis for Personalized Web Search. In: Zhang, Y., Tanaka, K., Yu, J.X., Wang, S., Li, M. (eds.) APWeb 2005. LNCS, vol. 3399, pp. 707–717. Springer, Heidelberg (2005)

45. Kim, Y.S., Oh, J.S., Lee, J.Y., Chang, J.H.: An intelligent grading system for descriptive examination papers based on probabilistic latent semantic analysis. In: Webb, G.I., Yu, X. (eds.) AI 2004. LNCS (LNAI), vol. 3339, pp. 1141–1146. Springer, Heidelberg (2004)

46. Dempster, A.P., Laird, N.M., Rubin, D.B.: Maximum likelihood from incomplete data via the EM algorithm. Journal of the Royal Statistical Society: Series B 39, 1–38 (1977)

47. Dobrokhotov, P.B., Goutte, C., Veuthey, A.L., Gaussier, R.: Assisting medical an-notation in swiss-prot using statistical classifiers. I. J. Medical Informatics 74(2-4), 317–324 (2005)

48. Srinivas, K., Rao, G., Govardhan, A.: Survey on prediction of heart morbidity using data mining techniques. International Journal of Data Mining & ... 1(3), 14–34 (2011)

49. Lu, Y., Zhang, P., Deng, S.: Exploring Health-Related Topics in Online Health Community Using Cluster Analysis. In: 2013 46th Hawaii International Confer-ence on System Sciences, pp. 802–811 (January 2013)

50. Masseroli, M., Chicco, D., Pinoli, P.: Probabilistic latent semantic analysis for pre-diction of gene ontology annotations. In: The 2012 International Joint Conference on Neural Networks (IJCNN), pp. 1–8 (2012)

51. Koehler, R.: Aspects of Automatic Text Analysis. Springer (2007)

52. Blei, D., Ng, A., Jordan, M.: Latent dirichlet allocation. The Journal of Machine Learning Research 3, 993–1022 (2003)

53. Kakkonen, T., Myller, N., Sutinen, E.: Applying latent Dirichlet allocation to automatic essay grading. In: Salakoski, T., Ginter, F., Pyysalo, S., Pahikkala, T. (eds.) FinTAL 2006. LNCS (LNAI), vol. 4139, pp. 110–120. Springer, Heidelberg (2006)

54. Xing, D., Girolami, M.: Employing latent dirichlet allocation for fraud detection in telecommunications. Pattern Recognition Letters 28(13), 1727–1734 (2007)

55. Girolami, M., Kaban, A.: Sequential activity profiling: Latent Dirichlet allocation of Markov chains. Data Mining and Knowledge Discovery 10(3), 175–196 (2005)

56. Minka, T., Lafferty, J.: Expectation-propagation for the generative aspect model. In: Proceedings of the Eighteenth Conference on Uncertainty in Artificial Intelli-gence, UAI 2002, pp. 352–359. Morgan Kaufmann Publishers Inc., San Francisco (2002)

57. Griffiths, T.L., Steyvers, M.: Finding scientific topics. Proceedings of the National Academy of Sciences 101(suppl. 1), 5228–5235 (2004)

58. Asou, T., Eguchi, K.: Predicting protein-protein relationships from literature us-ing collapsed variational latent dirichlet allocation. In: Proceedings of the 2nd International Workshop on Data and Text Mining in Bioinformatics, DTMBIO 2008, pp. 77–80. ACM, New York (2008)

59. Arnold, C.W., El-Saden, S.M., Bui, A.A.T., Taira, R.: Clinical case-based retrieval using latent topic analysis. In: AMIA Annu. Symp. Proc., vol. 2010, pp. 26–30 (2010)

60. Arnold, C., Speier, W.: A topic model of clinical reports. In: Proceedings of the 35th International ACM SIGIR Conference on Research and Development in Information Retrieval, SIGIR 2012, pp. 1031–1032. ACM, New York (2012)

61. Yao, L., Riedel, S., McCallum, A.: Unsupervised relation discovery with sense disambiguation. In: Proceedings of the 50th Annual Meeting of the Association for Computational Linguistics: Long Papers, ACL 2012, vol. 1, pp. 712–720. Association for Computational Linguistics, Stroudsburg (2012)

62. Dawson, J., Kendziorski, C.: Survival-supervised latent Dirichlet allocation models for genomic analysis of time-to-event outcomes. arXiv preprint arXiv:1202.5999, 1–21 (2012)

63. Hripcsak, G., Albers, D.J.: Next-generation phenotyping of electronic health records. JAMIA 20(1), 117–121 (2013)

64. Blei, D.M., Griffiths, T.L., Jordan, M.I.: The nested chinese restaurant process and bayesian nonparametric inference of topic hierarchies. J. ACM 57(2), 7:1–7:30 (2010)

65. Pitman, J.: Combinatorial stochastic processes. Springer Lecture Notes in Mathematics. Springer (2002); Lectures from the 32nd Summer School on Probability Theory held in Saint-Flour (2002)

66. Saria, S., Koller, D., Penn, A.: Discovering shared and individual latent structure in multiple time series. arXiv preprint arXiv:1008 (d), 1–9 (2028)

67. Bartlett, N., Wood, F., Perotte, A.: Hierarchically Supervised Latent Dirichlet Allocation. In: NIPS, pp. 1–9 (2011)

68. Hotelling, H.: Analysis of a complex of statistical variables into principal components. Journal of Educational Psychology 24(6), 417–441 (1933)

69. Pearson, K.: LIII. On lines and planes of closest fit to systems of points in space. Philosophical Magazine Series 6 2(11), 559–572 (1901)

70. Price, A.L., Patterson, N.J., Plenge, R.M., Weinblatt, M.E., Shadick, N.A., Reich, D.: Principal components analysis corrects for stratification in genome-wide association studies. Nat. Genet. 38(8), 904–909 (2006)

71. Robertson, M.M., Althoff, R.R., Hafez, A., Pauls, D.L.: Principal components analysis of a large cohort with Tourette syndrome. The British Journal of Psychiatry: the Journal of Mental Science 193(1), 31–36 (2008)

72. Himmel, W., Reincke, U., Michelmann, H.W.: Text mining and natural language processing approaches for automatic categorization of lay requests to web-based expert forums. Journal of Medical Internet Research 11(3), e25 (2009)

73. Oprea, T., Nielsen, S., Ursu, O.: Associating Drugs, Targets and Clinical Outcomes into an Integrated Network Affords a New Platform for Computer Aided Drug Repurposing. Molecular Informatics 30, 100–111 (2011)

74. Schölkopf, B., Smola, A., Müller, K.R.: Kernel principal component analysis. In: Gerstner, W., Hasler, M., Germond, A., Nicoud, J.-D. (eds.) ICANN 1997. LNCS, vol. 1327, pp. 583–588. Springer, Heidelberg (1997)

75. Cortes, C., Vapnik, V.: Support-vector networks. Mach. Learn. 20(3), 273–297 (1995)

76. Ben-Hur, A., Weston, J.: A user's guide to support vector machines. In: Carugo, O., Eisenhaber, F. (eds.) Data Mining Techniques for the Life Sciences. Methods in Molecular Biology, vol. 609, pp. 223–239. Humana Press (2010)

77. Crammer, K., Singer, Y.: On the algorithmic implementation of multiclass kernel-based vector machines. J. Mach. Learn. Res. 2, 265–292 (2002)

78. Guyon, I., Weston, J., Barnhill, S., Vapnik, V.: Gene selection for cancer classification using support vector machines. Mach. Learn. 46(1-3), 389–422 (2002)
79. Ghanem, M., Guo, Y., Lodhi, H., Zhang, Y.: Automatic scientific text classification using local patterns: Kdd cup 2002 (task 1). SIGKDD Explorations 4(2), 95–96 (2002)
80. Donaldson, I.M., Martin, J.D., de Bruijn, B., Wolting, C., Lay, V., Tuekam, B., Zhang, S., Baskin, B., Bader, G.D., Michalickova, K., Pawson, T., Hogue, C.W.V.: Prebind and textomy - mining the biomedical literature for protein-protein interactions using a support vector machine. BMC Bioinformatics 4, 11 (2003)
81. Eskin, E., Agichtein, E.: Combining text mining and sequence analysis to discover protein functional regions. In: Altman, R.B., Dunker, A.K., Hunter, L., Jung, T.A., Klein, T.E. (eds.) Pacific Symposium on Biocomputing, pp. 288–299. World Scientific (2004)
82. Joshi, M., Pedersen, T., Maclin, R.: A comparative study of support vector machines applied to the supervised word sense disambiguation problem in the medical domain. In: Prasad, B. (ed.) IICAI, pp. 3449–3468 (2005)
83. Uzuner, Z., Bodnari, A., Shen, S., Forbush, T., Pestian, J., South, B.R.: Evaluating the state of the art in coreference resolution for electronic medical records. JAMIA 19(5), 786–791 (2012)
84. Domingos, P., Pazzani, M.: On the optimality of the simple bayesian classifier under zero-one loss. Mach. Learn. 29(2-3), 103–130 (1997)
85. Quinlan, J.R.: C4.5: Programs for Machine Learning. Morgan Kaufmann Publishers Inc., San Francisco (1993)
86. Kim, J.D., Pyysalo, S.: Bionlp shared task. In: Dubitzky, W., Wolkenhauer, O., Cho, K.H., Yokota, H. (eds.) Encyclopedia of Systems Biology, pp. 138–141. Springer, New York (2013)
87. Arighi, C., Lu, Z., Krallinger, M., Cohen, K., Wilbur, W., Valencia, A., Hirschman, L., Wu, C.: Overview of the biocreative iii workshop. BMC Bioinformatics 12(suppl. 8), S1 (2011)
88. Hersh, W., Voorhees, E.: Trec genomics special issue overview. Information Retrieval 12(1), 1–15 (2009)
89. Kim, J.D., Ohta, T., Tateisi, Y., Tsujii, J.: Genia corpus: a semantically annotated corpus for bio-textmining. Bioinformatics 19(suppl. 1), i180–i182 (2003)
90. Bada, M., Eckert, M., Evans, D., Garcia, K., Shipley, K., Sitnikov, D., Baumgartner, W., Cohen, K., Verspoor, K., Blake, J., Hunter, L.: Concept annotation in the CRAFT corpus. BMC Bioinformatics 13(161) (2012)
91. Verspoor, K., Cohen, K., Lanfranchi, A., Warner, C., Johnson, H., Roeder, C., Choi, J., Funk, C., Malenkiy, Y., Eckert, M., Xue, N., Baumgartner, W., Bada, M., Palmer, M., Hunter, L.: A corpus of full-text journal articles is a robust evaluation tool for revealing differences in performance of biomedical natural language processing tools. BMC Bioinformatics 13, 207 (2012)
92. Klinger, R., Kolik, C., Fluck, J., Hofmann-Apitius, M., Friedrich, C.M.: Detection of iupac and iupac-like chemical names. Bioinformatics 24(13), i268–i276 (2008)
93. Verspoor, K., Jimeno Yepes, A., Cavedon, L., McIntosh, T., Herten-Crabb, A., Thomas, Z., Plazzer, J.P.: Annotating the biomedical literature for the human variome. Database 2013 (2013)
94. Voorhees, E., Tong, R.: Overview of the trec 2011 medical records track. In: Proceedings of the Text Retrieval Conference (2011)
95. Uzuner, O.: Second i2b2 workshop on natural language processing challenges for clinical records. In: Proceedings of the American Medical Informatics Association Annual Symposium, pp. 1252–1253 (2008)

96. Sun, W., Rumshisky, A., Uzuner, O.: Evaluating temporal relations in clinical text: 2012 i2b2 challenge. Journal of the American Medical Informatics Association 20(5), 806–813 (2013)

97. Suominen, H., et al.: Overview of the share/clef ehealth evaluation lab 2013. In: Forner, P., Müller, H., Paredes, R., Rosso, P., Stein, B. (eds.) CLEF 2013. LNCS, vol. 8138, pp. 212–231. Springer, Heidelberg (2013)

98. Cohen, A.M., Hersh, W.R.: A survey of current work in biomedical text mining. Briefings in Bioinformatics 6(1), 57–71 (2005)

99. Hirschman, L., Burns, G.A.P.C., Krallinger, M., Arighi, C., Cohen, K.B., Valencia, A., Wu, C.H., Chatr-Aryamontri, A., Dowell, K.G., Huala, E., Loureno, A., Nash, R., Veuthey, A.L., Wiegers, T., Winter, A.G.: Text mining for the biocuration workflow. Database 2012 (2012)

100. Ananiadou, S., Rea, B., Okazaki, N., Procter, R., Thomas, J.: Supporting systematic reviews using text mining. Social Science Computer Review 27(4), 509–523 (2009)

101. Dai, H.J., Chang, Y.C., Tsai, R.T.H., Hsu, W.L.: New challenges for biological text-mining in the next decade. J. Comput. Sci. Technol. 25(1), 169–179 (2009)

102. Tan, A.H.: Text mining: The state of the art and the challenges. In: Proceedings of the Pacific Asia Conf on Knowledge Discovery and Data Mining PAKDD 1999, Workshop on Knowledge Discovery from Advanced Databases, KDAD 1999, pp. 65–70 (1999)

103. Carrero, F., Cortizo, J., Gomez, J.: Testing concept indexing in crosslingual medical text classification. In: Third International Conference on Digital Information Management, ICDIM 2008, pp. 512–519 (November 2008)

104. Allvin, H., Carlsson, E., Dalianis, H., Danielsson-Ojala, R., Daudaravičius, V., Hassel, M., Kokkinakis, D., Lundgren-Laine, H., Nilsson, G., Nytrø, O., Salanterä, S., Skeppstedt, M., Suominen, H., Velupillai, S.: Characteristics and analysis of finnish and swedish clinical intensive care nursing narratives. In: Proceedings of the NAACL HLT 2010 Second Louhi Workshop on Text and Data Mining of Health Documents, Louhi 2010, pp. 53–60. Association for Computational Linguistics, Stroudsburg (2010)

105. Patrick, J., Sabbagh, M., Jain, S., Zheng, H.: Spelling correction in clinical notes with emphasis on first suggestion accuracy. In: 2nd Workshop on Building and Evaluating Resources for Biomedical Text Mining, pp. 2–8 (2010)

106. Holzinger, A., Yildirim, P., Geier, M., Simonic, K.M.: Quality-based knowledge discovery from medical text on the web. In: Pasi, G., Bordogna, G., Jain, L.C. (eds.) Quality Issues in the Management of Web Information, Intelligent Systems Reference Library. ISRL, vol. 50, pp. 145–158. Springer, Heidelberg (2013)

107. Wong, W., Martinez, D., Cavedon, L.: Extraction of named entities from tables in gene mutation literature. In: BioNLP 2009, p. 46 (2009)

108. Limaye, G., Sarawagi, S., Chakrabarti, S.: Annotating and searching web tables using entities, types and relationships. In: Proc. VLDB Endow., vol. 3(1-2), pp. 1338–1347 (September 2010)

109. Quercini, G., Reynaud, C.: Entity discovery and annotation in tables. In: Proceedings of the 16th International Conference on Extending Database Technology, EDBT 2013, pp. 693–704. ACM, New York (2013)

110. Zwicklbauer, S., Einsiedler, C., Granitzer, M., Seifert, C.: Towards disambiguating web tables. In: International Semantic Web Conference (Posters & Demos), pp. 205–208 (2013)

111. Jimeno Yepes, A., Verspoor, K.: Literature mining of genetic variants for curation: Quantifying the importance of supplementary material. Database: The Journal of Biological Databases and Curation 2013 (2013)

112. Liu, H., Johnson, S.B., Friedman, C.: Automatic Resolution of Ambiguous Terms Based on Machine Learning and Conceptual Relations in the UMLS. Journal of the American Medical Informatics Association 9(6), 621–636 (2002)

113. Aronson, A.R., Lang, F.M.: An overview of metamap: historical perspective and recent advances. Journal of the American Medical Informatics Association 17(3), 229–236 (2010)

114. Lu, Z., Kao, H.Y., Wei, C.H., Huang, M., Liu, J., Kuo, C.J., Hsu, C.N., Tsai, R., Dai, H.J., Okazaki, N., Cho, H.C., Gerner, M., Solt, I., Agarwal, S., Liu, F., Vishnyakova, D., Ruch, P., Romacker, M., Rinaldi, F., Bhattacharya, S., Srinivasan, P., Liu, H., Torii, M., Matos, S., Campos, D., Verspoor, K., Livingston, K., Wilbur, W.: The gene normalization task in biocreative iii. BMC Bioinformatics 12(suppl. 8), S2 (2011)

115. Zwicklbauer, S., Seifert, C., Granitzer, M.: Do we need entity-centric knowledge bases for entity disambiguation? In: Proceedings of the 13th International Conference on Knowledge Management and Knowledge Technologies, I-Know (2013)

116. Ogren, P.V.: Improving syntactic coordination resolution using language modeling. In: Proceedings of the NAACL HLT 2010 Student Research Workshop, HLT-SRWS 2010, pp. 1–6. Association for Computational Linguistics, Stroudsburg (2010)

117. Chae, J., Jung, Y., Lee, T., Jung, S., Huh, C., Kim, G., Kim, H., Oh, H.: Identifying non-elliptical entity mentions in a coordinated {NP} with ellipses. Journal of Biomedical Informatics 47, 139–152 (2014)

118. Gasperin, C., Briscoe, T.: Statistical anaphora resolution in biomedical texts. In: Proceedings of the 22nd International Conference on Computational Linguistics, COLING 2008, vol. 1, pp. 257–264. Association for Computational Linguistics, Stroudsburg (2008)

119. Jonnalagadda, S.R., Li, D., Sohn, S., Wu, S.T.I., Wagholikar, K., Torii, M., Liu, H.: Coreference analysis in clinical notes: a multi-pass sieve with alternate anaphora resolution modules. Journal of the American Medical Informatics Association 19(5), 867–874 (2012)

120. Kim, J.D., Nguyen, N., Wang, Y., Tsujii, J., Takagi, T., Yonezawa, A.: The genia event and protein coreference tasks of the bionlp shared task 2011. BMC Bioinformatics 13(suppl. 11), S1 (2012)

121. Yildirim, P., Ekmekci, I.O., Holzinger, A.: On knowledge discovery in open medical data on the example of the fda drug adverse event reporting system for alendronate (fosamax). In: Holzinger, A., Pasi, G. (eds.) HCI-KDD 2013. LNCS, vol. 7947, pp. 195–206. Springer, Heidelberg (2013)

122. Holzinger, A.: On topological data mining. In: Holzinger, A., Jurisica, I. (eds.) Knowledge Discovery and Data Mining. LNCS, vol. 8401, pp. 333–358. Springer, Heidelberg (2014)

123. Holzinger, K., Palade, V., Rabadan, R., Holzinger, A.: Darwin or lamarck? future challenges in evolutionary algorithms for knowledge discovery and data mining. In: Holzinger, A., Jurisica, I. (eds.) Knowledge Discovery and Data Mining. LNCS, vol. 8401, pp. 35–56. Springer, Heidelberg (2014)

124. Mukherjee, I., Al-Fayoumi, M., Mahanti, P., Jha, R., Al-Bidewi, I.: Content analysis based on text mining using genetic algorithm. In: 2nd International Conference on Computer Technology and Development (ICCTD), pp. 432–436. IEEE (2010)

125. Petz, G., Karpowicz, M., Fürschuß, H., Auinger, A., Stříteský, V., Holzinger, A.: Opinion mining on the web 2.0 – characteristics of user generated content and their impacts. In: Holzinger, A., Pasi, G. (eds.) HCI-KDD 2013. LNCS, vol. 7947, pp. 35–46. Springer, Heidelberg (2013)
126. Corley, C.D., Cook, D.J., Mikler, A.R., Singh, K.P.: Text and structural data mining of influenza mentions in Web and social media. International Journal of Environmental Research and Public Health 7(2), 596–615 (2010)
127. White, R.W., Tatonetti, N.P., Shah, N.H., Altman, R.B., Horvitz, E.: Web-scale pharmacovigilance: listening to signals from the crowd. Journal of the American Medical Informatics Association (2013)
128. Wu, H., Fang, H., Stanhope, S.J.: Exploiting online discussions to discover unrecognized drug side effects. Methods of Information in Medicine 52(2), 152–159 (2013)
129. Yildirim, P., Majnaric, L., Ekmekci, O., Holzinger, A.: Knowledge discovery of drug data on the example of adverse reaction prediction. BMC Bioinformatics 15(suppl. 6), S7 (2014)
130. Holzinger, A., Jurisica, I.: Knowledge discovery and data mining in biomedical informatics: The future is in integrative, interactive machine learning solutions. In: Holzinger, A., Jurisica, I. (eds.) Knowledge Discovery and Data Mining. LNCS, vol. 8401, pp. 1–18. Springer, Heidelberg (2014)
131. Holzinger, A., Stocker, C., Ofner, B., Prohaska, G., Brabenetz, A., Hofmann-Wellenhof, R.: Combining hci, natural language processing, and knowledge discovery - potential of ibm content analytics as an assistive technology in the biomedical domain. In: Holzinger, A., Pasi, G. (eds.) HCI-KDD 2013. LNCS, vol. 7947, pp. 13–24. Springer, Heidelberg (2013)

# Protecting Anonymity
# in Data-Driven Biomedical Science

Peter Kieseberg[1,2], Heidelinde Hobel[1], Sebastian Schrittwieser[3],
Edgar Weippl[1], and Andreas Holzinger[2]

[1] Secure Business Austria Research
[2] Research Unit HCI, Institute for Medical Informatics, Statistics & Documentation,
Medical University Graz
[3] University of Applied Sciences St. Pölten
{firstletteroffirstname,lastname}@sba-research.org,
andreas.holzinger@medunigraz.at
sebastian.schrittwieser@fhstp.ac.at

**Abstract.** With formidable recent improvements in data processing and
information retrieval, knowledge discovery/data mining, business intelligence, content analytics and other upcoming empirical approaches have
an enormous potential, particularly for the data intensive biomedical sciences. For results derived using empirical methods, the underlying data
set should be made available, at least during the review process for the
reviewers, to ensure the quality of the research done and to prevent fraud
or errors and to enable the replication of studies. However, in particular in the medicine and the life sciences, this leads to a discrepancy, as
the disclosure of research data raises considerable privacy concerns, as researchers have of course the full responsibility to protect their (volunteer)
subjects, hence must adhere to respective ethical policies. One solution
for this problem lies in the protection of sensitive information in medical
data sets by applying appropriate anonymization. This paper provides
an overview on the most important and well-researched approaches and
discusses open research problems in this area, with the goal to act as a
starting point for further investigation.

**Keywords:** Anonymization, pseudonymization, data-driven sciences, big
data, privacy, security, safety.

# 1 Introduction

New and advanced methods in statistical analysis and rapidly emerging technological improvements, e.g., in computation performance, data storage, cloud
computing and technologies that support worldwide collaborative work, have
laid the foundation for a new field of science that we call *data-driven sciences.*
In particular biomedical informatics is becoming such a data-driven science due
to the increasing trend toward personalized and precision medicine [1], [2], [3].
A recent example can be found in [4].

A. Holzinger, I. Jurisica (Eds.): Knowledge Discovery and Data Mining, LNCS 8401, pp. 301–316, 2014.
© Springer-Verlag Berlin Heidelberg 2014

Data-driven science uses these new resources to analyze enormous data sets, often called *big data* [5], and reasons based on the empirical findings and evidence from these analyses. The sources of big data can extremely vary, ranging from data gathered online from open sources to data sets provided by research partners, companies or volunteers, or coming from the own laboratories or hospitals; in the medical domain data can come from clinical patient treatment and/or from biomedical research, from hospital sources or from biobanks. The size and complexity of the data sets allows a large variety of inferences to be made, which makes big data very useful for research but can, at the same time, potentially be exploited to extract information that could be used in malicious ways or that might infringe on the privacy of the data subjects [6]. This especially concerns data-driven science in the medical sector, since, as a principle, most data in this field is sensitive and issues of privacy, security, safety and data protection are always an issue [7]. Even when access to the data is limited to a specific researcher or a research team  whose members might be from different organizations or universities  there is a high risk of disclosure. The more people have access to classified information, the higher the risk of it being exploited for malicious purposes.

However, research, particularly non-commercial research, is usually intended - or should be intended - for public dissemination through conferences or journals [8]. The peer-review procedure normally ensures the quality of such research, but without access to the underlying data, work in the field of data-driven medical science cannot be validated by reviewers. The result is an extremely problematic situation where authors either include the data only in a condensed or abstracted form, which protects privacy but means has the drawback the reader cannot validate the results or evaluate the data for a personal learning effect, or publish the data, even if only for the duration of the review process and with restricted access. The former solution is problematic in that the research cannot be properly reviewed, which results in chances for fraud and poor research, especially in the "publish or perish" atmosphere of pressure to publish frequently to gain the recognition of the academic field or funding institutions.

Furthermore, even in the absence of fraud, missing data can make perfectly valid results look debatable. The latter solution, while mitigating these problems, exposes data sets to potential misuse. Furthermore, especially regarding data-driven research in medical sciences, the publication of the raw data will most certainly result in legal issues. Recently, there is a strong movement towards the promotion of open data sets in biomedical research [9], but what to do in case the data *cannot* be made openly available?

We address the question of how to utilize and share research data without exposing it to risks by providing an overview on the latest anonymization and pseudonymization techniques, following previous work [10] and especially considering the biomedical sector. Furthermore, we will give an overview on open questions, again especially targeting this sensitive field of information processing.

## 2   Glossary and Key Terms

This section shall define the most important or ambiguous terms used in the paper to avoid any danger of misinterpretation and to ensure a common understanding.

**Anatomization:** An operation for achieving anonymization, this works by splitting the attributes of table records into QIs and sensitive columns which are stored in separate tables. Then the linking between the two tables in made ambiguous for providing anonymity (see Section 5.1).

**Anonymization:** A term denoting the removal of personal information from data including the ability to link the data to persons by utilizing characteristics.

**Big Data:** While this term is currently very popular, there exists no exact definition for it. Usually it is used to either describe the processing of large amounts of data, or as a paradigm for data processing, where information from several sources is mashed up in order to generate additional knowledge.

**Business Intelligence (BI):** This term describes a selection of methodologies, technologies and architectures for harvesting information relevant for business from raw data.

**Data Linkage:** The effort of constructing relationships between sensitive published data and data that is public or easily accessible for attackers is called *data linkage.*

**Data Precision Metric (DPM):** Metric or norm for measuring the information loss due to techniques for anonymization. Usually used in the context of *generalization.*

**Generalization:** This method replaces sensitive values with more general ones by grouping values in an interval or by using taxonomies and replacing the values with parent nodes, thus reducing the granularity of quasi identifiers (see Section 5.1).

**Identifier:** An attribute that uniquely identifies a person.

**$k$-anonymity:** A paradigm for anonymization. A more detailed description is given in Section 5.2.

**$l$-diversity:** This is an extension of the $k$-anonymity paradigm incorporating diversity into the equivalence classes (see Section 5.3).

**Permutation:** A concept similar to anatomization, this operation also splits records into QIs and sensitive attributes, stores them in different tables and makes the linkage ambiguous (see Section 5.1).

**Perturbation:** Distortion of data using mechanisms like adding noise or the introduction of synthetic values, further details can be found in Section 5.1.

**Pseudonymization:** Every identifier and all relevant quasi identifiers are exchanged for pseudonyms in order to cover the identity of the persons in questions.

**Quasi Identifier:** This are attributes which are not directly identifiers, but can be used in combination to identify persons.

**Rule Mining:** This keyword covers a multitude of techniques for the automatic extraction of rules in (often large) data sets. It constitutes an important set of techniques in the area of machine learning.

**Structured Data:** In general, a representation of information that is following fixed rules. Usually used for tables or structured file formats like XML.

**Suppression:** Single data elements, e.g. rows in a table, are removed from the set in order to get a higher level of anonymization. This technique is often used in order to achieve $k$-anonymity or related concepts, see Section 5.1.

**$t$-closeness:** An extension of $l$-diversity that is secure against skewness attacks, see Section 5.4.

## 3    Background

In [11–16] the authors claim that data-driven research is a paradigm that is constantly gaining popularity in most research areas. The term "big data" originated in the IT sector, where large data samples had to be analyzed, usually in order to evaluate proposed algorithms or prototypes, especially with regard to practical applicability and performance issues. They can also be analyzed to derive new empirical findings concerning general trends and characteristics. Health data publishing is a prime example of an area where sensitive data must be protected from leaking into the public [17, 18]. This field has shown that not only direct identifiers, such as social security numbers, can contribute to the threat of a privacy breach, but also so-called quasi-identifiers (QI), e.g., the triple ZIP-code, birth date and gender. It was shown in [17, 18] that this data triple alone allows the unambiguous identification of roughly 80% of the American citizens, resulting that private data, such as illnesses or treatment, can be inferred about them and used for malicious purposes. The effort of constructing relationships between sensitive published data and data that is public or easily accessible for attackers is called *data linkage* [19]. This is not only an issue in health care, either. For example, Dey et al. [13] analyzed approx. 1,400,000 Facebook account settings to infer privacy trends for several personal attributes. Although they used public accounts for their research, their results combined with the data they measured and recorded are highly sensitive and should not be published without applying appropriate anonymization or pseudonymization techniques. We, as researchers, are responsible for protecting the data we use and for preserving the privacy of our subjects, who are often volunteers. This protection includes ensuring the unlinkability of sensitive data so that data sets can be published to allow the validation of research, collaboration between several research groups, and learning by enabling the reader to repeat the described data analysis.

## 4    Privacy Threats in Data-Driven Science

The set of attributes that comprise research data can usually be divided into several categories: Identifiers, quasi identifiers, as well as sensitive and non-sensitive attributes and inferred knowledge obtained during research.

*Identifiers* are attributes that more or less uniquely identify a person. Typically, names are considered to be identifiers, even though they rarely "uniquely identify" a person in general (many popular names do not even uniquely identify a person in a small city), as well as addresses. While this definition does lack mathematical rigour, in general there is no big dispute on what is considered to be an identifier. Still, especially in medical data-driven research, we do see a problem with this definition when it comes to genome data, which should be classified as an identifier in our opinion. Considering the above-mentioned Facebook example, we assume that each data record comprising all required data of an account has been classified according to predefined privacy categories. This categorizes the links to the accounts into the *identifier*-category, which has to be removed before publishing.

*Quasi-Identifiers (QIs)* are a category initially proposed by Dalenius in [20] that includes all attributes that either themselves or in combination could also be used to identify persons. While this definition explicitly includes the identifier-category, these attributes are often removed in current literature, reducing this category to the set of attributes that do not uniquely identify a person themselves, but can pose a danger to privacy if combined with other quasi-identifiers. Common examples for QIs include birthdates or ZIP-codes.

*Inference Attacks* describe attacks, where background knowledge, a-priori-knowledge or public data sets are used to identify data record owners. This type of attacks is also called *linkage attacks*. In the Facebook example, identifying a person behind an account by mapping data derived from the list of friends to other sources, e.g. students-lists of universities, would result in an inference attack. Commonly, linkage attacks are categorized in four different types: Record linkage, attribute linkage, table linkage and probabilistic attacks [19]. In a *record linkage* attack, the QI is linked directly with additional information, as in the Facebook example described above. *Attribute linkage* looks for a correlation of QIs and inferred knowledge. For example, if an attacker knows a given individual is in a certain equivalence group, they can easily identify that persons sensitive attribute. *Table linkage* attacks determine the presence or absence of the record owner, while *probabilistic attacks* refer to the threat of a change in the general probabilistic belief of the attacker after seeing the published data.

In privacy-preserving data publishing, the identity of the record owners is usually hidden using anonymization [21] of the quasi-identifiers to prevent linkage without major information loss. There exist a number of ways in which data can be anonymized. The simplest method is the removal of attributes (quasi-identifiers) before publication in order to increase the difficulty of correctly re-identifying the individual. However, this can prevent the validation of the research method if the removed attributes influence the inferred knowledge. Additionally, the general objective of data-driven science is to find comprehensive knowledge, which means that a change in the "probabilistic belief" of an attacker is unavoidable. It can also be difficult to identify all attributes that constitute QIs, rendering anonymization efforts incomplete and, in the worst case, ineffectual.

Another closely related problem results from the new "Big Data" paradigm, where massive amounts of data from various sources are combined in order to mine correlations and/or derive rules. This is especially sensitive in case of open data initiatives, where data vaults are opened for the public and data from various sources can be combined through mashups, without prior verification of the resulting combination's sensitivity. A more detailed explanation of the inherent problems of this approach, together with a concept solution can be found in [22].

## 5   Anonymization Concepts

In this chapter we will discuss a selection of operations that can be used for achieving anonymization, followed by a selection of the most popular and well-researched models for defining anonymity.

### 5.1   Anonymization Operations

Methods of anonymization often relate to the removal or replacement of quasi-identifiers, making the relationship between QIs and sensitive values or inferred knowledge ambiguous, and distorte the data. Fung et al. [19] provided a survey on state-of-the-art anonymization techniques, which can be divided into the following categories: Suppression, generalization, anatomization, permutation and perturbation.

*Suppression* is the removal or replacement of data tuples, e.g. rows of a table, before publishing. While being the most basic method, it can help yielding good results and is often used together with generalization for achieving *k*-anonymity. Still, the removal of data rows may lead to a drastic change in the significance of the underlying data, especially when studying rare diseases. Thus, this method must be selected with great care and it must be made sure that the removed values do not change the distribution of relevant attributes significantly. Besides this basic definition of suppression, also called *Record Suppression*, that relies on the removal of whole records, some modified approaches have been proposed: Sometimes it is needed to suppress every appearance of a given value in a table (see [23]) or suppressing single cells (see [24]).

*Generalization* also replaces values, but seeks to preserve as much information as possible while meeting the requirements of the chosen privacy model. This method replaces sensitive values with more general ones by grouping values in an interval or by using taxonomies and replacing the values with parent nodes, e.g. classifying a date such as 01.01.1999 in the interval [1990 − 1999] or generalizing "Jane Doe" as "female". Figure 1 shows two possible generalization strategies for different kinds of attributes. The actual information loss is measured using so-called *Data Precision Metrics (DMPs)*[1]. While suppression is applied to single

---

[1] Despite the terminology, most DPMs are not metrics in a mathematical sense.

data elements (i.e. table rows), generalization affects entire attribute classes (i.e. table columns). In general, generalization is the method most often found in the literature on anonymization strategies. Still, there exist several extensions of this concept, e.g. *cell generalization* as introduced by LeFevre et. al. in [25] or *multi-dimensional generalization* (see [26, 27]).

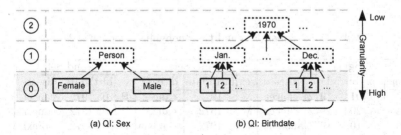

**Fig. 1.** Generalization of quasi-identifiers

*Anatomization* makes the relationship between QIs and inferred knowledge ambiguous by grouping, thereby solving the problem illustrated in Table 2. This works by splitting the quasi identifiers and the sensitive attributes into two tables $T_Q$, holding the quasi-identifiers, and $T_S$, containing the sensitive values, while adding a shared attribute *id* to both. Now the quasi identifiers are generalized in a way to make the linking between the two tables ambiguous - each characteristic of the sensitive data should then be linkable to each of the $l$ classes of quasi identifiers, where $l$ is a fixed threshold that determines the level of unlinkability. The main advantage of this concept is that the table holding the sensitive values can remain far more detailed compared to a pure generalization based approach, thus making them more valuable for statistic analysis.

*Permutation* is a concept rather similar to anatomization. It also relies on ambiguity, shuffling inferred knowledge tuples into predefined and generalized groups in a way that does not affect statistical evaluation, so that the results are the same before and after the permutation process.

*Perturbation* distorts data using different techniques, such as adding noise, swapping values or using synthetic values to replace real ones. Many of these methods can be seen as some kind of dual strategy to suppression. While the latter tries to achieve anonymization by removing records from the data set, many perturbation methods add new records. One advantage of many perturbation methods lies in the preservation of statistical information [19], especially when considering techniques that exchange real data for synthetic values, however, especially when searching for unexpected correlations e.g. by applying rule-mining, perturbation may influence the result.

## 5.2  k-anonymity

The anonymization concept called $k$-anonymity with its special consideration of quasi-identifiers was first introduced by Sweeney in [17]. She showed that it was possible to identify individuals even after uniquely identifying attributes such as the name or social security number were removed from health records by linking attributes such as ZIP code, birthdate, and sex.

**Table 1.** Original data and two anonymized sets ($k = 2$)

| Original data | | | | First Set | | | Second Set | | |
|------|-----|-----------|----------|-----|----------|----------|-----|----------|----------|
| name | sex | birthdate | disease  | sex | birthdate | disease | sex | birthdate | disease |
| Bill | m | 01.05.1972 | cancer   | M | 1972 | cancer   | P | 03.1972 | cancer   |
| Dan  | m | 20.05.1972 | cancer   | M | 1972 | cancer   | P | 03.1972 | cancer   |
| Anne | f | 10.03.1972 | anorexia | F | 1972 | anorexia | P | 04.1972 | anorexia |
| Jill | f | 31.03.1972 | typhlitis | F | 1972 | typhlitis | P | 04.1972 | typhlitis |

The criterion of $k$-anonymity is satisfied if each record is indistinguishable from at least $k-1$ other records with respect to the QIs. This means that quasi-identifying attributes must have the same values within a so-called equivalence class (which contains a minimum of $k$ records), so that it is no longer possible to uniquely link an individual to a specific record in that class. This criterion can, e.g., be achieved by generalizing data of quasi-identifiers, such as generalizing the birthdate attribute by giving only the month and the year, or even just the year or decade. High levels of anonymity are possible with this method by raising the value of the threshold $k$, but lower anonymity levels are often necessary to preserve the significance of the data.

Today, $k$-anonymity is a widely adopted anonymization method. Over the past years, several improvements have been proposed that introduce new, stricter criteria for $k$-anonymity, but do not replace the original idea.

## 5.3  l-diversity

Table 2 illustrates a major limitation of $k$-anonymity. In this example ($k = 3$), there are three male patients who were all born in 1972. The original $k$-anonymity algorithm creates an equivalence class for these three records to fulfill the $k = 3$ criterion, making them indistinguishable from each other with respect to the quasi-identifiers. The problem here, however, is that the sensitive attribute (disease) is identical for all three, which effectively negates the anonymization effort. If the sensitive attributes in an equivalence class lack diversity, $k$-anonymity cannot ensure privacy. This problem can be countered with $l$-diversity, which requires each equivalence class to have at least $l$ well-represented values for each sensitive attribute [28].

The definition of "well-represented" depends on the actual data. There are five different approaches, of which the most basic, "entropy $l$-diversity", requires each

**Table 2.** Original data and two anonymized sets ($k = 2$)

| Original data | | | | $k$-anonymity | | |
|---|---|---|---|---|---|---|
| name | sex | birthdate | disease | sex | birthdate | disease |
| Bill | m | 01.05.1974 | cancer | M | 1974 | cancer |
| Dan | m | 20.05.1974 | cancer | M | 1974 | cancer |
| Anne | f | 10.03.1972 | anorexia | F | 1972 | anorexia |
| Jill | f | 31.03.1972 | typhlitis | F | 1972 | typhlitis |
| William | m | 10.12.1974 | cancer | M | 1974 | cancer |
| Mary | f | 12.12.1973 | short breath | F | 1972 | short breath |

equivalence class to include at least $l$ different values for the sensitive attributes. Table 2 shows an example for data obeying entropy-$l$-diversity. To achieve higher levels of entropy diversity, the quasi-identifiers must be further generalized . The main problem of $l$-diversity is that it only prevents unique matching of an individual to a sensitive value while ignoring the overall distribution of sensitive values. This makes statistical analysis of equivalence classes possible (skewness attack): Consider a microdata set anonymized with entropy-2-diversity that has an equivalence class containing a sensitive attribute that applies only to a very small percentage (e.g., 1%) of a countrys population, e.g. a rare disease. The probability of a specific individual in this equivalence class suffering from this rare disease is up to 50%, which is much higher than the actual probability within the entire population.

### 5.4 $t$-closeness

The concept of $t$-closeness was developed as an improvement to $k$-anonymity and $l$-diversity in order to mitigate above mentioned skewness attacks. The basic principle lies in choosing the equivalence classes in a way that the distribution of any sensitive attribute in any class is similar to its distribution in the original table [29]. More precisely, let $D_{all}$ be the distribution of a sensitive attribute in the original table holding all data records and $D_i$ be the distribution of that same attribute in the $i^{th}$ equivalence class, for all classes $i = 1 \ldots n$ as defined in the $k$-anonymity paradigm. Then these equivalence classes are obeying the $t$-closeness criteria for a given value $t$ if and only if the the distance between $D_{all}$ and $D_i$ is at most $t, \forall i = 1 \ldots n$. However, the main questions is, how to measure this distance between equivalence classes, while including the semantic distance between values. The solution is the so-called *Earth Mover Distance EMD* as defined in [29].

The $t$-closeness paradigm has some drawbacks tough: (i) The first and most important drawback considers the impact of enforcing $t$-closeness on the data set: When assuming $t$-closeness, the sensitive values will have the same distribution in all equivalence classes with respect to the quasi identifiers, thus having a significant impact on the correlation between these attributes and the QIs. Since a lot of research in medical data-driven science is actually targeting at such correlations, $t$-closeness remains unusable in these cases. (ii) Another drawback is that $t$-closeness lacks the ability to specify separate protection levels for each quasi identifier. Furthermore, (iii) there still exist special attribute linkage attacks on $t$-closeness when utilizing it on sensitive numerical attributes as shown in [30].

## 5.5    Pseudonymization

Pseudonymization is a method related to anonymization that combines the advantages of anonymization and transparency for the publisher [21]. It is frequently employed in research that uses medical records and has the advantage of making it possible to reverse the anonymization process if necessary, e.g. for health care reasons. For example, in [31], pseudonyms are used to implement the link between individual and sensitive data, in this case medical health records. Cryptographic keys ensure that only authorized persons can re-identify the links. Related approaches can also be found in [32] and [33]. In [34], two solutions for protecting sensitive radiology data through pseudonymization are discussed: In the first approach the unique patient identification numbers are exchanged for reversible pseudonyms by using hashing and encryption techniques, the second one works by applying irreversible one-way pseudonyms. Both solutions lead to pseudonymized health records that can be used for research purposes while ensuring patient privacy.

# 6    Open Problems and Future Trends

Over the last years, a strong trend towards data-driven research methods has emerged in medical science. Results from the analysis of these data sets are improving constantly, which leads to the conclusion that data-driven research approaches will gain even more attention over the next years. For handling medical data there exist clear regulatory frameworks, e.g. the Health Insurance Portability and Accountability Act (HIPAA), which defines to what extent information can be released to third parties and forbids the disclosure of "individually identifiable health information". As medical data is complex and inhomogeneous, there exist many different potential anonymization approaches, while ongoing research in anonymization and pseudonymization promises even better privacy-preserving methods for the future.

Still, there are many problems to be solved in the realm of data protection in data-driven medical science. To begin with, many of the procedures currently in use only work with structured data, e.g. database records. This specially holds true for all techniques based on the $k$-anonymity concept, where each information particle falls into a well-defined category (column). But even for this heavily structured data, there exist several open research questions, which we will discuss in this chapter, grouped by their assets.

## 6.1    Questions Regarding Quasi Identifiers

The first group of concerns lies in the selection and treatment of the quasi identifiers. While this is rather straightforward in the standard examples (e.g. sex, birthdate), there are some inherent questions that need discussion, especially relating to the medical sector:

*Definition of quasi identifiers.* While sounding trivial and indeed very easy to decide in the standard example, this is not so trivial when considering medical data. A diagnose could, for example, be so rare that the field together with the ZIP-code results in deanonymization of the respective person. The diagnose would need to be treated as a QI in this example. Further examples include rare blood types and parts of genome sequences. The determination of QIs is an important research area for guaranteeing the privacy of patients in data-driven medical research.

*Generalization of non-trivial QIs.* Following the example in the previous paragraph, the field "diagnose", too, is a quasi identifier that a generalization strategy is needed for. While generalization is rather trivial for standard attributes like dates or numbers, it is rather difficult for free text fields. In the case of a diagnose, ontologies could help generating a generalization tree, still, when considering free text like it is found in notes from GPs, a lot of further research is needed.

*Independence of QIs.* Sometimes, QIs may not be as independent as they seem. E.g., considering the QI "sex", an entry in the field "diagnose" containing "breast cancer" leads to an approx. 99% chance of this record belonging to a female person, thus rendering the generalization of "sex" practically useless without the generalization of the field "diagnose". The research in this sector also includes the identification of such QIs, preferably without too much knowledge required on the respective field. One fruitful approach could be the utilization of rule mining in order to derive such dependencies.

## 6.2 Questions Regarding Collaboration

Collaborating with other research institutes again opens up several interesting research questions that need to be tackled in the close future.

*Data Precision Metrics.* Most metrics for measuring the information loss currently in use are rather trivially depending on the selected generalization strategies. While there exist examples for metrics depending on the actual data distribution, these are rather inefficient during the calculation. Finding efficient and expressive metrics seems to be a valuable research question to us. This also includes the question of fairness when using different strategies for different data recipients on the same source data.

*Leak Detection.* Even in case of perfect privacy protection, the leaking of research data may result in severe damage to the data owner, e.g. due to premature publication of results and the need for subsequent revision, or simply because of the value of the data set itself. While techniques for watermarking databases (e.g. see [35], [36] can be utilized, these are usually independent from the data (not the data storage, though) itself, thus making them removable without reducing the overall quality of the data sets. Thus, research on how to combine leak detection with privacy protection could enhance the willingness of data owners to share their data with other researchers. While there has been some research regarding this during the last years, these approaches (e.g. [37], [38]) currently only cover the basic $k$-anonymity concept.

## 6.3    General Research Questions

This Section contains some other research questions related to the topic of protecting privacy in data-driven medical science, which did not fit into the above categories.

*Structuring unstructured data.* While a lot of data used in medical research naturally possesses the form of structured data (e.g. derived from machines), there is also a wide variety of unstructured data found, e.g. notes and receipts from general practitioners, as well as simply older data. While there have been considerable efforts been spent on the topic of structuring this semi- and unstructured data vaults during the last years (e.g. by Heurix in [39] and [40]), a comparison of this research with a subsequent identification of the major weaknesses and research gaps is needed. Following this basic analysis, research into constructing a working mechanism needs to be conducted.

*Practical Considerations.* In order to spread these anonymization techniques, efficient implementations are needed, preferably open source in order to enable the researchers to optimize the algorithms with respect to the data. An example for a framework can be found in [41], with an outline for an optimization for biomedical datasets in [42]. This also includes research on the optimization of the algorithms, which e.g. has been conducted by El Emam et. al in [43] for basic $k$-anonymity. Furthermore, for review processes, an interface allowing the anonymous exchange of data sets in the course of the peer-review process would be a valuable addition.

## 6.4    Influencing Other Research Areas

In other research areas, the problem of privacy in data-driven science is rather new which results in a striking absence of specific laws or regulations. In classical IT security we are under the impression that currently research data is usually held back instead of released in an anonymized state. In our opinion this is largely due to a lack of rules for anonymous data publishing which pushes responsibility for privacy protection onto individual researchers, thus resulting in uncertainty. This poses a major problem for the reproducibility of results, which is one of the main pillars of modern science and it's underlying review paradigm. Furthermore, todays anonymization concepts mostly come from medical research and are therefore designed for highly structured data, thus often cannot be used for other types of data. This again opens up a new area for research into new methods. In view of the rapidly growing trend towards more data-driven research, these new methods will be needed rather sooner than later. Specific policies and guidelines governing the public availability of data in (data-driven) science would also be helpful in order to guarantee the validity of published research.

## 7 Conclusion

In this chapter, we discussed several important anonymization operations and models for ensuring privacy, especially relating to the medical sector, focussing on data-driven medical research. Anonymization methods aim to obfuscate the identity of the record owners, taking into account not only direct identifiers but also quasi-identifiers. The eligible anonymization methods depend on the internal structure of data and its external representation. Once the appropriate method has been identified, the requirements of the chosen privacy models can be satisfied, but each time a data set is anonymized, information is lost or the data may be distorted. Furthermore, we outlined several interesting research questions that need to be tackled in order to heighten the security margin for protecting privacy, as well as produce more significant anonymized data sets for analysis.

On related terms, an even more general problem concerning the reproducibility of research, lies in the authenticity of the used data. While this does not directly relate to the topic of anonymization as discussed in this work, it is vital to take into account that the data used in data-driven medical science must be trustworthy, may it be anonymized or not. Still, anonymization can hinder the inspection and/or validation of data, thus we see additional research questions arising from this antagonism of protecting privacy on the one side and providing means of validating data on the other. Furthermore, researchers in data driven-science must always have in mind that the proper validation of their data with respect to originality and authenticity, as well as of the algorithms in use is of the utmost importance.

**Acknowledgments.** The research was funded by COMET K1 and grant 840824 (KIRAS) by the FFG - Austrian Research Promotion Agency.

## References

1. Chawla, N.V., Davis, D.A.: Bringing big data to personalized healthcare: A patient-centered framework. Journal of General Internal Medicine 28, S660–S665
2. Holzinger, A.: Biomedical Informatics: Discovering Knowledge in Big Data. Springer, New York (2014)
3. Holzinger, A., Dehmer, M., Jurisica, I.: Knowledge discovery and interactive data mining in bioinformatics - state-of-the-art, future challenges and research directions. BMC Bioinformatics 15(suppl. 6), I1 (2014)

4. Emmert-Streib, F., de Matos Simoes, R., Glazko, G., McDade, S., Haibe-Kains, B., Holzinger, A., Dehmer, M., Campbell, F.: Functional and genetic analysis of the colon cancer network. BMC Bioinformatics 15(suppl. 6), S6 (2014)
5. Jacobs, A.: The pathologies of big data. Communications of the ACM 52(8), 36–44 (2009)
6. Craig, T., Ludloff, M.E.: Privacy and Big Data: The Players, Regulators and Stakeholders. Reilly Media, Inc., Beijing (2011)
7. Weippl, E., Holzinger, A., Tjoa, A.M.: Security aspects of ubiquitous computing in health care. Springer Elektrotechnik & Informationstechnik, e&i 123(4), 156–162 (2006)
8. Breivik, M., Hovland, G., From, P.J.: Trends in research and publication: Science 2.0 and open access. Modeling Identification and Control 30(3), 181–190 (2009)
9. Thompson, M., Heneghan, C.: Bmj open data campaign: We need to move the debate on open clinical trial data forward. British Medical Journal 345 (2012)
10. Hobel, H., Schrittwieser, S., Kieseberg, P., Weippl, E.: Privacy, Anonymity, Pseudonymity and Data Disclosure in Data-Driven Science (2013)
11. Bonneau, J.: The science of guessing: analyzing an anonymized corpus of 70 million passwords. In: 2012 IEEE Symposium on Security and Privacy (SP), pp. 538–552. IEEE (2012)
12. Chia, P.H., Yamamoto, Y., Asokan, N.: Is this app safe?: a large scale study on application permissions and risk signals. In: Proceedings of the 21st International Conference on World Wide Web, pp. 311–320. ACM (2012)
13. Dey, R., Jelveh, Z., Ross, K.: Facebook users have become much more private: A large-scale study. In: 2012 IEEE International Conference on Pervasive Computing and Communications Workshops (PERCOM Workshops), pp. 346–352. IEEE (2012)
14. Siersdorfer, S., Chelaru, S., Nejdl, W., San Pedro, J.: How useful are your comments?: analyzing and predicting youtube comments and comment ratings. In: Proceedings of the 19th International Conference on World Wide Web, pp. 891–900. ACM (2010)
15. West, R., Leskovec, J.: Human wayfinding in information networks. In: Proceedings of the 21st International Conference on World Wide Web, pp. 619–628. ACM (2012)
16. Zang, H., Bolot, J.: Anonymization of location data does not work: A large-scale measurement study. In: Proceedings of the 17th Annual International Conference on Mobile Computing and Networking, pp. 145–156. ACM (2011)
17. Sweeney, L.: Achieving k-anonymity privacy protection using generalization and suppression. International Journal of Uncertainty, Fuzziness and Knowledge-Based Systems 10(05), 571–588 (2002)
18. Sweeney, L.: k-anonymity: A model for protecting privacy. International Journal of Uncertainty, Fuzziness and Knowledge-Based Systems 10(05), 557–570 (2002)
19. Fung, B., Wang, K., Chen, R., Yu, P.S.: Privacy-preserving data publishing: A survey of recent developments. ACM Computing Surveys (CSUR) 42(4), 14 (2010)
20. Dalenius, T.: Finding a needle in a haystack-or identifying anonymous census record. Journal of Official Statistics 2(3), 329–336 (1986)
21. Pfitzmann, A., Köhntopp, M.: Anonymity, unobservability, and pseudonymity - A proposal for terminology. In: Federrath, H. (ed.) Anonymity 2000. LNCS, vol. 2009, pp. 1–9. Springer, Heidelberg (2001)
22. Hobel, H., Heurix, J., Anjomshoaa, A., Weippl, E.: Towards security-enhanced and privacy-preserving mashup compositions. In: Janczewski, L.J., Wolfe, H.B., Shenoi, S. (eds.) SEC 2013. IFIP AICT, vol. 405, pp. 286–299. Springer, Heidelberg (2013)

23. Wang, K., Fung, B.C., Philip, S.Y.: Handicapping attacker's confidence: an alternative to k-anonymization. Knowledge and Information Systems 11(3), 345–368 (2007)
24. Meyerson, A., Williams, R.: On the complexity of optimal k-anonymity. In: Proceedings of the Twenty-Third ACM SIGMOD-SIGACT-SIGART Symposium on Principles of Database Systems, pp. 223–228. ACM (2004)
25. LeFevre, K., DeWitt, D.J., Ramakrishnan, R.: Incognito: Efficient full-domain k-anonymity. In: Proceedings of the 2005 ACM SIGMOD International Conference on Management of Data, pp. 49–60. ACM (2005)
26. LeFevre, K., DeWitt, D.J., Ramakrishnan, R.: Mondrian multidimensional k-anonymity. In: Proceedings of the 22nd International Conference on Data Engineering, ICDE 2006, pp. 25–25. IEEE (2006)
27. LeFevre, K., DeWitt, D.J., Ramakrishnan, R.: Workload-aware anonymization. In: Proceedings of the 12th ACM SIGKDD International Conference on Knowledge Discovery and Data Mining, pp. 277–286. ACM (2006)
28. Machanavajjhala, A., Kifer, D., Gehrke, J., Venkitasubramaniam, M.: l-diversity: Privacy beyond k-anonymity. ACM Transactions on Knowledge Discovery from Data (TKDD) 1(1), 3 (2007)
29. Li, N., Li, T., Venkatasubramanian, S.: t-closeness: Privacy beyond k-anonymity and l-diversity. In: ICDE, vol. 7, pp. 106–115 (2007)
30. Li, J., Tao, Y., Xiao, X.: Preservation of proximity privacy in publishing numerical sensitive data. In: Proceedings of the 2008 ACM SIGMOD International Conference on Management of Data, pp. 473–486. ACM (2008)
31. Heurix, J., Karlinger, M., Neubauer, T.: Pseudonymization with metadata encryption for privacy-preserving searchable documents. In: 2012 45th Hawaii International Conference on System Science (HICSS), pp. 3011–3020. IEEE (2012)
32. Neubauer, T., Heurix, J.: A methodology for the pseudonymization of medical data. International Journal of Medical Informatics 80(3), 190–204 (2011)
33. Heurix, J., Neubauer, T.: Privacy-preserving storage and access of medical data through pseudonymization and encryption. In: Furnell, S., Lambrinoudakis, C., Pernul, G. (eds.) TrustBus 2011. LNCS, vol. 6863, pp. 186–197. Springer, Heidelberg (2011)
34. Noumeir, R., Lemay, A., Lina, J.M.: Pseudonymization of radiology data for research purposes. Journal of Digital Imaging 20(3), 284–295 (2007)
35. Agrawal, R., Kiernan, J.: Watermarking relational databases. In: Proceedings of the 28th International Conference on Very Large Data Bases, pp. 155–166. VLDB Endowment (2002)
36. Deshpande, A., Gadge, J.: New watermarking technique for relational databases. In: 2009 2nd International Conference on Emerging Trends in Engineering and Technology (ICETET), pp. 664–669 (2009)
37. Kieseberg, P., Schrittwieser, S., Mulazzani, M., Echizen, I., Weippl, E.: An algorithm for collusion-resistant anonymization and fingerprinting of sensitive microdata. Electronic Markets - The International Journal on Networked Business (2014)
38. Schrittwieser, S., Kieseberg, P., Echizen, I., Wohlgemuth, S., Sonehara, N., Weippl, E.: An algorithm for k-anonymity-based fingerprinting. In: Shi, Y.Q., Kim, H.-J., Perez-Gonzalez, F. (eds.) IWDW 2011. LNCS, vol. 7128, pp. 439–452. Springer, Heidelberg (2012)
39. Heurix, J., Rella, A., Fenz, S., Neubauer, T.: Automated transformation of semi-structured text elements. In: AMCIS 2012 Proceedings, pp. 1–11 (August 2012)

40. Heurix, J., Rella, A., Fenz, S., Neubauer, T.: A rule-based transformation system for converting semi-structured medical documents. Health and Technology, 1–13 (March 2013)

41. Kohlmayer, F., Prasser, F., Eckert, C., Kemper, A., Kuhn, K.A.: Flash: efficient, stable and optimal k-anonymity. In: 2012 International Conference on Privacy, Security, Risk and Trust (PASSAT), 2012 International Confernece on Social Computing (SocialCom), pp. 708–717. IEEE (2012)

42. Kohlmayer, F., Prasser, F., Eckert, C., Kemper, A., Kuhn, K.A.: Highly efficient optimal k-anonymity for biomedical datasets. In: 2012 25th International Symposium on Computer-Based Medical Systems (CBMS), pp. 1–6. IEEE (2012)

43. El Emam, K., Dankar, F.K., Issa, R., Jonker, E., Amyot, D., Cogo, E., Corriveau, J.P., Walker, M., Chowdhury, S., Vaillancourt, R., et al.: A globally optimal k-anonymity method for the de-identification of health data. Journal of the American Medical Informatics Association 16(5), 670–682 (2009)

# Biobanks – A Source of Large Biological Data Sets: Open Problems and Future Challenges

Berthold Huppertz[1] and Andreas Holzinger[2]

[1] Medical University of Graz, Biobank Graz, Neue Stiftingtalstraße 2a, 8036 Graz, Austria
berthold.huppertz@medunigraz.at
[2] Medical University of Graz, Institute for Medical Informatics, Statistics & Documentation,
Research Unit HCI, Auenbruggerplatz 2/V, 8036 Graz, Austria
andreas.holzinger@medunigraz.at

**Abstract.** Biobanks are collections of biological samples (e.g. tissues, blood and derivatives, other body fluids, cells, DNA, etc.) and their associated data. Consequently, human biobanks represent collections of human samples and data and are of fundamental importance for scientific research as they are an excellent resource to access and measure biological constituents that can be used to monitor the status and trends of both health and disease. Most -omics data trust on a secure access to these collections of stored human samples to provide the basis for establishing the ranges and frequencies of expression. However, there are many open questions and future challenges associated with the large amounts of heterogeneous data, ranging from pre-processing, data integration and data fusion to knowledge discovery and data mining along with a strong focus on privacy, data protection, safety and security.

**Keywords:** Biobank, Personalized Medicine, Big Data, Biological Data.

## 1 Introduction and Motivation

One of the grand challenges in our networked world are the large, complex, and often weakly structured data sets along with the increasing amount of unstructured information [1]. Often called "Big Data"[2], these challenges are most evident in the biomedical domain [3],[4] as the data sets are typically heterogeneous (Variety), time-sensitive (Velocity), of low quality (Veracity) and large (Volume) [5].

The trend towards **precision medicine** (P4 Medicine: Predictive, Preventive, Participatory, Personalized) [6] has resulted in an explosion in the amount of generated biomedical data sets – in particular -omics data (e.g. from genomics [7], [8], proteomics [9], metabolomics [10], lipidomics [11], transcriptomics [12], epigenetics [13], microbiomics [14], fluxomics [15], phenomics [16], etc.).

A good example in this respect is biomarker research [17]: Worldwide, health-care systems spend billions of dollars annually on biomarker research to foster personalized medicine. Success depends on the quality of specimens and data used to identify or validate biomarkers, but a lack of quality control for samples and data is polluting

A. Holzinger, I. Jurisica (Eds.): Knowledge Discovery and Data Mining, LNCS 8401, pp. 317–330, 2014.

the scientific literature with flawed information that will take a long time to be sorted out [18].

The word "Biobank" appeared only relatively recently in the biomedical literature, namely in a 1996 paper by Loft & Poulsen [19] and for the upcoming years it was mainly used to describe human population-based biobanks. In recent years, the term biobank has been used in a more general sense, including all types of **biological sample collection facilities** (samples from animals, plants, fungi, microbes, etc.). Unfortunately, there are currently various definitions that are used to define a biobank. Human biobanks are specific and limited to the collection of only human samples, sometimes even focusing on specific population-based or tissue-restricted collections.

Hewitt & Watson (2013) [20] carried out a survey of 303 questionnaires: The results show that there is consensus that the term biobank may be applied to biological collections of human, animal, plant or microbial samples; and that the term biobank should only be applied to **sample collections with associated sample data,** and to collections that are managed according to **professional standards.**

However, they found that there was no consensus on the purpose, size or level of access; consequently they argue that a general, broad definition of the term "biobank" is okay, but that now attention should be paid on the need for a universally-accepted, **systematic classification** of the different biobank types [20]. The same remark was made by Shaw, Elger & Colledge (2014) [21], who also confirm that there is agreement on what constitutes a biobank; however, that there is (still) much disagreement regarding a precise definition. Their results show that, in addition to the core concepts of biological samples and linked data, the planned use of samples (including sharing) is a key criterion, moreover it emerged that some researchers avoid the term to circumvent certain regulatory guidelines, including informed consent requirements [21]. All authors agree that biobanks are a multi-disciplinary facility and definitely important for the future of personalized, individualized and molecular medical approaches [22, 23].

Looking at the Swedish Act on Biobanks (SF 2002:297) one can find some interesting views on what a biobank can be. In this act it is defined that the size of a sample collection does not have any significance, rather even a single human sample may be a biobank. Moreover, the act defines that any human biological material that cannot be traced back to the donor (i.e. unidentified material) is not biobank material,

One of the major advantages of today's high-end technologies in the –omics field is the generation of huge amounts of data that – in combination with the medical data associated to the samples - open new avenues in personalized and stratified medicine. However, at the same time this is also one of the major challenges of these technologies. The respective data analysis has not been able to follow the speed of technological achievements and hence, large data sets are present that cannot be analyzed in a proper way and thus, important information cannot be used to further foster biomarker identification and stratification of diseases.

## 2     Glossary and Key Terms

*Biobank:* is a collection of biological samples (e.g. tissues, blood, body fluids, cells, DNA etc.) in combination with their associated data. Here this term is mostly used for collections of samples of human origin.

*Biomarker:* is a characteristic and quantifiable measure (e.g. "x" as a biomarker for the disease "y") used as an indicator for normal or pathogenic biological processes, or pharmacologic responses to a therapeutic intervention. Biomarkers can be physical measures (ultrasound, X-ray, blood pressure), proteins or other molecular indicators.

*Genomics:* is a branch of molecular biology, which focuses on the structure, function, mapping & evolution of the genome. Personal genomics analyses the genome of an individual.

*Metabolomics:* study /quantify short-lived metabolites. Today, a challenge is to integrate proteomic, transcriptomic, and metabolomic information to provide a more complete understanding of living organisms.

*Molecular Medicine:* emphasizes cellular and molecular phenomena and interventions rather than the previous conceptual and observational focus on patients and their organs.

*Omics data:* are derived from various sources, e.g. genomics, proteomics, metabolomics, lipidomics, transcriptomics, epigenetics, microbiomics, fluxomics, phenomics, foodomics, cytomics, embryomics, exposonomics, phytochemomics, etc. (all -omics technologies).

*Proteome:* describes the entire complex repertoire of proteins that is expressed by a cell, tissue, or organism at a specific time point and under specific environmental conditions.

*Proteomics:* is a field of molecular biology focusing on determining the proteins present in a cell/tissue/organ at a given time point, the proteome.

*P-Health Model:* Preventive, Participatory, Pre-emptive, Personalized, Predictive, Pervasive (= available to anybody, anytime, anywhere).

*Translational Medicine:* is based on interventional epidemiology. Progress of Evidence-Based Medicine (EBM) integrates research from basic science for patient care and prevention.

## 3     State-of-the-Art

### 3.1     Towards a Standardized Definition

Today, biobanks can be found all over the world. Due to the still unclear definition of biobanks (as outlined in the introduction), the term is widely used without any clear boundaries. Biobanks are heterogeneous constructs and mostly developed on demand in relation to a specific research question following local demands on annotation of the collected samples. Riegman et al. (2008) [24] classified biobanks into three categories:

1) Population-based biobanks to obtain biomarkers of susceptibility and population identity. Their operational substrate is mostly DNA from a huge number of healthy donors including large data sets including life style, environmental exposure etc., representative of a specific (e.g. regional) cohort.

2) Epidemiological, disease-oriented biobanks to focus on biomarkers of exposure, using a very large number of samples, following a healthy exposed cohort/case–control design. They study DNA or serum markers and a great amount of specifically designed and collected data.

3) Disease-oriented general biobanks (e.g. tumor banks) usually associated to clinical data and sometimes associated to clinical trials, where it is essential that the amount of clinical data linked to the sample determinate the availability and biological value of the sample (see [24] for more details).

There are biobanks such as Biobank Graz that represent a mixture of all three types of biobanks. Thus, such large and supra-regional biobanks offer samples and data for epidemiological as well as disease-based research studies.

A recent analysis from Korea by Kang et al. (2013) [25] revealed that in 60% of all biobanks there are samples of less than 100,000 donors and only very few biobanks (10%) store specimens of more than a million donors. Most of the biobanks today seem to be very small, and since the term biobank is not protected, even a single sample in a freezer may be called a biobank. It is anticipated that within the next few years a further clarification and refinement of what a biobank is all about will be achieved.

Parallel to the wide use of the term biobank, large and supra-regional biobanks are starting to connect to each other to enable not only easier access to samples and data world-wide, but also to speed-up harmonization of sample collection and storage conditions and protocols as well as data availability. The close interaction of those biobanks is also intended to harmonize ethical, legal and social issues that are still poorly defined, sometimes even within a single country. An example of emerging biobank networks is the recently established European infrastructure BBMRI-ERIC (Biobanking and Bio-Molecular resources Research Infrastructure - European Research Infrastructure Consortium). It is one of the first European infrastructures that is funded by member states of the EU and which aims at connecting all biobanks of the member states. BBMRI_ERIC started its action in January 2014 with its headquarter in Graz, Austria (bbmri-eric.eu).

The ongoing demands to define biobanks in a more rigorous way have led to the certification of biobanks according to the standards of ISO 2008:9001. Although this standard is not directly related to biobanking, it at least defines clear management tools to improve sample and data collection and storage. In the moment, there are actions under way, which aim to develop a **unique biobanking standard,** which then will be included into the ISO system to finally be used as a specific biobanking standard. As soon as this new standard will become available all biobanks will need to introduce this standard to become or maintain up-to-date.

## 3.2    Examples of Biobanks and Linkage to Medical Data

Roden et al. (2008) [26] developed a DNA biobank linked to phenotypic data derived directly from an electronic medical record (EMR) system: An "opt-out" model was implemented and their strategy included the development and maintenance of a **de-identified** mirror image of the EMR, which they named the "synthetic derivative" (SD). DNA extracted from discarded blood samples was then linked to the SD. Surveys of patients indicated a general acceptance of the concept, with only a minority (~5%) opposing it. They developed also algorithms for sample handling and procedures for de-identification and validated them in order to ensure acceptable error rates [26].

A non-European example is the national Biobank of Korea (NBK) aiming at consolidating various human-originated biomedical resources collected by individual hospitals nation-wide and integrating them with their donors' clinical information, which researchers can take advantage of. Kim et al. (2011) reported about their experiences in developing the Clinical Information Integration System (CIIS) for NBK: Their system automatically extracts clinical data from hospital information systems as much as possible to avoid errors from manual entry. It maintains the independence of individual hospitals by employing a two-layer approach, one of which takes care of all hospital-specific aspects. Interoperability is achieved by adopting HL7 v2.x messaging between the biobank and hospitals [27].

## 3.3    Example: Biobank Graz

Biobank Graz (www.medunigraz.at/biobank) is a central service facility of Medical University of Graz supporting investigations of the causes of diseases and the development of improvements in disease diagnosis and treatment. The goal is to contribute to the provision of improved healthcare for the general population and in particular to contribute towards the future of personalized health care. Biobank Graz is unique as it is the largest academic biobank in Europe, directly linked to the LKH University Hospital Graz. It houses nearly 6 million samples including formalin-fixed paraffin embedded (FFPE) tissue samples kept at room temperature, fresh frozen tissue samples kept in the vapor phase of liquid nitrogen and samples of body fluids (blood, serum, plasma, buffy coat, urine, liquor) kept at minus 80°C. All standard procedures run at Biobank Graz are based on standard operating procedures (SOPs), consistent with its certification according to ISO 2008:9001.

The maintenance of **sample quality** during pre-analytics is one of the major challenges biobanks have to face. As soon as a sample is taken from a human, this sample will start to change and the content will undergo degradative processes. Hence, at any biobank protocols need to be in place that minimize handling times and temperature changes of any given sample. At Biobank Graz a typical example shows how this problem can be solved. Blood samples from any cooperating clinic at LKH University

Hospital Graz are sent to the central laboratory of the hospital, where a unique pipetting robot of Biobank Graz is located. Any blood sample reaching the central lab will be automatically screened for its inclusion into the collection of Biobank Graz and if so, will be directly transferred to the respective robot. This robot is unique in that it identifies the sample (serum, plasma, buffy coat, etc.) and its volume, opens the respective number of tubes for aliquoting, aliquots the samples and transfers single tubes to an integrated freezing unit. Hence, the whole process from identification of the primary tube to freezing of the aliquots takes maximally five minutes. This way, sample quality is maintained as good as possible.

Recently, Biobank Graz has become member of the Austrian (BBMRI.AT) as well as the European network of biobanks (BBMRI-ERIC), see Figure 1. These networks have been established as infrastructures to intensify crosstalk between biobanks enabling biomarker research on a much higher level. The headquarters of both networks, the national and the European network of biobanks, are located in close vicinity to Biobank Graz, allowing a direct interaction and exchange between the networks and the biobank.

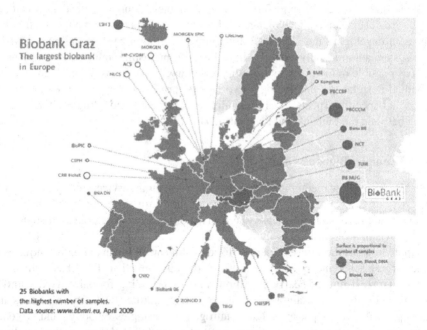

**Fig. 1.** In 2009 the 25 European biobanks with the largest numbers of samples cooperated to establish a European network of biobanks. This lead to the development of BBMRI-ERIC which started its action in January 2014.

## 3.4    Minimal Data Set

Samples stored in a biobank always need to be linked to the respective data of the donor. Without this information, a sample is of no value since a simple piece of tissue or a simple aliquot of blood without any further information on the donor cannot be used for any research study. It may only be used to test a specific method where for example a test kit or an antibody is tested. Even then, information on the sample itself is important.

On the BBMRI Wiki homepage (bbmri-wiki.com) the MIABIS 2.0 site gives detailed information on the minimum information required to initiate collaboration between biobanks and between biobanks and researchers. At the same time, each and every biobank has its own definition of the minimal data set. At Biobank Graz, the minimal data set comprises the following data:

- Age (age of donor at time of sample collection),
- Gender (male, female, other),
- Date of death (if applicable),
- Pathological diagnosis (type of tumor etc.),
- Sample type (DNA, blood cells, serum etc.),
- Data on processing and storage of sample (time, temperature etc.).

For specific sample sets more detailed sets of data can be offered. For example, tumor samples are further connected to a standard data set at Biobank Graz, comprising the following additional data:

- ICD-10 / ICD-0 code,
- TNM classification,
- Staging,
- Grading,
- Receptor status,
- Residual tumor,
- Affection of lymph nodes,
- Metastases.

Of course, such standard data set can be extended dependent on the amount of clinical information available for each sample. If a biobank is directly connected to a hospital, it may be possible to retrieve all clinical information of a donor and link them to a sample. In these cases even longitudinal information on disease and treatment progresses may become available.

## 3.5    From a Sample to Big Data

Following the data flow from obtaining a human biological sample to a research study, one can easily identify the accumulation of data (Figure 2). If a patient approaching a hospital signs an informed consent and allows the use of his/her samples for research studies, this person becomes a donor of a biobank (Figure 2B). The newly derived clinical data plus the data from the clinical labs from the current stay at the hospital are added to the already existing clinical data. If the samples are used in a research project additional data are added. This research data may be derived from a variety of methods including all the –omics technologies. Hence, huge data sets may be generated that add to the already existing data.

This way, clinical data over time (including diagnoses, images etc.) are linked to clinical lab data (over time), different sample types (again over time) and a large variety of lab data from research projects. So far, this data sets are not directly linked to each other and hence, the benefit of large data integration and analysis still awaits its use. A typical workflow can be seen in figure 2.

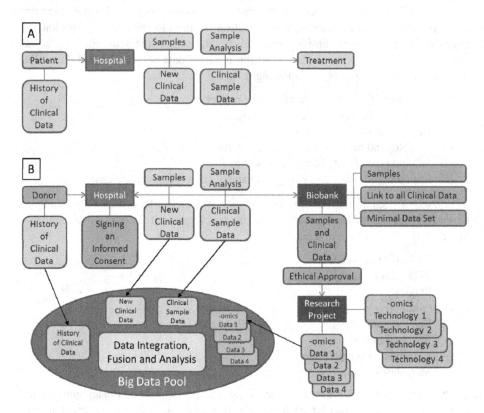

**Fig. 2.** (A) Typical sample workflow in the hospital; (B) Data integration, data fusion and analysis as main future challenges in the cross-disciplinary workflows of hospitals and biobanks

## 4     Open Challenges

Today, sample and data quality in biobanks shows an astonishing level of heterogeneity. As outlined above, so far, harmonization of sample and data collection and storage protocols has not been achieved yet. At the same time, any agreement on a minimal quality level is not acceptable as it would produce another mass of suboptimal scientific data and publications. Hence, it will be the task of large biobanks such as Biobank Graz, networks such as BBMRI-ERIC and societies such as ISBER (International Society for Biological and Environmental Repositories) to develop standards and definitions for best practice in biobanking.

A typical example and use case of the heterogeneity and quality differences in biobanks today is presented as follows: A scientific study has asked for a collection of a specific set of samples and approached a number of biobanks to result in a sufficient number of cases. The scientists received the samples from the different biobanks and evaluated the samples according to their protocols. Looking for their marker of interest the scientists identified differences in the samples and thought it would relate to cases and controls. However, a thorough analysis of their data revealed that the differences they detected were *not* related to cases and controls but rather to the biobank the samples were collected from. The data they achieved with their methods could be clustered into groups directly representing the different biobanks. This example clearly illustrates the paramount importance of collecting and storing samples and data at the highest quality level. Taken together, the establishment and maintenance of biobanks is demanding and surveillance systems are mandatory to ensure trustworthy samples for future research [28]. Besides quality of samples, biobanks have to face further challenges in the following years. Some open challenges include but are not limited to:

**Challenge 1:** Systematic assessment and use of clinical data associated with samples. Problem: Most of the clinical data are available only as unstructured information, partly in free text [29] or at least in semi-structured form.

**Challenge 2:** Data integration and fusion of the heterogeneous data sets from various data banks (e.g. business enterprise hospital information systems and biobank). Problem: Heterogeneity of data, weakly structured data, complexity of data, massive amount of unstructured information, lack of data quality etc.

**Challenge 3:** Integration of other medical data including, e.g. data from imaging systems [30] such as ultrasound or radiology. Problem: Complexity and heterogeneity of data, new approaches for data integration needed.

**Challenge 4:** Integration and association of scientific data with clinical data and samples. Problem: On the scientific side huge amounts of scientific data are produced by -omics technologies, which so far cannot be easily linked to medical data in a wider range.

**Challenge 5:** A major issue is the general underuse of biobanks [31]. Biobanks are housing millions and millions of samples while use of such samples is very limited due to various reasons. Problem: Lack of awareness in the communities, lack of exchange standards, lack of open data initiatives.

**Challenge 6:** To support research on an international level, the availability of open data sets would be required. Problem: Privacy, data protection, safety and security issues.

Moreover, ethical and legal issues remain a big challenge [32]. Different biobanks follow different strategies how to deal with information of donors, specificity of the informed consent and acceptance of studies by local ethical committees. Accordingly, access to samples from different biobanks is restricted due to the various policies that are embedded in different ethical and legal frameworks.

Public awareness and information of the general population on the importance and possibilities of biobanks are still lacking [33]. Hundreds of biobanks are currently in operation across Europe. And although scientists routinely use the phrase "biobank", the wider public is still confused when the word 'bank' is being connected with the collection of their biological samples.

Lack of data quality regarding pre-analytical procedures remains one of the major challenges associated with biobanking. Simeon-Dubach & Perren (2011) [18] analyzed 125 papers retrieved in a PubMed search of open-access articles using the key words *biomarker discovery* for the years 2004 and 2009. Astonishingly, more than half of the papers contained no information about the bio-specimens used, and even four papers on biomarker discoveries published in Nature in 2009 contained insufficient specimen data. Leading journals are trendsetters when it comes to defining publication criteria. For example, for some 15 years they have required statements on ethical review boards and informed consent; today for most journals a biomedical paper without this information would be unthinkable. To uphold standards, all journals should insist on full details of biobanked specimens (including pre-analytical procedures such as collection, processing and storage). Thousands of potential biomarkers are reported every year, consequently the responsible biobank managers should collect *complete data sets* on specimens and pass it on to researchers to include the source data in their publications [18].

## 5     Conclusion and Future Work

A recent article in Nature Medicine [34] proposed a number of solutions to the problem of **sample underuse in biospecimen repositories**, but the article failed to address one important source of underuse: the lack of access to biobank resources by researchers working in the biomedical domain [35]. This results in the fact that scientific data generated by analyzing samples from biobanks are not flowing back to the biobanks – and hence cannot be linked to medical data or other scientific data.

Consequently, a grand challenge today can be identified in data fusion and data integration, fusing clinical data (e.g. patient records, medical reports, pathological data, etc.) with scientific data such as -omics data derived from biobank samples. To reach this goal cooperation is needed between advanced knowledge discovery experts and data mining specialists, biobanking experts and clinicians, -omics data producers and business experts. This concerted action will bring research results into daily practice seeking the advice of international experts and with full consideration of data protection, security, safety and privacy protection.

Marko-Varga et al. (2012) emphasized that biobanks are a major resource to access and measure biological constituents that can be used to monitor the status of health and disease, both in unique individual samples and within populations. Moreover, most -omics-related activities rely on the access to these collections to provide the basis for establishing the ranges and frequencies of expression. Furthermore, information about the relative abundance and form of protein constituents found in stored samples provides an important historical index for comparative studies of inherited, epidemic and developing diseases. Standardization of sample quality including handling, storage and analysis is an important unmet need and requirement for gaining the full benefit from collected samples.

Coupled to this standard is the provision of annotation describing clinical status and metadata of measurements of clinical phenotype that characterizes the sample.

Today, we have not yet achieved consensus on how to collect, manage, and build biobank repositories to reach the goal where these efforts are translated into value for the patient. Several initiatives (OBBR, ISBER, BBMRI) that disseminate best practice examples for biobanking are expected to play an important role in ensuring the need to preserve sample integrity of biosamples stored for periods that reach one or several decades. These developments will be of great value and importance to programs such as the Chromosome Human Protein Project (C-HPP) that will associate protein expression in healthy and disease states with genetic foci along each of the human chromosomes [36].

LaBaer (2012) [37] reported that the increasing interest in translational research has created a large demand for blood, tissue and other clinical samples, which find use in a broad variety of research including genomics, proteomics and metabolomics. Hundreds of millions of dollars have been invested internationally on the collection, storage and distribution of samples. Nevertheless, many researchers complain in frustration about their inability to obtain relevant and/or useful samples for their research. Lack of access to samples, poor conditions of samples and unavailability of appropriate control samples have slowed our progress in studying diseases and biomarkers. The five major challenges that hinder use of clinical samples for translational research are: (1) Define own biobanking needs. (2) Increase using and accessing standard operating procedures (SOPs). (3) Recognize interobserver differences to normalize diagnoses. (4) Identify appropriate internal controls to normalize differences due to different biobanks. (5) Redefine clinical sample paradigms by establishing partnerships with the general population [37].

The author states, that for each challenge, the respective tools are already available to achieve the objective soon. However, it remains that the future of proteomics and other –omics technologies strongly depends on access to high quality samples, collected under standardized conditions, accurately annotated and shared under conditions that promote research that is needed [37].

Finally, Norlin et al. (2012) reported on numerous successful scientific results which have emerged from projects using biobanks. They emphasized that in order to facilitate the discovery of underutilized biobank samples, it would be helpful to establish a global biobank register, containing descriptive information about existing samples. However, for shared data to be comparable, data needs to be harmonized first. It is the aim of BBMRI-ERIC to harmonize biobanking across Europe and to move towards a universal information infrastructure for biobanking. This is directly connected to the issues of interoperability through standardized message formats and controlled terminologies. Therefore, the authors have developed a minimal data set for biobanks and studies using human biospecimens. The data set is called MIABIS (Minimum Information About BIobank data Sharing) and consists of 52 attributes describing a biobank content. The authors aim to facilitate data discovery through harmonization of data elements describing a biobank at an aggregated level. As many biobanks across Europe possess a tremendous amount of samples that are underutilized, this would help pave the way for biobank networking on a national and international level, resulting in time and cost savings and faster emergence of new scientific results [38].

Within the HORIZON 2020 program, where "big data" generally, and personalized medicine specifically are major issues [39] there are numerous calls open that ask for actions on big data and open data innovation as well as big data research. The latter calls address fundamental research problems related to the scalability and responsiveness of analytics capabilities always basing on biobank samples and data.

Today, the grand challenge is to make the data useable and useful for the medical professional. To reach such a goal it needs a concerted effort of various research areas ranging from the very physical handling of complex and weakly-structured data, i.e. data fusion, pre-processing, data mapping and interactive data mining to interactive data visualization at the clinical workplace ensuring privacy, data protection, safety and security at every time [40]. Due to the complexity of biomedical data sets, a manual analysis will no longer be possible, hence we must make use of sophisticated machine learning algorithms [41], [42], [43]; and a more effective approach is in putting the human users in control, since human experts have the abilities to identify patterns which machines cannot [44], [45]. To bring together these different worlds the international expert network "HCI-KDD" has been established [46].

# References

1. Holzinger, A.: On Knowledge Discovery and Interactive Intelligent Visualization of Biomedical Data - Challenges in Human–Computer Interaction & Biomedical Informatics. In: DATA 2012, pp. 9–20. INSTICC (2012)
2. Howe, D., Costanzo, M., Fey, P., Gojobori, T., Hannick, L., Hide, W., Hill, D.P., Kania, R., Schaeffer, M., St Pierre, S., Twigger, S., White, O., Rhee, S.Y.: Big data: The future of biocuration. Nature 455(7209), 47–50 (2008)
3. Holzinger, A.: Biomedical Informatics: Computational Sciences meets Life Sciences. BoD, Norderstedt (2012)
4. Holzinger, A.: Biomedical Informatics: Discovering Knowledge in Big Data. Springer, New York (2014)
5. Fan, W.: Querying big social data. In: Gottlob, G., Grasso, G., Olteanu, D., Schallhart, C. (eds.) BNCOD 2013. LNCS, vol. 7968, pp. 14–28. Springer, Heidelberg (2013)
6. Hood, L., Friend, S.H.: Predictive, personalized, preventive, participatory (P4) cancer medicine. Nature Reviews Clinical Oncology 8(3), 184–187 (2011)
7. Emmert-Streib, F., de Matos Simoes, R., Glazko, G., McDade, S., Haibe-Kains, B., Holzinger, A., Dehmer, M., Campbell, F.: Functional and genetic analysis of the colon cancer network. BMC Bioinformatics 15(suppl. 6), S6 (2014)
8. Pennisi, E.: Human genome 10th anniversary. Will computers crash genomics? Science 331, 666–668 (2011)
9. Boguski, M.S., McIntosh, M.W.: Biomedical informatics for proteomics. Nature 422(6928), 233–237 (2003)
10. Tomita, M., Kami, K.: Systems Biology, Metabolomics, and Cancer Metabolism. Science 336(6084), 990–991 (2012)
11. Wenk, M.R.: The emerging field of lipidomics. Nature Reviews Drug Discovery 4(7), 594–610 (2005)
12. Wang, Z., Gerstein, M., Snyder, M.: RNA-Seq: a revolutionary tool for transcriptomics. Nature Reviews Genetics 10(1), 57–63 (2009)

13. Egger, G., Liang, G.N., Aparicio, A., Jones, P.A.: Epigenetics in human disease and prospects for epigenetic therapy. Nature 429(6990), 457–463 (2004)
14. Egert, M., de Graaf, A.A., Smidt, H., de Vos, W.M., Venema, K.: Beyond diversity: functional microbiomics of the human colon. Trends in Microbiology 14(2), 86–91 (2006)
15. Winter, G., Kromer, J.O.: Fluxomics - connecting 'omics analysis and phenotypes. Environmental Microbiology 15(7), 1901–1916 (2013)
16. Houle, D., Govindaraju, D.R., Omholt, S.: Phenomics: the next challenge. Nature Reviews Genetics 11(12), 855–866 (2010)
17. Sawyers, C.L.: The cancer biomarker problem. Nature 452(7187), 548–552 (2008)
18. Simeon-Dubach, D., Perren, A.: Better provenance for biobank samples. Nature 475(7357), 454–455 (2011)
19. Loft, S., Poulsen, H.E.: Cancer risk and oxidative DNA damage in man. Journal of Molecular Medicine 74(6), 297–312 (1996)
20. Hewitt, R., Watson, P.: Defining Biobank. Biopreservation and Biobanking 11(5), 309–315 (2013)
21. Shaw, D.M., Elger, B.S., Colledge, F.: What is a biobank? Differing definitions among biobank stakeholders. Clinical Genetics 85(3), 223–227 (2014)
22. Olson, J.E., Ryu, E., Johnson, K.J., Koenig, B.A., Maschke, K.J., Morrisette, J.A., Liebow, M., Takahashi, P.Y., Fredericksen, Z.S., Sharma, R.G., Anderson, K.S., Hathcock, M.A., Carnahan, J.A., Pathak, J., Lindor, N.M., Beebe, T.J., Thibodeau, S.N., Cerhan, J.R.: The Mayo Clinic Biobank: A Building Block for Individualized Medicine. Mayo Clinic Proceedings 88(9), 952–962 (2013)
23. Akervall, J., Pruetz, B.L., Geddes, T.J., Larson, D., Felten, D.J., Wilson, G.D.: Beaumont Health System BioBank: A Multidisciplinary Biorepository and Translational Research Facility. Biopreservation and Biobanking 11(4), 221–228 (2013)
24. Riegman, P.H.J., Morente, M.M., Betsou, F., de Blasio, P., Geary, P.: Biobanking for better healthcare. Molecular Oncology 2(3), 213–222 (2008)
25. Kang, B., Park, J., Cho, S., Lee, M., Kim, N., Min, H., Lee, S., Park, O., Han, B.: Current Status, Challenges, Policies, and Bioethics of Biobanks. Genomics & Informatics 11(4), 211–217 (2013)
26. Roden, D.M., Pulley, J.M., Basford, M.A., Bernard, G.R., Clayton, E.W., Balser, J.R., Masys, D.R.: Development of a Large-Scale De-Identified DNA Biobank to Enable Personalized Medicine. Clin. Pharmacol. Ther. 84(3), 362–369 (2008)
27. Kim, H., Yi, B.K., Kim, I.K., Kwak, Y.S.: Integrating Clinical Information in National Biobank of Korea. Journal of Medical Systems 35(4), 647–656 (2011)
28. Norling, M., Kihara, A., Kemp, S.: Web-Based Biobank System Infrastructure Monitoring Using Python, Perl, and PHP. Biopreservation and Biobanking 11(6), 355–358 (2013)
29. Holzinger, A., Geierhofer, R., Modritscher, F., Tatzl, R.: Semantic Information in Medical Information Systems: Utilization of Text Mining Techniques to Analyze Medical Diagnoses. J. Univers. Comput. Sci. 14(22), 3781–3795 (2008)
30. Woodbridge, M., Fagiolo, G., O'Regan, D.P.: MRIdb: Medical Image Management for Biobank Research. J. Digit. Imaging 26(5), 886–890 (2013)
31. Scudellari, M.: Biobank managers bemoan underuse of collected samples. Nature Medicine 19(3), 253–253 (2013)
32. Wolf, S.M.: Return of results in genomic biobank research: ethics matters. Genetics in Medicine 15(2), 157–159 (2013)
33. Sandor, J., Bard, P., Tamburrini, C., Tannsjo, T.: The case of biobank with the law: between a legal and scientific fiction. Journal of Medical Ethics 38(6), 347–350 (2012)

34. Puchois, P.: Finding ways to improve the use of biobanks. Nat. Med. 19(7), 814–815 (2013)
35. Paradiso, A., Hansson, M.: Finding ways to improve the use of biobanks. Nat. Med. 19(7), 815–815 (2013)
36. Marko-Varga, G., Vegvari, A., Welinder, C., Lindberg, H., Rezeli, M., Edula, G., Svensson, K.J., Belting, M., Laurell, T., Fehniger, T.E.: Standardization and Utilization of Biobank Resources in Clinical Protein Science with Examples of Emerging Applications. Journal of Proteome Research 11(11), 5124–5134 (2012)
37. LaBaer, J.: Improving International Research with Clinical Specimens: 5 Achievable Objectives. Journal of Proteome Research 11(12), 5592–5601 (2012)
38. Norlin, L., Fransson, M.N., Eriksson, M., Merino-Martinez, R., Anderberg, M., Kurtovic, S., Litton, J.E.: A Minimum Data Set for Sharing Biobank Samples, Information, and Data: MIABIS. Biopreservation and Biobanking 10(4), 343–348 (2012)
39. Norstedt, I.: Horizon 2020: European perspectives in healthcare sciences and implementation. EPMA Journal 5(suppl. 1), A1 (2014)
40. Kieseberg, P., Hobel, H., Schrittwieser, S., Weippl, E., Holzinger, A.: Protecting Anonymity in the Data-Driven Medical Sciences. In: Holzinger, A., Jurisica, I. (eds.) Knowledge Discovery and Data Mining. LNCS, vol. 8401, pp. 303–318. Springer, Heidelberg (2014)
41. Holzinger, A., Stocker, C., Ofner, B., Prohaska, G., Brabenetz, A., Hofmann-Wellenhof, R.: Combining HCI, Natural Language Processing, and Knowledge Discovery - Potential of IBM Content Analytics as an assistive technology in the biomedical field. In: Holzinger, A., Pasi, G. (eds.) HCI-KDD 2013. LNCS, vol. 7947, pp. 13–24. Springer, Heidelberg (2013)
42. Holzinger, A., Dehmer, M., Jurisica, I.: Knowledge Discovery and Interactive Data Mining in Bioinformatics – State-of-the-Art, Future challenges and Research Directions. BMC Bioinformatics 15(suppl. 6) (I1) (2014)
43. Holzinger, A., Jurisica, I.: Knowledge Discovery and Data Mining in Biomedical Informatics: The future is in Integrative, Interactive Machine Learning Solutions. In: Holzinger, A., Jurisica, I. (eds.) Knowledge Discovery and Data Mining. LNCS, vol. 8401, pp. 1–18. Springer, Berlin (2014)
44. Shneiderman, B.: The Big Picture for Big Data: Visualization. Science 343(6172), 730–730 (2014)
45. Jeanquartier, F., Holzinger, A.: On Visual Analytics and Evaluation In Cell Physiology: A Case Study. In: Cuzzocrea, A., Kittl, C., Simos, D.E., Weippl, E., Xu, L. (eds.) CD-ARES 2013. LNCS, vol. 8127, pp. 495–502. Springer, Heidelberg (2013)
46. hci4all.at, http://www.hci4all.at/expert-network-hci-kdd/

# On Topological Data Mining

Andreas Holzinger[1,2]

[1] Research Unit Human-Computer Interaction, Institute for Medical Informatics,
Statistics & Documentation, Medical University Graz, Austria
`a.holzinger@hci4all.at`
[2] Institute for Information Systems and Computer Media, Graz University of
Technology, Austria
`a.holzinger@tugraz.at`

**Abstract.** Humans are very good at pattern recognition in dimensions
of $\leq 3$. However, most of data, e.g. in the biomedical domain, is in dimensions much higher than 3, which makes manual analyses awkward,
sometimes practically impossible. Actually, mapping higher dimensional
data into lower dimensions is a major task in Human–Computer Interaction and Interactive Data Visualization, and a concerted effort including
recent advances in computational topology may contribute to make sense
of such data. Topology has its roots in the works of Euler and Gauss,
however, for a long time was part of theoretical mathematics. Within
the last ten years computational topology rapidly gains much interest
amongst computer scientists. Topology is basically the study of abstract
shapes and spaces and mappings between them. It originated from the
study of geometry and set theory. Topological methods can be applied
to data represented by point clouds, that is, finite subsets of the $n$-
dimensional Euclidean space. We can think of the input as a sample of
some unknown space which one wishes to reconstruct and understand,
and we must distinguish between the ambient (embedding) dimension
$n$, and the intrinsic dimension of the data. Whilst $n$ is usually high, the
intrinsic dimension, being of primary interest, is typically small. Therefore, knowing the intrinsic dimensionality of data can be seen as one first
step towards understanding its structure. Consequently, applying topological techniques to data mining and knowledge discovery is a hot and
promising future research area.

**Keywords:** Computational Topology, Data Mining, Topological Data
Mining, Topological Text Mining, Graph-based Text Mining.

# 1 Introduction and Motivation

Medicine, Biology and health care of today is challenged with complex, high-
dimensional, heterogenous, noisy, and weakly structured data sets from various
sources [1]. Within such data, relevant *structural* patterns and/or *temporal* patterns ("knowledge") are often hidden, difficult to extract, hence not accessible
to a biomedical expert.

A. Holzinger, I. Jurisica (Eds.): Knowledge Discovery and Data Mining, LNCS 8401, pp. 331–356, 2014.
© Springer-Verlag Berlin Heidelberg 2014

Consequently, a grand challenge is to interactively discover unknown patterns within such large data sets. Computational geometry and algebraic topology may be of great help here [2] embedded in understanding large and complex data sets. Vin de Silva (2004) [3] in his research statement brought the basic idea straight to the point: Let $M$ be a topological space, known as the hidden parameter space; let $\mathbb{R}^D$ be an Euclidean space, defined as observation space, and let $f : M \to \mathbb{R}^D$ be a continuous embedding; $X \subset M$, be a finite set of data points, and $Y = f(X) \subset \mathbb{R}^D$ be the image of these points under the mapping $f$. Consequently, we may refer to $X$ as the hidden data, and $Y$ as the observed data. The central question then is: Suppose $M$, $f$ and $X$ are unknown, but $Y$ is known: can we identify $M$?

This paper of course can only be a scratch on the sheer endless surface, however, the main intention is in motivation and stimulation of further research and to provide a rough guide to the concepts of topology for the non-mathematician, with open eyes on applicability in knowledge discovery and data mining. The paper is organized as follows: In section 2 some key terms are explained to ensure a common and mutual understanding. It is always good to know a bit about who was working in the past in these areas and who are the current leading researchers, consequently in section 3 a very short look on the past is given, followed by section 4 with a brief look on the present. Section 5 provides a nutshell-like overview on the basics of topology, introducing the concepts of point clouds and spaces, manifolds, simplicial complexes and the alpha complex. In chapter 6 a short view on the state-of-the-art in topological data mining, and topological data analysis, respectively, is given; followed by topological text mining in chapter 7. A few software packages are listed in chapter 8, and a few open problems are described in chapter 9. The paper finishes with a section on future challenges and a conclusion with a one-sentence outlook into the future.

## 2     Glossary and Key Terms

*Algebraic Topology:* the older name was combinatorial topology, is the field of algebra concerned with computations of homologies and homotopies and other algebraic models in topological spaces [4]. Note: *Geometric topology* is the study of manifolds and embeddings of manifolds.

*Alpha Shapes:* is a family of piecewise linear simple curves in the Euclidean plane associated with the shape of a finite set of points [5]; i.e. $\alpha$-shapes are a generalization of the convex hull of a point set: Let $\mathbf{S}$ be a finite set in $\mathbb{R}^3$ and $\alpha$ a real number $0 \leq \alpha \leq \infty$; the u-shape of $\mathbf{S}$ is a polytope that is neither necessarily convex nor necessarily connected. For $\alpha \to \infty$ the $\alpha$-shape is identical to the convex hull of $\mathbf{S}$ [6]. $\alpha$-shapes are important e.g. in the study of protein-related interactions [7].

*Betti Number:* can be used to distinguish topological spaces based on the connectivity of $n$-dimensional simplicial complexes: In dimension $k$, the rank of the $k$-th homology group is denoted $\beta_k$, useful e.g. in content-based image retrieval in the presence of noisy shapes, because Betti numbers can be used as shape descriptor admitting dissimilarity distances stable under continuous shape deformations [8].

*Computational geometry:* A field concerned with algorithms that can be defined in terms of geometry (line segments, polyhedra, etc.) [9].

*Contour:* ia a connected component of a level set $h - 1(c)$ of a Morse function $h : M \to R$ defined on a manifold $M$.

*Delaunay triangulation:* Given a set of points in a plane $P = p_1, ..., p_n$, a Delaunay triangulation separates the set into triangles with $p's \in P$ as their corners, such that no circumcircle of any triangle contains any other point in its interior [10].

*Euler characteristic $\chi$:* is an integer associated to a manifold, e.g. $\chi$ of a surface is given by the number of faces minus edges plus vertices [11].

*Gromov-Norm:* is an invariant associated with the homology of a topological space that measures how many simplices are needed to represent a given homology class.

*Hausdorff-Space:* is a topologically separated space. Let $x$ and $y$ be two distinct points in a topological space $X$. Let $U$ be the neighbourhood of $x$ and $V$ be the neighborhood of $y$. $x$ and $y$ are said to be separable if $U \cap V = \emptyset$. Then $X$ is a Hausdorff-Space if every possible pair of points $x, y$ it contains are separable. A Hausdorff space is defined by the property that every two distinct points have disjoint neighborhoods.

*Homomorphism:* is a function that preserve the operators associated with the specified structure.

*Homological algebra:* is the study of homology and cohomology of manifolds. Homological algebra is a grand generalization of linear algebra.

*Homotopy:* Given two maps $f, g : X \to Y$ of topological spaces, $f$ and $g$ are homotopic, $f \simeq g$, if there is a continuous map $H : X \times [0, 1] \to Y$ so that $H(x, 0) = f(x)$ and $H(x, 1) = g(x)$ for all $x \in X$ [12].

*Homology:* Homology and cohomology are algebraic objects associated to a manifold, which give one measure of the number of holes of the object. Computation of the homology groups of topological spaces is a central topic in classic algebraic topology [13]; if the simplicial complex is small, the homology group computations can be done manually; to solve such problems generally a classic algorithm exists, see: [14].

*Isometry:* is a mapping of metric spaces which preserves the metric.

*Metric space:* A space in which a distance measure between pairs of elements (points) exists. Note: a metric is a distance function on a space or set; an assignment of distance to every unordered pair of points that satisfies the triangle inequality.

*Manifold:* is a fundamental mathematical object which locally resembles a line, a plane, or space.

*Persistent Homology:* Persistent homology is an algebraic tool for measuring topological features of shapes and functions. It casts the multi-scale organization we frequently observe in nature into a mathematical formalism. Here we give a record of the short history of persistent homology and present its basic concepts. Besides the mathematics we focus on algorithms and mention the various connections to applications, including to biomolecules, biological networks, data analysis, and geometric modeling [15]. The concept of persistence emerged independently in the work of Frosini, Ferri et al., and in the thesis of Robins at Boulder, Colorado, and within the biogeometry project of Edelsbrunner at Duke, North Carolina.

*Point clouds:* are finite sets equipped with a family of *proximity* (or *similarity measure*) functions $sim_q: S^{q+1} \to [0, 1]$, which measure how "close" or "similar" $(q + 1)$-tuples of elements of $S$ are (a value of 0 means totally different objects, while 1 corresponds to essentially equivalent items).

*Reeb graph:* is a graph that captures the connectivity of contours; when not having cycles, it is called a contour tree [16]. The Reeb graph is a useful tool in visualizing real-valued data obtained from computational simulations of physical processes [17], [18].

*Simplex:* is an $n$-dimensional generalization of the triangle and the tetrahedron: a polytope in $n$ dimensions with $n + 1$ vertices.

*Simplicial Complex:* is made up of simplices, e.g. a simplicial polytope has simplices as faces and a simplicial complex is a collection of simplices pasted together in any reasonable vertex-to-vertex and edge-to-edge arrangement. A graph is a 1-dim simplicial complex.

*Space:* is generally a set of points $a \in \mathbb{S}$ which satisfy some geometric postulate.

*Sphere:* is any manifold equivalent (homeomorphic) to the usual round hollow shell in some dimension: a sphere in $n + 1$-dimension is called an $n$-sphere.

*Topological Space:* is a pair $(\mathbb{X}, \mathbb{T})$ with $\emptyset \in \mathbb{T}$, $\mathbb{X} \in \mathbb{T}$ and a collection of subspaces, so that the union and intersections of subspaces are also in $\mathbb{T}$, in other words, it is a set of points, along with a set of neighbourhoods for each point, that satisfy a set of axioms relating points and neighbourhoods. The definition of a topological space relies only upon set theory and is the most general notion of a mathematical space that allows for the definition of concepts such as continuity, connectedness, and convergence. Other spaces, such as manifolds and metric spaces, are specializations of topological spaces with extra structures or constraints.

*Voronoi region:* Given a set of points in a plane $p_1, ..., p_n$, a Voronoi diagram erects regions around a point $p_i$ such that all points $q$ within its region are closer to $p_i$ (with regard to some distance measure) than to any other point $p_j$.

*Knowledge Discovery:* Exploratory analysis and modeling of data and the organized process of identifying valid, novel, useful and understandable patterns from these data sets.

*Minimum Spanning Tree:* Given a graph $G = (V, E, \omega)$ with $V$ being the set of vertices, $E$ being the set of edges and $\omega$ being the sets of edge weights, a Minimum Spanning tree is the connected acyclic subgraph defined by the subset $E' \subseteq E$ reaching all vertices $v \in V$ with the minimal sum of edge weights possible.

*weak/weakly:* in mathematics an object is called weak if it is of a generalized kind with fewer properties, and a property holds weakly if it holds in a lesser sense; e.g. a weak solution to an equation might be a discontinuous solution if a straightforward interpretation implies continuity.

## 3   Topology - The Past

If we want to look into the future, we always should at first look into the past. Topology has its roots in the work on graph theory by Leonhard Euler (1707–1783) [19]. The first book on topology titled "Vorstudien zur Topologie" was published 1848 by Johann Benedict Listing (1808–1882), who emphasized that the term "analysis geometria situs" used by Gottfried Wilhelm Leibniz (1646–1716) was a different geometric concept, hence topology did *not* start before the time of Euler [20]. Listing was very advanced at his time, which can be seen in his 1862 work (see Fig. 1) "Census raeumlicher Complexe" [21]. Significant contributions were made by Carl Friedrich Gauss (1777–1855) and August Ferdinand Moebius (1790–1868), who started with the first steps in set theoretic topology with his 1863 work "Theorie der elementaren Verwandtschaft" [22]. However, topology was not established as own discipline before the formal introduction of *set theory* by Georg Cantor (1845–1918) and Richard Dedekind (1831–1916), the latter was the last student of Gauss.

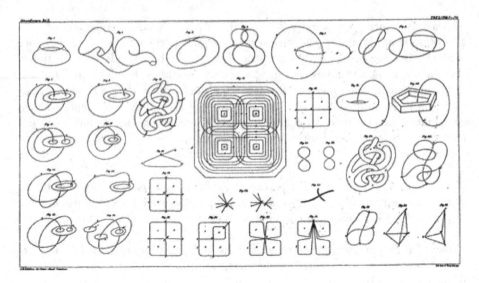

**Fig. 1.** From the book of Listing (1862)[21]; the image is already in the public domain

Consequently, actual pioneers of (combinatorial, the later algebraic) topology include Henri Poincare (1854–1912), but also Felix Klein (1849–1925), Enrico Betti (1823–1892), Bernhard Riemann (1826–1866) and last but not least Emmi Noether (1882–1935). After these pioneering years the field did not gain much interest, until the discovery of the concept of a *topological space* in 1914 by Felix Hausdorff (1868–1942). In the period after world war I, a collective of mainly French mathematicians pursued these topics amongst others, and they published from 1935 on under a pseudonym called Nicolas Bourbaki. The topics were continued by many meanwhile famous mathematicians, to mention only a few of the "big names": Edwin Evariste Moise (1918–1998), Georges Henri Reeb (1920–1993), Boris Nikolaevich Delaunay (1890–1980), Pavel Sergeyevich Alexandrov (1896–1982) to mention only a few.

According to Blackmore & Peters (2007) [23] the term "computational topology" occurred first in the dissertation of Maentylae in 1983, but there is a journal paper by Tourlakis & Mylopoulus called "Some results in Computational Topology" from 1973 [24] preceded by a conference paper.

## 4    Computational Topology - The Present

As it is important to look at the past, it is even more important to know some current experts in the field (in alphabetical order, list *not* complete - please forgive shortness and missing names):

*Peter Bubenik* from the department of mathematics at the Cleveland State University is combining ideas from topology and statistics [25].

*Benjamin A Burton* from the School of Mathematics and Physics at the University of Queensland, Brisbane, Australia, is the developer of Regina, which is a suite of mathematical software for 3-manifold topologists [26].

*Gunnar Carlsson* from the Stanford Topology Group, USA, is working in this area for a long time and got famous with his work on "topology and data" and "data has shape" [27].

*Tamal K. Dey* at the Ohio State University, Columbus, is together with Edelsbrunner and Guha one of the early promoters of computational topology [28].

*Nathan Dunfield* at the University of Illinois at Urbana-Champaign is working on Topology and geometry of 3-manifolds and related topics and maintaining the CompuTop.org Software Archive (see chapter software) [29].

*Herbert Edelsbrunner* born in Graz, long time at Duke, North Carolina, is one of the early pioneers in the field and currently at the Institute of Science and Technology Austria in Maria Gugging (near Vienna) [2].

*Massimo Ferri* , University of Bologna, Italy, was contributing to the concept of persistence, which emerged independently in the work of Cerri, Frosini et al. in Bologna, in the doctoral work of Robins at Boulder, Colorado, and within the biogeometry project of Edelsbrunner at Duke, North Carolina [30].

*Robert W. Ghrist* at the department of mathematics of the University of Pennsylvania, is particulary working on applied topology in sensor networks [31].

*John L. Harer* Duke University, Durham, North Carolina, USA, worked a long time together with Edelsbrunner at Duke [2].

*Dmitriy Morozov* at the Visualization group of the Lawrence Berkeley National Lab, is working on persistent homology [32].

*Marian Mrozek* is mathematician at the Computer Science Department, Jagiellonian University, Krakw, Poland [33].

*Valerio Pascucci* at the Center for Extreme Data Analysis and Visualization, University of Utah, applies topological methods to Visualization [34].

*Vanessa Robins* from the Applied Mathematics department at the Australian National University [35].

*Vin de Silva* worked with Tenenbaum and Carlsson and is now at Pomona College [36].

*Joshua B. Tenenbaum* from the Department of Brain and Cognitive Sciences, MIT, Cambridge, Massachusetts, gained much popularity (7097 citations in Google Scholar as of April,18,2014) with the paper in Science on "A Global Geometric Framework for Nonlinear Dimensionality Reduction" [36].

*Afra Zomorodian* currently working with the D.E. Shaw Group, New York, USA, formerly Department of Computer Science at Dartmouth College, Hanover, New Hamsphire is author of the book "Topology for Computing" [37].

# 5    Topology in a Nutshell

## 5.1    Benefits of Topology

Let us start with a thought on our human visual system: We do not see in three spatial dimensions directly, but rather via sequences of planar projections integrated in a manner that is sensed if not comprehended. A newborn does not know what "Google" is, well this is a very abstract example, but the newborn does also not know what an "apple" is. We spend a significant portion of the first decade of our life to learn how to infer three-dimensional spatial data from paired planar projections. Years of practice have tuned a remarkable ability to extract global structure from representations in a strictly lower dimension. Ghrist (2007) [31] starts in the beginning of his paper with summarizing three benefits of topology:

1. It is beneficial to replace a set of data points with a family of simplicial complexes, indexed by a proximity parameter. This converts the data set into global topological objects.
2. It is beneficial to view these topological complexes through the lens of algebraic topology - specifically, via the theory of persistent homology adapted to parameterized families.
3. It is beneficial to encode the persistent homology of a data set in the form of a parameterized version of a Betti number: a barcode.

Algebra and Topology are axiomatic fields, hence would need many definitions, which is impossible to present here, however, before continuing with the main part of this paper, topological data mining, it is necessary to briefly present two fundamental concepts: manifolds and simplicial complexes. Even before, we introduce the primitives of topology: point sets.

## 5.2    Primitives of Topology: Point Cloud Data Sets

Point cloud data sets (PCD) are the primitives of topology. Consequently, the first question is: "How to get point sets?", or "How to get a graph structure?". Apart from "naturally available" point clouds as discussed below, the answer to this question is not trivial; for some solutions see [38]. In Fig. 2 we see point sets

in the plane, resulting from a continuous handwriting input signal given by an
input device as

$$X(t) = (x(t), y(t), p(t))^T \tag{1}$$

It contains the coordinates $x(t)$ and $y(t)$ as well as the pressure $p(t)$ of the
stylus. After the digitalization process, $X(t)$ is considered as a discrete time
series sampled at different points $t \in T$ over time. Let the sampling times be
$t_0, t_1, ..., t_n$, satisfying $0 \le t_0 < t_1 < ... < t_n$. If the time points are equally
spaced (i.e., $|t_{i+1} - t_i| = \tau$ for all $i = 0, 1, ..., n - 1$, $\tau > 0$ some constant), we
call the input signal *regularly* sampled.

Let $d(X(t_i), X(t_{i+1})) = \left( (x(t_{i+1}) - x(t_i))^2 + (y(t_{i+1}) - y(t_i))^2 \right)^{1/2}$ be the Eu-
clidian distance with respect to the coordinates $x(t)$ and $y(t)$. A sampling of the
handwriting trajectory satisfying $d(X(t_i), X(t_{i+1})) = \delta$, for some constant $\delta > 0$
and $i = 0, 1, ..., m - 1$, is referred as the *equidistant* re-sampling of the time
series $X(t)$. We also notice that $t_m \le t_n$ holds and in general the equidistant
re-sampling is not regular (see Fig. 2 on the right).

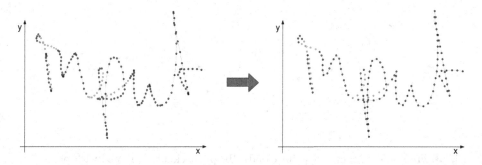

**Fig. 2.** Point Cloud in $\mathbb{R}^2$ from an handwriting example [39]

Another "natural" source for such point cloud data sets are 3-D Laser scanners (for example the Kinect device). Medical images in nuclear medicine are
usually represented in 3D, where a point cloud is a set of points in $\mathbb{R}^3$, whose
vertices are characterized by their position and intensity. In dimensions higher
than three, point clouds (feature vectors) can be found in the representation of
high-dimensional manifolds (see next chapter), where it is usual to work directly
with this type of data [40], resulting from protein structures or protein interaction networks [41]. Also in the representation of text data, point clouds appear:
Based on the vector space model, which is a standard tool in text mining for a
long time [42], a collection of text documents (corpus) can be mapped into a set
of points (vectors) in $\mathbb{R}^n$. Each word can also be mapped into vectors, resulting
in a very high dimensional vector space. These vectors are the so-called term
vectors, with each vector representing a single word. If there, for example, are
$n$ keywords extracted from all the documents then each document is mapped to

a point (*term vector*) in $\mathbb{R}^n$ with coordinates corresponding to the weights. In this way the whole corpus can be transformed into a point cloud set. Usually, instead of the Euclidean metric, using a specialized similarity (proximity) measure is more convenient. The *cosine similarity measure* is one example which is now a standard tool in text mining, see for example [43]. The cosine of the angle between two vectors (points in the cloud) reflects how "similar" the underlying weighted combinations of keywords are [44].

A set of such primitive points forms a space (see Fig. 3a), and if we have finite sets equipped with proximity or similarity measure functions $sim_q : S^{q+1} \rightarrow [0,1]$, which measure how "close" or "similar" $(q+1)$-tuples of elements of $S$ are we have a topological space (see Fig. 3b). A value of 0 means totally different objects, while 1 corresponds to essentially equivalent items. In Fig. 2 we see a good example of a direct source for point clouds in an space which we can easily perceive in $\mathbb{R}^2$. A metric space (see Fig. 3c) has an associated metric (see Fig. 3d the Euclidean distance), enabling to measure distances between points in that space and to define their neighborhoods. Consequently, a metric provides a space with a topology, and a metric space is a topological space.

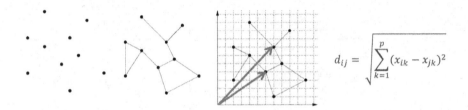

$$d_{ij} = \sqrt{\sum_{k=1}^{p} (x_{ik} - x_{jk})^2}$$

**Fig. 3.** From left to right: (a) point clouds, (b) point clouds equipped with proximity in a graph structure, (c) points in a metric space $\mathbb{R}$, this is practical because we can (d) measure in this space with the Euclidean distance

### 5.3 Manifolds

A manifold is a topological space, which is locally homeomorphic (has a continuous function with an inverse function) to a real $n$-dimensional space (e.g. Euclidean space as in Fig. 3). In other words: $X$ is a $d$-manifold if every point of $X$ has a neighborhood homeomorphic to $\mathbb{B}^d$; **with boundary** if every point has a neighborhood homeomorphic to $\mathbb{B}$ or $\mathbb{B}^d_+$, in other words it is a topological space which is locally homeomorphic (has a continuous function with an inverse function) to a real $n$-dimensional space (e.g. Euclidean space) [45].

A topological space may be viewed as an abstraction of a metric space, and similarly, manifolds generalize the connectivity of $d$-dimensional Euclidean spaces $\mathbb{B}^d$ by being locally similar, but globally different. A $d$-dimensional chart at $p \in X$ is a homeomorphism $\phi : U \rightarrow \mathbb{R}^d$ onto an open subset of $\mathbb{R}^d$, where $U$ is a neighborhood of $p$ and open is defined using the metric. A $d$-dimensional manifold ($d$-manifold) is a topological space $X$ with a $d$-dimensional chart at every point $x \in X$.

The circle or 1-sphere $S^1$ in Fig. 4(a) is a 1-manifold as every point has a neighborhood homeomorphic to an open interval in $\mathbb{R}^1$. All neighborhoods on the 2-sphere $S^2$ in Fig. 4(b) are homeomorphic to open disks, so $S^2$ is a 2-manifold, also called a surface. The boundary $\partial X$ of a $d$-manifold $X$ is the set of points in $X$ with neighborhoods homeomorphic to $H^d = x \in \mathbb{R}^d | x_1 \geq 0$. If the boundary is nonempty, we say $X$ is a manifold with boundary. The boundary of a $d$-manifold with boundary is always a $(d-1)$-manifold without boundary. Figure 4(c) displays a torus with boundary, the boundary being two circles [46].

**Fig. 4.** Manifolds. From left to right: (a) a circle $S$ is a 1-manifold; (b) The sphere $S^2$ is a 2-manifold; (c) The torus is also a 2-manifold with boundaries; (d) A Boys surface is a geometric immersion of the projective plane $P^2$, thus a non-orientable 2-manifold; (e) The famous Klein bottle is a non-orientable 2-manifold [46].

### 5.4 Simplicial Complexes

Simplicial complexes are spaces described in a very particular way, the basis is in Homology. The reason is that it is not possible to represent surfaces precisely in a computer system due to limited computational storage. Consequently, surfaces are sampled and represented with triangulations. Such a triangulation is called a simplicial complex, and is a combinatorial space that can represent a space. With such simplicial complexes, the topology of a space from its geometry can be separated, and Zomorodian compares it with the separation of syntax and semantics in logic [46].

Carlsson emphasizes that not every space can be described as a simplicial complex and that each space can be described as a simplicial complex in many different ways and that calculations of homology for simplicial complexes remains the best method for explicit calculation. Because most spaces of interest are either explicitly simplicial complexes or homotopy equivalent to such, it turns out that simplicial calculation is sufficient for most situations.

Let $S = \{x_0, x_1, \ldots, x_n\}$ denote a subset of a Euclidean space $\mathbb{R}^k$. We say $S$ is in general position if it is not contained in any affine hyperplane of $\mathbb{R}^k$ of dimension less than $n$. When $S$ is in general position, we define the *simplex spanned by* $S$ to be the convex hull $\sigma = \sigma(S)$ of $S$ in $\mathbb{R}^k$. The points $x_i$ are called *vertices*, and the simplices $\sigma(T)$ spanned by non-empty subsets of $T \subseteq S$ are called *faces* of $\sigma$ By a (finite) *simplicial complex*, we will mean a finite collection $\mathcal{X}$ of simplices in a Euclidean space so that the following conditions hold.

1. For any simplex $\sigma$ of $\mathcal{X}$, all faces of $\sigma$ are also contained in $\mathcal{X}$
2. For any two simplices $\sigma$ and $\tau$ of $\mathcal{X}$, the intersection $\sigma \cap \tau$ is a simplex, which is a face of both $\sigma$ and $\tau$ .

**Definition 1.** *By an abstract simplicial complex $X$, we will mean a pair $X = (V(X), \Sigma(X))$, where $V(X)$ is a finite set called the vertices of $X$, and where $\Sigma(X)$ is a subset (called the simplices) of the collection of all non-empty subsets of $V(X)$, satisfying the conditions that if $\sigma \in \Sigma(X)$, and $\emptyset \neq \tau \subseteq \sigma$, then $\tau \in \Sigma(X)$. Simplices consisting of exactly two vertices are called edges.*

Figure 5 shows some examples; for more details and background please refer to the excellent recent notes of Carlsson (2013) [47], and to the books of Zomorodian (2009) [46] and the book of Edelsbrunner & Harer (2010) [2].

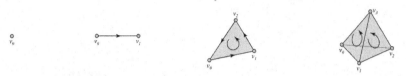

**Fig. 5.** Oriented $k$-simplices, $0 \leq k \leq 3$. An oriented simplex induces orientation on its faces, as shown for the edges of the triangle and two faces of the tetrahedron [46].

Topological techniques originated in pure mathematics, but have been adapted to the study and analysis of data during the past two decades. The two most popular topological techniques in the study of data are *homology* and *persistence*. The connectivity of a space is determined by its cycles of different dimensions. These cycles are organized into groups, called homology groups. Given a reasonably explicit description of a space, the homology groups can be computed with linear algebra. Homology groups have a relatively strong discriminative power and a clear meaning, while having low computational cost. In the study of persistent homology the invariants are in the form of persistence diagrams or barcodes [48].

Carlsson [47] defines the persistence vector space as follows:

**Definition 2.** *Let $k$ be any field. Then by a* persistence vector space *over $k$, we will mean a family of $k$-vector spaces $\{V_r\}_{r \in [0,+\infty)}$, together with linear transformations $L_V(r, r') : V_r \to V_{r'}$ whenever $r \leq r'$, so that $L_V(r', r'') \cdot L_V(r, r') = L_V(r, r'')$ for all $r \leq r' \leq r''$. A linear transformation $f$ of persistence vector spaces over $k$ from $\{V_r\}$ to $\{W_r\}$ is a family of linear transformations $f_r : V_r \to W_r$, so that for all $r \leq r'$, all the diagrams*

$$
\begin{array}{ccc}
V_r & \xrightarrow{L_V(r,r')} & V_{r'} \\
\downarrow{f_r} & & \downarrow{f_{r'}} \\
W_r & \xrightarrow{L_W(r,r')} & W_{r'}
\end{array}
$$

*commute in the sense that*

$$f_{r'} \circ L_V(r, r') = L_W(r, r') \circ f_r$$

*A linear transformation is an* isomorphism *if it admits a two sided inverse. A sub-persistence vector space of $\{V_r\}$ is a choice of $k$-subspaces $U_r \subseteq V_r$, for all $r \in [0, +\infty)$, so that $L_V(r, r')(U_r) \subseteq U_{r'}$ for all $r \leq r'$. If $f : \{V_r\} \to \{W_r\}$ is a linear transformation, then the image of $f$, denoted by $im(f)$, is the sub-persistence vector space $\{im(f_r)\}$.*

In data mining it is important to extract significant features, and exactly for this, topological methods are useful, since they provide robust and general feature definitions with emphasis on global information.

## 5.5  Alpha complex

A very important concept which should be mentioned is the so-called $\alpha$-**complex**: This construction is performed on a metric space $X$ which is a subspace of a metric space $Y$. Typically $Y$ is a Euclidean space $\mathbb{R}^N$, and most often $N$ is small, i.e. $= 2, 3,$ or $4$. For any point $x \in X$, we define the *Voronoi* cell of $x$, denoted by $V(x)$, by

$$V(x) = \{y \in Y | d(x, y) \leq d(x', y) \text{ for all } x' \in X\}$$

The collection of all Voronoi cells for a finite subset of Euclidean space is called its Voronoi diagram (see Fig. 6).

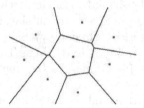

**Fig. 6.** A picture of part of a Voronoi diagram in $\mathbb{R}^2$ [47], for more details on Voronoi please refer to [49]

For each $x \in X$, we also denote by $B_\epsilon(x)$ the set $\{y \in Y | d(x, y) \leq \epsilon\}$. By the $\alpha$-cell of $x \in V(x)$ with scale parameter $\epsilon$, we will mean the set $A_\epsilon(x) = B_\epsilon(x) \cap V(x)$. The $\alpha$-*complex with scale parameter* $\epsilon$ of a subset $x \in X$, denoted by $\alpha_\epsilon(X)$ will be the abstract simplicial complex with vertex set $X$, and where the set $\{x_0, \ldots, x_k\}$ spans a $k$-simplex iff

$$\bigcap_{i=0}^{k} A_\epsilon(x_i) \neq \emptyset$$

An example might look as shown in Figure 7.

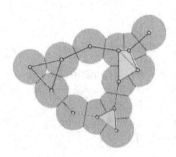

**Fig. 7.** A typical alpha complex [47], for more details please refer to [6]

## 6    Topological Data Mining - State-of-the-Art

The term "topological data mining" is still rarely used to date: A Google search as of 30.03.2014 returned only 18 hits in total, a Google Scholar search only 13 hits and a Web of Science search returned *none*. A better known term is "Topological Data Analysis (TDA)", which returns many hits on Google - but on Google Scholar still only 23 results and on the Web of Science 5 hits, however, only three of them are relevant: 1) The editorial on a 2011 special issue in the journal "Inverse Problems" [50] where the editors Charles Epstein, Gunnar Carlsson and Herbert Edelsbrunner emphasize the importance of persistent homology for data analysis;

2) An overview chapter by Afra Zomorodian (2012) [51] in the book "Algorithms and Theory of Computation Handbook, Second Edition, Volume 2: Special Topics and Techniques" by Attalah & Blanton, where he provides on 31 pages a concise overview on Topological Spaces (manifolds, data structures), Topological Invariants (Euler Characteristic, Homotopy), Simplicial Homology, Persistent Homology (and he provides an Algorithm), Morse Theory (Reeb Graph, Morse-Smale Complex), Structures for Point Sets (Geometric Complexes, Persistent Homology);

3) A paper by Blumberg & Mandell (2013) [52] where the authors lay the foundations for an approach to apply the ideas of Michail Gromov on quantitative topology to data analysis. For this purpose they introduce a so-called "contiguity complex", which is a simplicial complex of maps between simplicial complexes defined in terms of the combinatorial notion of contiguity. Moreover, they generalize the Simplicial Approximation Theorem in order to show that the contiguity complex approximates the homotopy type of the mapping space as they subdivide the domain; consequently the authors describe algorithms for approximating the rate of growth of the components of the contiguity complex under subdivision of the domain, which allows to computationally distinguish spaces with isomorphic homology but different homotopy types.

A search with title = "computational topology" resulted also in only 22 hits, the most recent paper, indeed a very good hit: Computational Topology with Regina: Algorithms, Heuristics and Implementations by Burton (2013) [26], where the author documents for the first time in the literature some of the key algorithms, heuristics and implementations that are central to the performance of his software called REGINA; including the simplification heuristics, key choices of data structures and algorithms to alleviate bottlenecks in normal surface enumeration, modern implementations of 3-sphere recognition and connected sum decomposition. The oldest paper is from Tourlaki & Mylopoul (1973) [53], where the authors study topological properties of finite graphs that can be embedded in the $n$-dimensional integral lattice; they show that two different methods of approximating an $n$-dimensional closed manifold with boundary by a graph of the type studied in this paper lead to graphs whose corresponding homology groups are isomorphic. This is at the same time the paper with the highest citations, however only 17 (as of April, 18, 2014). A highly cited paper (504 times in the web of science, 1008 in Google Scholar (as of April, 18, 2014) is a survey paper by Kong & Rosenfeld (1989) [54], Digital Topology: Introduction and Survey, however, this is dealing with topological properties of digital images, which is the study of image arrays, not the study of algebraic topology; this must not be mixed up.

# 7   Topological Text Mining - State-of-the-Art

Maybe the first work on the application of computational topology in text mining was presented at the Computational Topology in *Image* Context conference (CTIC 2012) by [44]. The background is in the vector space model, which is a standard tool in text mining [42]. A collection of text documents (corpus) is mapped into points (=vectors) in $\mathbb{R}^n$. And each word can also be mapped into vectors, resulting in a very high dimensional vector space. These vectors are the so-called term vectors, each vector is representing e.g. a single word. If there are $n$ keywords extracted from all the documents then each document is mapped to a point (*term vector*) in $\mathbb{R}^\times$ with coordinates corresponding to the weights. In this way the whole corpus can be transformed into a point cloud set. Usually, instead of the Euclidean metric, using a specialized similarity (proximity) measure is more convenient. The *cosine similarity measure* is one example which is now a standard tool in text mining, see e.g. [43]. Namely, the cosine of the angle between two vectors (points in the cloud) reflects how "similar" the underlying weighted combinations of keywords are. Amongst the many different text mining methods (for a recent overview refer to [55]), a topological approach is very promising, but needs a lot of further research; let us first look on graph-based approaches.

## 7.1   Graph-Based Approaches for Text Mining

Graph-theoretical approaches for Text Mining emerged from the combination of the fields of data mining and topology, especially graph theory [56]. Graphs are intuitively more informative as example words/phrase representations [57]. Moreover graphs are the best studied data structure in computer science and mathematics and they also have a strong relation with logical languages [56].

Its structure of data is suitable for various fields like biology, chemistry, material science and communication networking [56]. Furthermore, graphs are often used for representing text information in natural language processing [57]. Dependency graphs have been proposed as a representation of syntactic relations between lexical constituents of a sentence. This structure is argued to more closely capture the underlying semantic relationships, such as subject or object of a verb, among those constituents [58].

The beginning of graph-theoretical approaches in the field of data mining was in the middle of the 1990's [56] and there are some pioneering studies such as [59,60,61]. According to [56] there are five theoretical bases of graph-based data mining approaches such as (1) subgraph categories, (2) subgraph isomorphism, (3) graph invariants, (4) mining measures and (5) solution methods. Furthermore, there are five groups of different graph-theoretical approaches for data mining such as (1) greedy search based approach, (2) inductive logic programming based approach, (3) inductive database based approach, (4) mathematical graph theory based approach and (5) kernel function based approach [56].

There remain many unsolved questions about the graph characteristics and the isomorphism complexity [56]. Moreover the main disadvantage of graph-theoretical text mining is the computational complexity of the graph representation. The goal of future research in the field of graph-theoretical approaches for text mining is to develop efficient graph mining algorithms which implement effective search strategies and data structures [57].

**Examples in the Biomedical Domain:** Graph-based approaches in text mining have many applications from biology and chemistry to internet applications [62]. According to Morales et al [63] graph-based text mining approach combined with an ontology (e.g. the Unified Medical Language System - UMLS) can lead to better automatic summarization results. In [64] a graph-based data mining approach was used to systematically identify frequent co-expression gene clusters. A graph-based approach was used to disambiguate word sense in biomedical documents in Agirre et al. [65]. Liu [66] proposed a supervised learning method for extraction of biomedical events and relations, based directly on subgraph isomorphism of syntactic dependency graphs. The method extended earlier work [67] that required sentence subgraphs to exactly match a training example, and introduced a strategy to enable approximate subgraph matching. These method have resulted in high-precision extraction of biomedical events from the literature.

**Discussion:** While graph-based approaches have the *disadvantage* of being computationally expensive, they have the following *advantages*:

- It offers a far more expressive document encoding than other methods [57].
- Data which is graph structured widely occurs in different fields such as biology, chemistry, material science and communication networking [56].

## 7.2   Topological Text Data Mining

Very closely related to graph-based methods are topological data mining methods, due to the fact that for both we need point cloud data sets as input, which can e.g. be achieved by the vector space model, where the tips of the vectors in an arbitrarily high dimensional space can be seen as point data sets [38].

Due to finding meaningful topological patterns greater information depth can be achieved from the same data input [44]. However, with increasing complexity of the data to process also the need to find a scalable shape characteristic is greater [68]. Therefore methods of the mathematical field of topology are used for complex data areas like the biomedical field [68], [48]. Topology as the mathematical study of shapes and spaces that are not rigid [68], pose a lot of possibilities for the application in knowledge discovery and data mining, as topology is the study of connectivity information and it deals with qualitative geometric properties [69].

**Functionality:** One of the main tasks of applied topology is to find and analyse higher dimensional topological structures in lower dimensional spaces (e.g. point cloud from vector space model [44]). A common way to describe topological spaces is to first create simplicial complexes. A simplicial complex structure on a topological space is an expression of the space as a union of simplices such as points, intervals, triangles, and higher dimensional analogues. Simplicial complexes provide an easy combinatorial way to define certain topological spaces [69]. A simplicial complex $K$ is defined as a finite collection of simplices such that $\sigma \in K$ and $\tau$, which is a face of $\sigma$, implies $\tau \in K$, and $\sigma, \sigma' \in K$ implies $\sigma \cap \sigma'$ can either be a face of both $\sigma$ and $\sigma'$ or empty[70]. One way to create a simplicial complex is to examine all subsets of points, and if any subsets of points are close enough, a p-simplex (e.g. line) is added to the complex with those points as vertices. For instance, a Vietoris-Rips complex of diameter $\epsilon$ is defined as $VR(\epsilon) = \sigma | diam(\sigma) \leq \epsilon$, where $diam(\epsilon)$ is defined as the largest distance between two points in $\sigma$ [70]. Figure 8 shows the Vietoris-Rips complex with varying $\epsilon$ for four points with coordinates (0,0), (0,1), (2,1), (2,0). A common way a analyse the topological structure is to use persistent homology, which identifies cluster, holes and voids therein. It is assumed that more robust topological structures are the one which persist with increasing $\epsilon$. For detailed information about persistent homology, it is referred to [70].

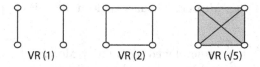

VR (1)     VR (2)     VR (√5)

**Fig. 8.** Vietoris-Rips complex of four points with varying $\epsilon$ [70]

**Examples in the Biomedical Domain:** In [71] a graph-theoretical approach for Text Mining is used to extract relation information between terms in free-text electronic health care records that are semantically or syntactically related. Another field of application is the text analysis of web and social media for detecting influenza-like illnesses [72].

Moreover there can be content-rich relationship networks among biological concepts, genes, proteins and drugs developed with topological text data mining like shown in [73]. According to [74] network medicine describes the clinical application field of topological text mining due to adressing the complexity of human diseases with molecular and phenotypic network maps.

**Discussion:** A clear *advantage* of topological text mining is that here can be greater information depth achieved through understanding the global structure of the data [44]. The *disadvantages* include

- The Complexity of the graph representation itself is a problem [57].
- There is a performance limitation in handling large datasets in high dimensions [44].

# 8    Computational Topology: Software

Maybe the most famous algorithm is the one by Delfinado & Edelsbrunner (1995) [75], where the authors present an incremental method for computing the Betti numbers of a topological space represented by a simplicial complex. The algorithm, which has been presented two years earlier at the 9th symposium on computational geometry [76], is an good example of how algorithmic graph techniques can be applied and extended to complexes of dimension higher than one, which was an important step in raising interest for algebraic topology.

Besides from available geometry software, whole software packages in computational topology are rare to date. A good starting point is the CompuTop.org Software Archive maintained by Nathan Dunfield, enlisting prominent packages for computing the homology and cohomology of simplicial complexes and groups; another good source is the CompTop page from Stanford.

*Computational Homology Project (CHomP):* provides a set of tools for computing the homology of a collection of $n$-dimensional cubes, with a view towards applied applications in dynamical systems, chaos theory, and pattern characterization, developed by Pawel Pilarczyk and supported by Konsantin Mischaikow, Hiroshi Kokubu, Marian Mrozek, Thomas Gedeon, Jean-Philippe Lessard and Marcio Gameiro.

*Dionysus:* is a C++ library developed by Dmitriy Morozov for computing persistent homology, distributed together with thin Python bindings. It currently implements persistent homology, vineyards, persistent cohomology, zigzag, alpha shapes, Vietoris-Rips complexes, Čech complexes, circle valued coordinatization, and piecewise linear vineyards.

*Homological Algebra Programming (HAP):* is a homological algebra library (current version 1.10.15 from November,21, 2013), also for use with GAP with initial focus on computations related to the cohomology of finite and infinite groups [77].

*Linbox:* is a C++ library with GAP and Maple interfaces for exact, high-performance linear algebra computation with dense, sparse, and structured matrices over the integers and over finite fields [78]. (GAP is a system for computational discrete algebra, with particular emphasis on Computational Group Theory, the current version GAP 4.7.4 released on February, 20, 2014; Maple is the well-known computer algebra system, version 18 released in March 2014).

*Mapper:* is a software (cf. Patent US20100313157A1) developed by the Stanford Carlsson group (Sexton, Singh, Memoli) [79] for extracting simple descriptions of high dimensional data sets in the form of simplicial complexes, and is based on the idea of partial clustering of the data guided by a set of functions defined on the data. Mapper is the basis of Ayasdi, the company offering the so-called Insight Discovery Platform using Topological Data Analysis (TDA) to allow people to discover insights in data.

*Persistent Homology in R (PHOM):* is a package by Andrew P Tausz, who graduated in 2013 from the Carlsson Group in Stanford, who also developed JavaPlex. PHPOM is an R package [80] that computes the persistent homology of geometric data sets, to make persistent homology available to the statistics community.

*Persistent homology computations (JavaPlex):* is a library that implements persistent homology and related techniques from computational and applied topology, enabling extensions for further research projects and approaches. It was developed in 2010/11 by the Stanford CompTop Group to improve JPlex, which is a package for computing persistent homology of finite simplicial complexes, often generated from point cloud data [81].

*Regina:* is a suite of software for 3-manifold topologists. It focuses on the study of 3-manifold triangulations and normal surfaces. Other highlights of Regina include angle structures, census enumeration, combinatorial recognition of triangulations, and high-level tasks such as 3-sphere recognition and connected sum decomposition. Regina comes with a full graphical user interface, and also offers Python bindings and a low-level C++ programming interface [26].

## 9  Open Problems

There are many topological algorithms having exponential time complexity and the quest for developing efficient algorithms has started only recently and most of the problems in computational topology still wait for efficient solutions [82]. Some unsolved problems include, for example:

*Problem 1.* Point cloud data sets or at least distances are the primitives for the application of topological approaches, so unless you do not have direct point data input (e.g. from scanners) the first problem to be solved is in preprocessing, i.e. in transforming data, e.g. natural images into point cloud data sets, which is not a trivial task and poses a lot of problems [38].

*Problem 2.* Volodin, Kuznetsov and Fomenko (1974) [83] stated the problem of discriminating algorithmically the standard three-dimensional sphere, so an algorithm would be sought that determines whether a simplicial 3-manifold is topological equivalent to $\mathbb{S}^3$, this is a hard problem.

*Problem 3.* A further open problem is in the design of an algorithm that computes all minimal triangulations for a surface of genus $g$, or the determination of the minimal size of a triangulation for a triangulable $d$-manifold; here Vegter provides some pointers to Brehm and Khnel (1987) [84] and Sarkaria (1987) [85].

*Problem 4.* To date none of our known methods, algorithms and tools scale to the massive amount and dimensionalities of data we are confronted in practice; we need much more research efforts towards making computational topology successful as a general method for data mining and knowledge discovery [46].

*Problem 5.* A big problem is to compute Reeb graphs for spaces of dimension higher than 3, which would be necessary for knowledge discovery from high-dimensional data [18].

Whilst computational topology has much potential for the analysis of arbitrarily high-dimensional data sets, humans are very good at pattern recognition in dimensions of $\leq 3$, this immediately suggests a combination of the "best of the two worlds" towards integrated and interactive solutions [1],[86]. Scientifically, this can be addressed by the HCI-KDD approach: while Human–Computer Interaction (HCI) puts its emphasis on human issues, including perception, cognition, interaction and human intelligence and is tightly connected with Visualization and Interactive Visual Analytics, Knowledge Discovery &Data Mining (KDD) is dealing with computational methodologies, methods, algorithms and tools to discover new, previously insights into data, hence we may speak of supporting human learning with machine learning [87]; the HCI-KDD network of excellence (see www.hci4all.at) is proactively supporting this approach in bringing together people with diverse background but sharing a common goal.

Suppose we were given a million points in 100 dimensions and we wish to recover the topology of the space from which these points were sampled. Currently, none of our tools either scale to these many points or extend to this high a dimension. Yet, we are currently inundated with massive data sets from acquisition devices and computer simulations. Computational topology could provide powerful tools for understanding the structure of this data. However, we need both theoretical results as well as practical algorithms tailored to massive data sets for computational topology to become successful as a general method for data analysis.

# 10    Conclusion and Future Outlook

Topology is basically the study of shapes, in particular of properties that are preserved when a shape is deformed. Topological techniques originated in pure mathematics in the last 200+ years, and for quite a time it was the playing field of some quirky mathematicians interested in differences between a donut and a dumpling. Meanwhile, topology as mathematical study of shapes and spaces is a mature and established mathematical field, and in the past two decades the principles of topology have been adapted and applied to the study and analysis of data sets, emerging into a very young discipline: *computational* topology. A very popular topological technique related to the study of data sets is homology. The connectivity of a space is determined by its cycles of different dimensions, and these cycles can be organized into groups, so-called homology groups. Given a reasonably description of a space, these homology groups can be computed e.g. by help of linear algebra. Homology groups have a relatively strong discriminative power and a clear meaning at relatively low computational effort. In the study of persistent homology the invariants are in the form of persistence diagrams or so-called barcodes [48].

For knowledge discovery and data mining it is important to visualize and comprehend complex data sets, i.e. to find and extract significant features. Exactly for this reason, topological methods are very useful, since they provide robust and general feature definitions. They emphasize a "global information", although this can lead to problems during parallelization [88]. Rieck et al. (2012) [89] presented a novel method for exploring high-dimensional data sets by coupling topologically-based clustering algorithms with the calculation of topological signatures. Future challenges are in achieving better localization (i.e. assigning a geometrical meaning) of features when using topological signatures. Rieck et al. also suggested that in future research the different ways of creating simplicial complexes should be examined and several metrics for the Rips graph (or neighbourhood graph) should be further investigated. Recently, Morozov (2013) [88] presented a parallel algorithm for merging two trees. They realized that new ideas in this domain will be necessary. Future architectures will have many more cores with non-uniform memory access, hence, an important future research direction is developing data structures that explicitly take asymmetry into account.

A large area of future research is in graph-theoretical approaches for text mining, in particular to develop efficient graph mining algorithms which implement robust and efficient search strategies and data structures [57]. However, there remain much unsolved questions about the graph characteristics and the isomorphism complexity [56], so there are plenty of interesting research lines in the future.

The grand challenge is in the *integration* of methods, algorithms and tools from computational topology into useable and useful solutions for *interactive* knowledge discovery and data mining in high-dimensional and complex data sets.

**Acknowledgments.** The author is very grateful for fruitful discussions with the hci4all.at Team and with members of the HCI-KDD network of excellence,

I thank my Institutes both at Graz University of Technology and the Medical University of Graz, my colleagues and my students for the enjoyable academic freedom, the intellectual environment, and the opportunity to think about crazy ideas following my motto: "Science is to test ideas!".

# References

1. Holzinger, A., Dehmer, M., Jurisica, I.: Knowledge discovery and interactive data mining in bioinformatics state-of-the-art, future challenges and research directions. BMC Bioinformatics 15(suppl. 6), I1 (2014)
2. Edelsbrunner, H., Harer, J.L.: Computational Topology: An Introduction. American Mathematical Society, Providence (2010)
3. De Silva, V.: Geometry and topology of point cloud data sets: a statement of my research interests (2004), http://pomona.edu
4. Hatcher, A.: Algebraic Topology. Cambridge University Press, Cambridge (2002)
5. Edelsbrunner, H., Kirkpatrick, D., Seidel, R.: On the shape of a set of points in the plane. IEEE Transactions on Information Theory 29(4), 551–559 (1983)
6. Edelsbrunner, H., Mucke, E.P.: 3-dimensional alpha-shapes. ACM Transactions on Graphics 13(1), 43–72 (1994)
7. Albou, L.P., Schwarz, B., Poch, O., Wurtz, J.M., Moras, D.: Defining and characterizing protein surface using alpha shapes. Proteins-Structure Function and Bioinformatics 76(1), 1–12 (2009)
8. Frosini, P., Landi, C.: Persistent betti numbers for a noise tolerant shape-based approach to image retrieval. Pattern Recognition Letters 34(8), 863–872 (2013)
9. Goodman, J.E., O'Rourke, J.: Handbook of Discrete and Computational Geometry. Chapman and Hall/CRC, Boca Raton (2010)
10. Cignoni, P., Montani, C., Scopigno, R.: Dewall: A fast divide and conquer delaunay triangulation algorithm in ed. Computer-Aided Design 30(5), 333–341 (1998)
11. Bass, H.: Euler characteristics and characters of discrete groups. Inventiones Mathematicae 35(1), 155–196 (1976)
12. Whitehead, G.W.: Elements of homotopy theory. Springer (1978)
13. Alexandroff, P., Hopf, H.: Topologie I. Springer, Berlin (1935)
14. Munkres, J.R.: Elements of algebraic topology, vol. 2. Addison-Wesley, Reading (1984)
15. Edelsbrunner, H., Harer, J.: Persistent Homology - a Survey. Contemporary Mathematics Series, vol. 453, pp. 257–282. Amer Mathematical Soc., Providence (2008)
16. Doraiswamy, H., Natarajan, V.: Efficient algorithms for computing reeb graphs. Computational Geometry 42(67), 606–616 (2009)
17. Edelsbrunner, H., Harer, J., Mascarenhas, A., Pascucci, V., Snoeyink, J.: Time-varying reeb graphs for continuous space-time data. Computational Geometry-Theory and Applications 41(3), 149–166 (2008)
18. Biasotti, S., Giorgi, D., Spagnuolo, M., Falcidieno, B.: Reeb graphs for shape analysis and applications. Theoretical Computer Science 392(13), 5–22 (2008)
19. Euler, L.: Solutio problematis ad geometriam situs pertinentis. Commentarii Academiae Scientiarum Petropolitanae 8(1741), 128–140
20. Listing, J.B.: Vorstudien zur Topologie. Vandenhoeck und Ruprecht, Goettingen (1848)
21. Listing, J.B.: Der Census rauumlicher Complexe: oder Verallgemeinerung des euler'schen Satzes von den Polyedern, vol. 10. Dieterich, Goettingen (1862)

22. Moebius, A.F.: Theorie der elementaren verwandtschaft. Berichte der Saechsischen Akademie der Wissensschaften 15, 18–57 (1863)
23. Blackmore, D., Peters, T.J.: Computational topology, pp. 491–545. Elsevier, Amsterdam (2007)
24. Tourlakis, G., Mylopoulos, J.: Some results in computational topology. Journal of the ACM (JACM) 20(3), 439–455 (1973)
25. Bubenik, P., Kim, P.T.: A statistical approach to persistent homology. Homology, Homotopy and Applications 9(2), 337–362 (2007)
26. Burton, B.A.: Computational topology with Regina: Algorithms, heuristics and implementations, vol. 597, pp. 195–224. American Mathematical Society, Providence (2013)
27. Carlsson, G.: Topology and data. Bulletin of the American Mathematical Society 46(2), 255–308 (2009)
28. Dey, T.K., Edelsbrunner, H., Guha, S.: Computational topology. Contemporary Mathematics 223, 109–144 (1999)
29. Dunfield, N.M., Gukov, S., Rasmussen, J.: The superpolynomial for knot homologies. Experimental Mathematics 15(2), 129–159 (2006)
30. Cerri, A., Fabio, B.D., Ferri, M., Frosini, P., Landi, C.: Betti numbers in multidimensional persistent homology are stable functions. Mathematical Methods in the Applied Sciences 36(12), 1543–1557 (2013)
31. Ghrist, R.: Barcodes: the persistent topology of data. Bulletin of the American Mathematical Society 45(1), 61–75 (2008)
32. Edelsbrunner, H., Morozov, D., Pascucci, V.: Persistence-sensitive simplification functions on 2-manifolds. In: Proceedings of the Twenty-Second Annual Symposium on Computational Geometry, pp. 127–134. ACM (2006)
33. Kaczynski, T., Mischaikow, K., Mrozek, M.: Computational homology, vol. 157. Springer (2004)
34. Pascucci, V., Tricoche, X., Hagen, H., Tierny, J.: Topological Methods in Data Analysis and Visualization: Theory, Algorithms, and Applications (Mathematics+Visualization). Springer, Heidelberg (2011)
35. Robins, V., Abernethy, J., Rooney, N., Bradley, E.: Topology and intelligent data analysis. In: Berthold, M., Lenz, H.-J., Bradley, E., Kruse, R., Borgelt, C. (eds.) IDA 2003. LNCS, vol. 2810, pp. 111–122. Springer, Heidelberg (2003)
36. Tenenbaum, J.B., de Silva, V., Langford, J.C.: A global geometric framework for nonlinear dimensionality reduction. Science 290(5500), 2319–2323 (2000)
37. Zomorodian, A.: Topology for computing, vol. 16. Cambridge University Press, Cambridge (2005)
38. Holzinger, A., Malle, B., Bloice, M., Wiltgen, M., Ferri, M., Stanganelli, I., Hofmann-Wellenhof, R.: On the generation of point cloud data sets: the first step in the knowledge discovery process. In: Holzinger, A., Jurisica, I. (eds.) Knowledge Discovery and Data Mining. LNCS, vol. 8401, pp. 57–80. Springer, Heidelberg (2014)
39. Holzinger, A., Stocker, C., Peischl, B., Simonic, K.M.: On using entropy for enhancing handwriting preprocessing. Entropy 14(11), 2324–2350 (2012)
40. Mémoli, F., Sapiro, G.: A theoretical and computational framework for isometry invariant recognition of point cloud data. Foundations of Computational Mathematics 5(3), 313–347 (2005)
41. Canutescu, A.A., Shelenkov, A.A., Dunbrack, R.L.: A graph-theory algorithm for rapid protein side-chain prediction. Protein Science 12(9), 2001–2014 (2003)
42. Salton, G., Wong, A., Yang, C.: A vector space model for automatic indexing. Communications of the ACM 18(11), 620 (1975)

43. Holzinger, A.: Biomedical Informatics: Computational Sciences meets Life Sciences. BoD, Norderstedt (2012)
44. Wagner, H., Dłotko, P., Mrozek, M.: Computational topology in text mining. In: Ferri, M., Frosini, P., Landi, C., Cerri, A., Di Fabio, B. (eds.) CTIC 2012. LNCS, vol. 7309, pp. 68–78. Springer, Heidelberg (2012)
45. Cannon, J.W.: The recognition problem: what is a topological manifold? Bulletin of the American Mathematical Society 84(5), 832–866 (1978)
46. Zomorodian, A.: Chapman & Hall/CRC Applied Algorithms and Data Structures series. In: Computational Topology, pp. 1–31. Chapman and Hall/CRC, Boca Raton (2010), doi:10.1201/9781584888215-c3.
47. Carlsson, G.: Topological pattern recognition for point cloud data (2013)
48. Epstein, C., Carlsson, G., Edelsbrunner, H.: Topological data analysis. Inverse Problems 27(12), 120201 (2011)
49. Aurenhammer, F.: Voronoi diagrams a survey of a fundamental geometric data structure. ACM Computing Surveys (CSUR) 23(3), 345–405 (1991)
50. Epstein, C., Carlsson, G., Edelsbrunner, H.: Topological data analysis. Inverse Problems 27(12) (2011)
51. Zomorodian, A.: Topological Data Analysis, vol. 70, pp. 1–39 (2012)
52. Blumberg, A., Mandell, M.: Quantitative homotopy theory in topological data analysis. Foundations of Computational Mathematics 13(6), 885–911 (2013)
53. Tourlaki, G., Mylopoul, J.: Some results in computational topology. Journal of the ACM (JACM) 20(3), 439–455 (1973)
54. Kong, T.Y., Rosenfeld, A.: Digtial topology - introduction and survey. Computer Vision Graphics and Image Processing 48(3), 357–393 (1989)
55. Holzinger, A., Schantl, J., Schroettner, M., Seifert, C., Verspoor, K.: Biomedical text mining: State-of-the-art, open problems and future challenges. In: Holzinger, A., Jurisica, I. (eds.) Knowledge Discovery and Data Mining. LNCS, vol. 8401, pp. 271–300. Springer, Berlin (2014)
56. Washio, T., Motoda, H.: State of the art of graph-based data mining. ACM SIGKDD Explorations Newsletter 5(1), 59 (2003)
57. Jiang, C., Coenen, F., Sanderson, R., Zito, M.: Text classification using graph mining-based feature extraction. Knowledge-Based Systems 23(4), 302–308 (2010)
58. Melcuk, I.: Dependency Syntax: Theory and Practice. State University of New York Press (1988)
59. Cook, D.J., Holder, L.B.: Substructure discovery using minimum description length and background knowledge. J. Artif. Int. Res. 1(1), 231–255 (1994)
60. Yoshida, K., Motoda, H., Indurkhya, N.: Graph-based induction as a unified learning framework. Applied Intelligence 4(3), 297–316 (1994)
61. Dehaspe, L., Toivonen, H.: Discovery of frequent DATALOG patterns. Data Mining and Knowledge Discovery 3(1), 7–36 (1999)
62. Fischer, I., Meinl, T.: Graph based molecular data mining – an overview. In: SMC, vol. 5, pp. 4578–4582. IEEE (2004)
63. Morales, L.P., Esteban, A.D., Gervás, P.: Concept-graph based biomedical automatic summarization using ontologies. In: Proceedings of the 3rd Textgraphs Workshop on Graph-Based Algorithms for Natural Language Processing. TextGraphs-3, pp. 53–56. Association for Computational Linguistics, Stroudsburg (2008)
64. Yan, X., Mehan, M.R., Huang, Y., Waterman, M.S., Yu, P.S., Zhou, X.J.: A graph-based approach to systematically reconstruct human transcriptional regulatory modules. Bioinformatics 23(13), i577–i586 (2007)
65. Agirre, E., Soroa, A., Stevenson, M.: Graph-based word sense disambiguation of biomedical documents. Bioinformatics 26(22), 2889–2896 (2010)

66. Liu, H., Hunter, L., Keselj, V., Verspoor, K.: Approximate subgraph matching-based literature mining for biomedical events and relations. PLoS One 8(4) (April 2013)
67. Liu, H., Komandur, R., Verspoor, K.: From graphs to events: A subgraph matching approach for information extraction from biomedical text. In: Proceedings of BioNLP Shared Task 2011 Workshop, pp. 164–172. Association for Computational Linguistics (2011)
68. Nicolau, M., Levine, A.J., Carlsson, G.: Topology based data analysis identifies a subgroup of breast cancers with a unique mutational profile and excellent survival. Proceedings of the National Academy of Sciences of the United States of America 108(17), 7265–7270 (2011)
69. Carlsson, G.: Topology and Data. Bull. Amer. Math. Soc. 46, 255–308 (2009)
70. Zhu, X.: Persistent homology: An introduction and a new text representation for natural language processing. In: Proceedings of the Twenty-Third International Joint Conference on Artificial Intelligence, pp. 1953–1959. AAAI Press (2013)
71. Zhou, X., Han, H., Chankai, I., Prestrud, A., Brooks, A.: Approaches to text mining for clinical medical records. In: Proceedings of the 2006 ACM Symposium on Applied Computing, SAC 2006, p. 235–239. ACM Press, New York (2006)
72. Corley, C.D., Cook, D.J., Mikler, A.R., Singh, K.P.: Text and structural data mining of influenza mentions in Web and social media. International Journal of Environmental Research and Public Health 7(2), 596–615 (2010)
73. Chen, H., Sharp, B.M.: Content-rich biological network constructed by mining PubMed abstracts. BMC Bioinformatics 5(1), 147 (2004)
74. Barabási, A., Gulbahce, N., Loscalzo, J.: Network medicine: a network-based approach to human disease. Nature Reviews Genetics 12(1), 56–68 (2011)
75. Delfinado, C.J.A., Edelsbrunner, H.: An incremental algorithm for betti numbers of simplicial complexes on the 3-sphere. Computer Aided Geometric Design 12(7), 771–784 (1995)
76. Delfinado, C.J.A., Edelsbrunner, H.: An incremental algorithm for betti numbers of simplicial complexes. In: Proceedings of the Ninth Annual Symposium on Computational Geometry, pp. 232–239. ACM (1993)
77. Ellis, G.: Homological Algebra Programming. Contemporary Mathematics Series, vol. 470, pp. 63–74. Amer Mathematical Soc., Providence (2008)
78. Dumas, J.G., Gautier, T., Giesbrecht, M., Giorgi, P., Hovinen, B., Kaltofen, E., Saunders, B.D., Turner, W.J., Villard, G.: Linbox: A generic library for exact linear algebra. In: Cohen, A.M., Gao, X.S., Takayama, N. (eds.) 1st International Congress of Mathematical Software (ICMS 2002), pp. 40–50. World Scientific (2002)
79. Singh, G., Memoli, F., Carlsson, G.: Topological methods for the analysis of high dimensional data sets and 3d object recognition. In: Botsch, M., Pajarola, R. (eds.) Eurographics Symposium on Point-Based Graphics, vol. 22, pp. 91–100. Euro Graphics (2007)
80. Kobayashi, M.: Resources for studying statistical analysis of biomedical data and R. In: Holzinger, A., Jurisica, I. (eds.) Knowledge Discovery and Data Mining. LNCS, vol. 8401, pp. 183–195. Springer, Heidelberg (2014)
81. Tausz, A., Vejdemo-Johansson, M., Adams, H.: Javaplex: A research software package for persistent (co) homology (2011), http://code.google.com/javaplex
82. Vegter, G.: Computational topology, pp. 517–536. CRC Press, Inc., Boca Raton (2004)
83. Volodin, I., Kuznetsov, V., Fomenko, A.T.: The problem of discriminating algorithmically the standard three-dimensional sphere. Russian Mathematical Surveys 29(5), 71 (1974)

84. Brehm, U., Khnel, W.: Combinatorial manifolds with few vertices. Topology 26(4), 465–473 (1987)
85. Sarkaria, K.S.: Heawood inequalities. Journal of Combinatorial Theory, Series A 46(1), 50–78 (1987)
86. Otasek, D., Pastrello, C., Holzinger, A., Jurisica, I.: Visual Data Mining: Effective Exploration ofthe Biological Universe. In: Holzinger, A., Jurisica, I. (eds.) Knowledge Discovery and Data Mining. LNCS, vol. 8401, pp. 19–33. Springer, Heidelberg (2014)
87. Holzinger, A.: Human Computer Interaction & Knowledge Discovery (HCI-KDD): What is the benefit of bringing those two fields to work together? In: Cuzzocrea, A., Kittl, C., Simos, D.E., Weippl, E., Xu, L. (eds.) CD-ARES 2013. LNCS, vol. 8127, pp. 319–328. Springer, Heidelberg (2013)
88. Morozov, D., Weber, G.: Distributed merge trees. In: Proceedings of the 18th ACM SIGPLAN Symposium on Principles and Practice of Parallel Programming, vol. 48, pp. 93–102 (August 2013)
89. Rieck, B., Mara, H., Leitte, H.: Multivariate data analysis using persistence-based filtering and topological signatures. IEEE Transactions on Visualization and Computer Graphics 18(12), 2382–2391 (2012)

# Author Index

Bachler, Martin   209
Bloice, Marcus   57, 101
Bober, Miroslaw   197
Boselli, Roberto   141

Cesarini, Mirko   141

Dehmer, Matthias   241

Ferri, Massimo   57

Hauser, Helwig   117
Hobel, Heidelinde   301
Hofmann-Wellenhof, Rainer   57
Holzinger, Andreas   1, 19, 35, 57, 101,
   117, 209, 241, 271, 301, 317, 331
Holzinger, Katharina   35
Hörtenhuber, Matthias   209
Huppertz, Berthold   317

Jeanquartier, Fleur   117
Jurisica, Igor   1, 19

Katz, Gilad   81
Kieseberg, Peter   301
Kobayashi, Mei   183
Koslicki, David   209

Lee, Sangkyun   227

Malle, Bernd   57
Mayer, Christopher   209
Mercorio, Fabio   141
Mezzanzanica, Mario   141

Nguyen, Hoan   255

Ofner, Bernhard   241
Otasek, David   19

Palade, Vasile   35
Pastrello, Chiara   19
Pinho, Armando J.   209
Poch, Olivier   255

Rabadan, Raul   35
Rokach, Lior   81

Schantl, Johannes   271
Schrittwieser, Sebastian   301
Schroettner, Miriam   271
Schutz, Patrick   255
Seifert, Christin   271
Shabtai, Asaf   81
Stanganelli, Ignazio   57

Thompson, Julie D.   255
Turkay, Cagatay   117

van Leeuwen, Matthijs   169
Verspoor, Karin   271

Wassertheurer, Siegfried   209
Weippl, Edgar   301
Wiltgen, Marco   57
Windridge, David   197

Yildirim, Pinar   101